Central Nervous System Cancer Rehabilitation

Central Nervous System Cancer Rehabilitation

ADRIAN CRISTIAN, MD, MHCM
Chief
Cancer Rehabilitation
Miami Cancer Institute,
Miami, Florida, United States

ELSEVIER

ELSEVIER

3251 Riverport Lane
St. Louis, Missouri 63043

Central Nervous System Cancer Rehabilitation ISBN: 978-0-323-54829-8

Content Strategist: Kayla Wolfe
Content Development Manager: Christine McElvenny
Content Development Specialist: Jennifer Horigan
Publishing Services Manager: Shereen Jameel
Project Manager: Nadhiya Sekar
Designer: Gopalakrishnan Venkatraman

Printed in United States of America

Last digit is the print number: 9 8 7 6 5 4 3 2 1

List of Contributors

Mohammad Aalai, MD
Attending Physician
Interventional Pain Medicine
Unique Pain Medicine
New York, NY, United States

Ruth E. Alejandro, MD
TBI Inpatient and Day Hospital Attending Physiatrist
Rehabilitation Medicine Department
Blythedale Children's Hospital
Valhalla, NY, United States

Residency Site Program Director for NYPH-University Hospital of Columbia & Cornell PM&R Residency Program and New York Medical College PM&R Residency Program
Rehabilitation Medicine Department
Blythedale Children's Hospital
Valhalla, NY, United States

Assistant Clinical Professor
Department of Rehabilitation and Regenerative Medicine
Columbia College of Physicians and Surgeons/New York Presbyterian Hospital
New York City, NY, United States

Hilary Berlin, MD
Clinical Assistant Professor
Department of Rehabilitation Medicine
Donald and Barbara Zucker School of Medicine at Hofstra Northwell
Hempstead, NY, United States

Department of Physical Medicine and Rehabilitation
Nothwell-Long Island Jewish Medical Center
New Hyde Park, NY, United States

Ravi Bhargava, MD
Physician and Corporate Manager of Research
Department of Corporate Research
William Osler Health System
Brampton, ON, Canada

Division of Palliative Care
William Osler Health System
Brampton, ON, Canada

Thomas N. Bryce, MD
Professor
Rehabilitation Medicine
Icahn School of Medicine at Mount Sinai
New York, NY, United States

Martin R. Chasen, MBChB, FCP (SA), MPhil (PALL MED)
Medical director Palliative Care
Palliative Care
William Osler Health Services
Brampton, ON, Canada

Veronica J. Chehata, BSBiology, MD
Resident Physician
Physical Medicine and Rehabilitation
Northwell Health
Manhasset, NY, United States

Adrian Cristian, MD, MHCM
Chief, Cancer Rehabilitation
Miami Cancer Institute
Miami, FL, United States

Joanna Edeker, DPT
Carolinas Healthcare System
NC, United States

Miguel Xavier Escalon, MD, MPH
Assistant Professor
Department of Rehabilitation Medicine
Icahn School of Medicine
New York, NY, United States

Jack Fu, MD
Associate Professor, Palliative, Rehabilitation & Integrative Medicine
University of Texas MD Anderson Cancer Center
Houston, TX, United States

Kathryn Gibbs, DO
Spinal Cord Injury Fellow
Kessler Institute for Rehabilitation
West Orange, NJ, United States

Daniel T. Ginat, MD, MS
Director of Head and Neck Imaging
Radiology
University of Chicago
Chicago, IL, United States

Gary Goldberg, BASc, MD, FABPMR (BIM)
Professor
Physical Medicine and Rehabilitation
Medical College of Virginia / Virginia Commonwealth University Health System
Richmond, VA, United States

Staff Physician
Physcial Medicine and Rehabilitation Service
Hunter Holmes McGuire VA Medical Center
Richmond, VA, United States

A. Iannicello, MD
Pain Management Fellow
Unique Pain Management
New York, United States

Naomi Kaplan, BSc (Hons), MBBS
Resident Physician
Physical Medicine & Rehabilitation
Zucker School of Medicine at Hofstra/Northwell
Hempstead, NY, United States

Sarah Khan, DO
Assistant Professor
Physical Medicine and Rehabilitation
Northwell Health
Glen Cove
New York
United States

Assistant Professor
Physical Medicine and Rehabilitation
Northwell Health
Bethpage
NY
United States

Ashish Khanna, MD
Attending Physician
Department of Cancer Rehabilitation
Kessler Institute for Rehabilitation
West Orange, NJ, United States

Clinical Assistant Professor
Department of Physical Medicine and Rehabilitation
Rutgers New Jersey Medical School
Newark, NJ, United States

Cosmo Kwok, MD
Pediatric Rehabilitation Medicine Fellow
University of Colorado
School of Medicine and Children's Hospital Colorado
CO, United States

T. Lefkowitz, DO, DABPMR
Vice Chairman & Program Director
Department of Rehabilitation Medicine
Kingsbrook Jewish Medical Center
Brooklyn, NY, United States

Brittany Lorden, OT
Carolinas Healthcare System
NC, United States

Terrence MacArthur Pugh, MD
Assistant Professor
Physical Medicine and Rehabilitation
Carolinas Medical Center
Charlotte, NC, United States

Vice-Chief
Section of Rehabilitation
Supportive Care
Levine Cancer Institute
Charlotte, NC, United States

Associate Director of Oncology Rehabilitation
Physical Medicine and Rehabilitation
Carolinas Rehabilitation
Charlotte, NC, United States

Susan Maltser, DO
Assistant Professor
Department of Rehabilitation Medicine
Donald and Barbara Zucker School of Medicine at Hofstra Northwell
Hempstead, NY, United States

Director Cancer Rehabilitation Northwell Health
Manhasset, NY, United States

Marc D. Moisi, MD, MS
Assistant Professor
Department of Neurosurgery
Wayne State University
Chief of Neurosurgery
Detroit Receiving Hospital
Dettroit, MI, United States

Seong-Jin Moon, MD
Resident Physician
Department of Neurological Surgery
Wayne State University
MI, United States

N. Ozurumba, MD
Attending Physician
Department of Rehabilitation Medicine
Jacoby Hospital Medical Center
New York, United States

Komal Patel, MD
Brain Injury Fellow
Department of Rehabilitation Medicine
Donald and Barbara Zucker School of Medicine at Hofstra Northwell
Hempstead, NY, United States

Vishwa S. Raj, MD
Director of Oncology Rehabilitation
PM&R
Levine Cancer Institute
Carolinas Rehabilitation
Charlotte, NC, United States

Brittany Schenke-Reilly, MA, CCC-SLP, CBIS
Speech Pathologist
Rehabilitation Services
Northwell-Glen Cove Hospital
Glen Cove, NY, United States

Marilyn Frost Rubenstein, MA, CCC-SLP
Speech Pathologist
Rehabilitation Services
Glen Cove Hospital
Glen Cove, NY, United States

Supervisor
Rehabilitation Services
Glen Cove Hospital
Glen Cove, NY, United States

Lisa Marie Ruppert, MD
Assistant Attending
Rehabilitation Medicine Service
Memorial Sloan Kettering Cancer Center
New York, NY, United States

Matthew Shatzer, DO
Residency Program Director
Physical Medicine and Rehabilitation
Donald and Barbara School of Medicine at Hofstra-Northwell
Hempstead, NY, United States

Chief
Physical Medicine and Rehabilitation
North Shore University Hospital
Manhasset, NY, United States

Assistant Professor
Physical Medicine and Rehabilitation
Donald and Barbara School of Medicine at Hofstra-Northwell
Hempstead, NY, United States

R. Shane Tubbs, MS, PA-C, PhD
Chief Scientific Officer
Seattle Science Foundation
SSF
Seattle
Washington
United States

Adjunct Professor
University of Dundee
Dundee, United Kingdom

Gonzalo A. Vazquez-Casals, PhD
Neuropsychologist
Rehabilitation Services
Northwell-Glen Cove Hospital
Glen Cove, NY, United States

Blake Walker, MD
Resident Physician
Department of Neurological Surgery
Wayne State University
MI, United States

Nadia N. Zaman, DO
Resident Physician
Department of Physical Medicine & Rehabilitation
Donald and Barbara Zucker School of Medicine at Hofstra/Northwell
Manhasset, NY, United States

Preface

Rehabilitation of a person with cancer of the brain and spinal cord requires individualized care by a team of specialists from time of initial diagnosis through active treatment, survivorship, and advanced stages of the disease.

The purpose of this book is to provide useful information to assist these clinicians in the noble endeavor of rehabilitating individuals diagnosed and treated for cancer of the central nervous system with the goal of maximizing the level of function and quality of life.

This book begins with a description of the cancer rehabilitation continuum of care, safety considerations, and functional outcomes. The section on brain cancer provides content on neurosurgical management, rehabilitation, cognitive deficits, communication, and swallowing impairments. The section on spinal cord cancer provides the reader with information on characteristics of spinal cord tumors, neurosurgical management, and rehabilitation. A chapter on rehabilitation of the child with brain and spinal cord cancer addresses the unique needs of this population. Pain and fatigue are very common concerns raised by persons with cancer of the central nervous system, and these topics are covered as well. The final chapter covers the equally important topic of the role of palliative rehabilitation in advanced cancer.

I would like to thank all of the authors for their meaningful contribution to this book. Their hard work, expertise, and enthusiasm for this project helped make it a reality.

Adrian Cristian, MD, MHCM
Chief, Cancer Rehabilitation
Miami Cancer Institute
Florida, USA

I dedicate

To my family, who is my source of love, joy, strength, and support

To my teachers, students, and patients with deep gratitude for all they have taught me

To Holli Hupart, an outstanding educator, wife, mother, and daughter

Contents

CHAPTER 1

Cancer Rehabilitation Continuum of Care and Delivery Models

JACK FU, MD • ADRIAN CRISTIAN, MD, MHCM

INTRODUCTION

Cancer rehabilitation has been defined as "medical care that should be integrated throughout the oncology care continuum and delivered by trained rehabilitation professionals who have it within their scope of practice to diagnose and treat patients' physical, psychologic, and cognitive impairments in an effort to maintain or restore function, reduce symptom burden, maximize independence, and improve quality of life in this medically complex population."[1]

Persons with cancer often receive their oncologic care in a variety of settings such as acute care hospitals, long-term healthcare facilities, outpatient clinics, and the person's home. This parallels the types of locations where they also receive their rehabilitative care. It is therefore important to have fully integrated oncologic and rehabilitative care across this continuum of care. The fundamental goal of rehabilitation of the person with brain or spinal cord cancer is to maximize function and to improve the quality of life regardless of the setting where they receive their healthcare.

To accomplish this goal, the person should first be evaluated for functional deficits by a rehabilitation specialist. This is meant to establish a baseline functional level and serves as the foundation for an individualized rehabilitation plan of care. The person should subsequently be screened periodically and treated for cancer-related impairments throughout their life across the rehabilitation continuum. The rehabilitative treatments need to be provided by an experienced clinical staff, in the most appropriate setting, and at the most appropriate time in the person's cancer care. The management of functionally relevant impairments should be holistic and person-centered, addressing physical impairments, nutrition, emotional well-being, sexuality, spirituality, and the role of the individual in their family and society.[2]

The aim of this chapter is to describe the components of the rehabilitative continuum of care and the advantages and challenges faced by each of these components in the provision of rehabilitative services to the person with cancer.

Barriers to the Provision of Rehabilitation Services to Persons With Brain and Spinal Cord Cancer

This current delivery model of rehabilitative care is hindered by several barriers as follows: (1) patients, their families, and medical providers may have a limited knowledge about the benefits of rehabilitation; (2) the families and significant others of persons with cancer are often overwhelmed by the complexity, cost, and limited resources and cannot fit rehabilitation into an already busy schedule; (3) a limited workforce of rehabilitation providers that has the necessary working knowledge and expertise to provide cancer rehabilitation services to persons with brain or spinal cord cancer; (4) a fragmented carryover of a rehabilitation treatment plan across the continuum of care; (5) lack of a coordinated plan of care that incorporates both cancer treatment and rehabilitation; (6) lack of use of standardized rehabilitation clinical protocols and outcome measures across the rehabilitation continuum; (7) lack of standardization of cancer rehabilitation programs across the United States; and (8) limited coverage for rehabilitation services by health insurance companies.[2,3]

THE CONTINUUM OF CARE FOR ONCOLOGIC REHABILITATION

Dietz classified cancer rehabilitation using four distinct roles: preventive, restorative, supportive, and palliative.[4] These fundamental roles can be applied and used to guide rehabilitative treatment from time of diagnosis, through acute cancer treatment and survivorship, and in the advanced stages of cancer. Preventive rehabilitation begins at the time of diagnosis when preexisting impairments are identified and treated. It is also an opportunity to optimize the individual's level of physical and mental fitness using exercise, nutrition, and psychosocial interventions. Restorative rehabilitation focuses on maximizing the person's level of function by addressing their impairments. For example, a person with cancer affecting the spinal cord and paralysis of the extremities would benefit from acute inpatient rehabilitation to address the corresponding deficits. Supportive rehabilitation focuses on improving self-care and mobility and maximizing function in persons with progressing cancer. Palliative rehabilitation aims to improve the level of function of the person with cancer in the advanced stages of the disease by managing symptoms such as pain and fatigue and addressing physical impairments that can limit function. It can also be used to minimize the risk of developing potentially preventable conditions such as pressure ulcers and contractures.

Acute Hospitalization

During the acute hospitalization period, the person with cancer often moves from one setting to another depending on their underlying condition and medical stability. It is not uncommon to have the person be admitted through the emergency room and spend time on a medical and/or surgical floor and/or in an intensive care unit in one hospitalization. As a result they can become deconditioned very quickly due to prolonged bed rest and use of steroid medications.

The goals of rehabilitation in this setting include the following: (1) minimize the deleterious effects of prolonged immobilization; (2) maximize patient safety (i.e., minimize risk of falls, development of aspiration pneumonia, pressure ulcers, contractures, and medication side effects); (3) maximize level of function for activities of daily living; (4) mobilize the patient if they are able to ambulate; (5) maximize nutritional intake; (6) educate the person and their significant others about cancer-related physical impairments; (7) address psychosocial stressors; and (8) assist the primary treatment team with discharge recommendations to the most appropriate setting.

The physiatrist has a significant role in the coordination of rehabilitative services during an acute hospitalization. Through close communication with members of the rehabilitation team and referring physicians, the physiatrist can address the physical impairments of the person with cancer of the brain and spinal cord. In addition, he/she can make recommendations for discharge to the most appropriate setting for the patient. Rehabilitative services are typically provided at the bed side or in an inpatient gym in the institution. Under-referral of cancer patients to rehabilitation has been a chronic problem for the cancer rehabilitation specialty[5–7] and has also been noted in the inpatient setting specifically.[8,9] A recent Italian study by Pace et al. evaluated the rehabilitation referrals of brain tumors patients. Only 12.8% received inpatient rehabilitation, 3.1% received intensive outpatient rehabilitation, and 11.8% received traditional outpatient rehabilitation.[10] Like traditional brain injury populations, neurologic deficits can include hemiplegia, spasticity, aphasia, dysphagia, ataxia, cognitive deficits, bowel/bladder dysfunction, visual symptoms including diplopia and dysarthria. Given that 75% of brain tumor patients have 3 or more neurologic deficits and 39% have more than 5 neurologic deficits, these low referral rates to rehabilitation for this patient group appear grossly inadequate.[11] Some referring oncology services have been shown to lack understanding of what rehabilitation does and fail to identify impairments that rehabilitation can help treat.[12–14]

A consult-based inpatient cancer rehabilitation program has been used at the Mayo Clinic—Rochester called the Cancer Adaptation Team (CAT) and MD Anderson Cancer Center called the Mobile Team. The CAT consists of a nurse, physiatrist, physical therapists, occupational therapist, social worker, nutritionist, and chaplain who meet daily to coordinate rehabilitation care.[15] The MD Anderson Mobile Team enabled patients to receive up to 1 h of physical and 1 h of occupational therapy daily while still on the acute care service and met weekly. The idea was to provide a mobile acute inpatient rehabilitation type program for cancer patients. These rehabilitation models allow more intensive coordinated team-based rehabilitation led by a physiatrist while the patient is still on the acute care oncology service. The services have been particularly useful for medical fragile hematologic cancer patients but could also be used in a neurologic tumor population. Barriers to this model of consult-based rehabilitation include the Prospective Payment System and therapy resource availability.[16]

The challenges of providing rehabilitative services in this setting include the following: (1) rapid changes in the person's medical condition; (2) lack of knowledge about the role of physiatry and rehabilitation among oncologists and other healthcare providers involved in the person's care; (3) delay in the identification and initiation of rehabilitative services; and (4) gaps in communication between the oncology and rehabilitation teams.

Postacute Care

Postacute rehabilitative care is most commonly provided in acute inpatient rehabilitation facilities (IRFs) as well as subacute and skilled nursing facilities. Common challenges to the provision of rehabilitative services in these settings include the following: (1) the rehabilitation plan not fully integrated into the oncology treatment plan; (2) significant variability in the type of rehabilitative services available in each of these settings; (3) lack of standardization in the treatment protocols for cancer-related impairments across the United States; (4) variable provider awareness of the benefits of rehabilitation for persons with cancer across the continuum; and (5) payer limitations.[3]

Acute Inpatient Rehabilitation

Brain tumors are the second highest cause of neurologic disease and neurologic tumors account for over half of all cancer patient admissions to American acute IRFs.[17,18] They are also the largest group of IRF patients at Shirley Ryan AbilityLab (formerly known as the Rehabilitation Institute of Chicago)[19] and MD Anderson Cancer Center.[20] However, cancer patients are only 2.4% of all US IRF patients and half of IRFs admit fewer than 10 brain tumor patients annually.[18,21]

Neurologic tumors may be the largest group of IRF cancer patients for several reasons. First, the Medicare 60 percent rule mandates that, in order to participate in the Medicare Prospective Payment System, 60% of an IRF's admissions have 1 of 13 diagnoses. Cancer and deconditioning are not 1 of the 13, which may discourage the acceptance of many cancer patients. However, brain injury is a 60 percent rule diagnosis and brain tumor patients would be considered brain injury.[16,22] Because it is housed within a National Cancer Institute Comprehensive Cancer Center that is exempt from the Medicare Prospective Payment System, the MD Anderson acute inpatient rehabilitation unit does not have to adhere to the 60 percent rule. While lower than the proportions reported in the American national data or Shirley Ryan AbilityLab, neurologic tumors are the largest group of patients admitted to the acute inpatient rehabilitation service (17%) at MD Anderson.[20]

In an IRF, patients are required to participate in at least 3 h of therapy per day for 5 days a week. They are also required to be seen by a physician at least three times a week but are typically seen more frequently. The vast majority of inpatient rehabilitation research in neurologic tumor patients has been in the IRF setting.

The medical fragility of cancer patients may discourage their acceptance to IRFs. It has been shown that general cancer patients are transferred back to the primary more frequently than noncancer patients.[23] The hematologic cancer populations can be among the most medically fragile cancer patients with rates of return to the primary acute care service reported between 26% and 38%.[24–27] However, the brain cancer rates of return to the primary acute care service (reported between 7.5% and 24%)[11,28–30] are substantially lower and close to their traumatic brain injury (TBI) (20%)[31] and stroke (7.1%)[32] counterparts.

Logistical and regulatory barriers exist for IRF brain cancer patients receiving concurrent chemotherapy and/or radiation therapy. From a regulatory standpoint, the cost of concurrent radiation or chemotherapy can be significant and can cut into margins or make patient acceptance a money-losing proposition under the Medicare Prospective Payment System. This is an important consideration that is different from stroke and TBI patients who are usually finished with all diagnostic and treatment procedures prior to inpatient rehabilitation transfer.

Logistical considerations also exist. First, rehabilitation facilities may be unable to give chemotherapy due to lack of chemotherapy trained nurses and medical staff, pharmacy restrictions, hospital policy, or lack of accompanying monitoring such as telemetry (if needed). Radiation treatments can interfere with inpatient rehabilitation therapy times. While the radiation treatment is relatively quick (usually only 10–20 min.), the transportation to and from radiation can add up to a large part of the day gone from rehabilitation. Transportation often consists of ambulance transportation to a facility miles away. This may present challenges for therapists to provide the 3 h daily of therapy required in an IRF. Radiation-related fatigue, which typically occurs after the first few treatments, may interfere with rehabilitation therapy performance and tolerance. It may be beneficial to ask to schedule inpatient rehabilitation patients for the last radiation sessions of the day after they have completed their rehabilitation. By doing so, patients are able to sleep after the radiation and then wake up more refreshed in the morning while also eliminating the return trip transportation time from cutting into potential therapy time.[33,34]

Patients with neurologic tumors often suffer from a number of cancer-related symptoms which can impact function and therapy tolerance. They can include fatigue, poor appetite, insomnia, cognitive deficits, depression, and anxiety. These patients are at risk for cognitive deficits not only due to the brain tumor and treatment itself but also exacerbating concomitant symptoms. Owing to their high risk, a screening speech therapy cognitive evaluation at inpatient rehabilitation may be of benefit because these deficits may not be obvious on casual conversation. Cognitive deficits can have discharge planning implications as well. Postacute brain injury rehabilitation programs may be a useful resource; however, they are only covered by some private insurance policies and not Medicare/Medicaid.

The substantial cancer symptom burden of inpatient rehabilitation cancer patients can impact function and therapy tolerance. Because of this, inpatient cancer physiatrists treat cancer symptoms and have been shown to make statistically significant improvements in symptoms likely from physical activity but also medication management.[35,36] Owing to a cancer-related hyperinflammatory state, pain, fatigue, nausea, and insomnia can develop and make physical activity difficult. Cancer-related fatigue is experienced by over 80% of brain tumor patients during treatment.[37] Neurostimulants have shown some benefit for cancer-related fatigue although their effects are less pronounced in placebo-controlled trials.[38] Poor appetite may respond to appetite stimulants such as dronabinol and mirtazapine. Megestrol may be effective but also has a side effect of hypercoagulability which may increase the already high risk of venous thromboembolic disease. Depression and anxiety are treated much like the noncancer population. Psychotherapy may be of benefit.[39] Mirtazapine is an antidepressant with weight gain effects and may be useful in patients with both cachexia and depression. Constipation is common among cancer rehabilitation inpatients due to immobility, neurogenic contributors, and frequent opiate use. Constipation can also contribute to nausea and poor appetite. Daily monitoring of bowel movements is encouraged. Patients with new-onset nausea or abdominal distension may benefit from an abdominal X-ray to evaluate the degree of constipation present. Aggressive use of laxatives may be required. Sexuality issues should be explored with a thorough history to determine contributing factors beyond just the neurologic but also cancer symptom—related contributors like depression and fatigue.

After a neurosurgical biopsy or craniotomy with resection, a specimen is sent for pathologic evaluation to confirm the diagnosis. Typically, the final pathology results are not completed until another week after the operation. By that time, many patients are on inpatient rehabilitation. Patients and their families are understandably eager to find out the pathologic diagnosis and then what prognosis is associated with it. Oncologists and neurosurgeons may be unable to visit with the patient and family in a freestanding rehabilitation hospital due to a lack of hospital privileges or distance. Because the physiatrist is often the only physician caring for a freestanding inpatient rehabilitation hospital patient, questions about the cancer diagnosis and prognosis may be directed at them. These conversations may be uncomfortable for a physiatrist due to unfamiliarity with the latest oncologic research and treatments but also their mortal nature. The oncologist is the most qualified person to answer these questions, but patients may have to wait until an oncology clinic after discharge to discuss them.[33]

Subacute Rehabilitation and Long-Term Care Facilities

Persons with brain or spinal cord cancer who cannot tolerate the intensity of an IRF program as well as persons who completed such a program and are not ready to return back to their homes are often referred to rehabilitation programs in subacute or skilled nursing facilities.

The goals of rehabilitation in these facilities are similar to the ones mentioned earlier, which are as follows: (1) minimize the deleterious effects of prolonged immobilization; (2) maximize patient safety (i.e., minimize risk of falls, development of aspiration pneumonia, pressure ulcers, contractures, and medication side effects); (3) continue and modify as necessary the rehabilitation treatment plan initiated at the previous facility; (4) maximize level of function for activities of daily living; (5) mobilize the patient if they are able to ambulate; (6) maximize nutritional intake; (7) educate the person and their significant others about cancer-related physical impairments; (8) address psychosocial stressors.

The rehabilitation at these types of facilities is usually less intense on a daily basis than in IRFs; however, the person typically spends more days in these facilities. The physician in charge of the person's care may or may not be a physiatrist, and their knowledge about the treatment of impairments commonly seen in brain and spinal cord cancer may be limited. Team members often include physical therapists, occupational therapists, and speech pathologists. However, these therapists may or may not have significant experience and education in cancer rehabilitation principles. It should be noted that there are facilities that have a focus on neurologic rehabilitation and as such will have a clinical staff that is better versed in the care of persons with these types of cancer. Another challenge is in care coordination between the referring facility and the subacute/skilled nursing facility with respect to the rehabilitation plan. A physiatrist can be very instrumental in facilitating the communication between these facilities with respect to the rehabilitation treatment plan.

Some subacute rehabilitation facilities are unable to administer chemotherapy due to lack of qualified staff. Also they may be reluctant to accept patients who require additional chemotherapy and radiation therapy because these often expensive treatments may come out of a Prospective Payment System payment. Skilled nursing facilities typically do not have blood bank transfusion capabilities, which may be an issue with pancytopenic chemotherapy patients.

Postacute Brain Injury Residential Rehabilitation

Some patients after completing an inpatient rehabilitation program may require additional rehabilitation in a residential type setting. Postacute brain injury rehabilitation facilities were designed for such patients and may be useful for patients with significant cognitive, behavioral, or social limitations.[40,41] There has been little published regarding the experiences of brain tumor patients in these settings. Unfortunately, postacute brain injury rehabilitation facilities are not covered by traditional Medicare/Medicaid.

Home Rehabilitation

Once discharged from an acute IRF, a subacute rehabilitation program, or an acute hospitalization, the person with brain or spinal cord cancer often requires continued rehabilitative services, however, cannot attend an outpatient rehabilitation program. The reasons often include (1) limited access to transportation to and from the outpatient program; (2) an inability to tolerate the intensity of an outpatient program; or (3) limited health insurance coverage for rehabilitative services. The availability of home rehabilitative services can vary by geographic region as well as frequency and intensity; however, the goal is to make the person more independent in their home environment and to educate them and their significant others on strategies to maximize level of function. The main advantage to the home therapy program is the convenience of having the services provided in the home. The main disadvantage is the limited type of exercises and equipment that can be provided in the home setting by the treating therapist. The rehabilitation program is typically initiated by a referring physician who can then monitor the patient's progress. As technology improves, telerehabilitative services could potentially be of benefit in both the education and the monitoring of the person with brain and spinal cord cancer at home.

Outpatient Rehabilitation

Persons with brain and spinal cord cancer often need multiple rehabilitative disciplines working together closely to address the complexity of impairments commonly seen in this population. This often includes physical therapy, occupational therapy, and speech pathology; however, there are occasions when the services of an orthotist, neuropsychologist, vocational rehabilitation specialist, and driving trainer may be required. The physiatrist is best suited to coordinate the rehabilitation team efforts in the outpatient setting. The advantages to a comprehensive outpatient program include more focused rehabilitation interventions for gait and balance training, wheelchair transfers, and manual dexterity just to name a few, compared with those that can be accomplished in the home. The use of additional equipment commonly available in the gym setting is an added advantage over home therapy. Rehabilitation interventions in this population are often reimbursable by payers (task force). Challenges to the provision of outpatient rehabilitative services include (1) a rapid deterioration in the person's medical condition secondary to the tumor often requires changes to the treatment plan and prioritization of goals (i.e., progression of cancer, seizures, newly identified impairments, etc.); (2) limited health insurance coverage for rehabilitation services; (3) access and transportation barriers to receiving rehabilitative services; (4) geographic variability in the availability of necessary rehabilitation services and in providers with experience in brain and spinal cord cancer rehabilitation; and (5) communication barriers between rehabilitation clinicians and their oncology colleagues.

During outpatient supportive rehabilitation, patients may experience significant cancer symptoms related to radiation, chemotherapy, or other medications such as antiepileptics and analgesics. Glioblastoma multiforme (GBM) patients receiving the Stupp regimen's 6 weeks of radiation therapy may experience significant fatigue after their radiation session. If possible, scheduling radiation sessions later in the day after rehabilitation therapy may be useful. Patients will have an opportunity to sleep/rest and hopefully have more energy the next morning for additional rehabilitation. During the Stupp regimen, GBM patients receive oral temozolomide chemotherapy cycles for 5 days with 23 days off.[42] During the 5 days of temozolomide, patients may experience increased fatigue and nausea, which may affect rehabilitation performance and tolerance. It may be best to reduce or temporarily suspend therapy during these 5-day periods.

An important distinction between brain tumor patients and the more typical brain injury rehabilitation populations of stroke and TBI are that brain tumors are dynamic lesions. The lesions can grow or recur over time, which can lead to further weakness and neurologic changes. Furthermore, cancer treatments can cause additional brain injury. Radiation late effects can cause new neurologic deficits typically months to years after radiation completion. It is not uncommon for brain tumor patients to require inpatient or outpatient rehabilitation multiple times over the course of their cancer due to declines in function from the cancer or its treatment. For high-grade astrocytoma patients, it is not a question of if these patients will experience neurologic decline in the future, but when. Therefore, continued outpatient physiatry follow-up is recommended.[33,34] Also due to the dynamic nature of brain cancer, it is common over time for brain tumor patients to accumulate a number of brain injuries due to repeated surgical resections, cancer progression/recurrence, and radiation necrosis. The rate and degree of functional improvement is often reduced after each repeated bout of functional decline.[33]

CONCLUSION

As the number of persons actively treated for cancer and cancer survivors continues to grow, it is imperative that rehabilitative care be an integral part of the person's healthcare plan. Each of the settings described in this chapter has both advantages and challenges in provision of rehabilitative services to persons with CNS cancer. The physiatrist is well equipped to coordinate care for, advocate for, and treat the cancer-related impairments of the person with cancer across the cancer rehabilitation continuum of care.

REFERENCES

1. Silver JK, Raj VS, Fu JB, Wisotzky EM, Smith SR, Kirch RA. Cancer rehabilitation and palliative care: critical components in the delivery of high-quality oncology services. *Support Care Cancer*. 2015;23:3633–3643.
2. Cheville AL, Mustian K, Winters-Stone K, Zucker DS, Gamble GL, Alfano CM. Cancer rehabilitation: an overview of current need, delivery models, and levels of care. *Phys Med Rehabil Clin N Am*. 2017.
3. Stout NL, Silver JK, Raj VS, et al. Toward a national initiative in cancer rehabilitation: recommendations from a subject matter expert group. *Arch Phys Med Rehabil*. November 2016;97(11):2006–2015.
4. Dietz JH. Rehabilitation of cancer patient. *Med Clin North Am*. 1969;53(3):607–624.
5. Cheville AL, Troxel AB, Basford JR, Kornblith AB. Prevalence and treatment patterns of physical impairments in patients with metastatic breast cancer. *J Clin Oncol*. 2008;26(16):2621–2629.
6. Cheville AL, Beck LA, Petersen TL, Marks RS, Gamble GL. The detection and treatment of cancer-related functional problems in an outpatient setting. *Support Care Cancer*. 2009;17(1):61–67.
7. Cheville AL, Rhudy L, Basford JR, Griffin JM, Flores AM. How receptive are patients with late stage cancer to rehabilitation services and what are the sources of their resistance? *Arch Phys Med Rehabil*. 2017;98(2):203–210.
8. Lin HF, Wu YT, Tsauo JY. Utilization of rehabilitation services for inpatient with cancer in Taiwan: a descriptive analysis from national health insurance database. *BMC Health Serv Res*. 2012;12:255.
9. Movsas SB, Chang VT, Tunkel RS, Shah VV, Ryan LS, Millis SR. Rehabilitation needs of an inpatient medical oncology unit. *Arch Phys Med Rehabil*. 2003;84:1642–1646.
10. Pace A, Villani V, Parisi C, et al. Rehabilitation pathways in adult brain tumor patients in the first 12 months of disease. A retrospective analysis of services utilization in 719 patients. *Support Care Cancer*. 2016;24(11):4801–4806.
11. Mukand JA, Blackinton DD, Crincoli MG, Lee JJ, Santos BB. Incidence of neurological deficits and rehabilitation of patients with brain tumours. *Am J Rehab Med*. 2001;80(5):346–350.
12. Piil K, Juhler M, Jakobsen J, Jarden M. Controlled rehabilitative and supportive care intervention trials in patients with high-grade gliomas and their caregivers: a systematic review. *BMJ Support Palliat Care*. 2016;6(1):27–34.
13. Cheville AL. Cancer rehabilitation. *Semin Oncol*. 2005;32:219–224.
14. Lehmann JF, DeLisa JA, Warren CG, deLateur BJ, Bryant PL, Nicholson CG. Cancer rehabilitation: assessment of need, development, and evaluation of a model of care. *Arch Phys Med Rehabil*. 1978;59(9):410–419.
15. Sabers SR, Kokal JE, Girardi JC, et al. Evaluation of consultation-based rehabilitation for hospitalized cancer patients with functional impairment. *Mayo Clin Proc*. 1999;74(9):855–861.
16. Fu JB, Raj VS, Guo Y. A guide to inpatient cancer rehabilitation: focusing on patient selection and evidence-based outcomes. *PM R*. 2017;9(9S2):S324–S334.
17. Radhakrishan K, Bohnen NI, Kurland LT. Epidermiology of brain tumors. In: Morantz RA, Walsh JW, eds. *Brain Tumors: A Comprehensive Text*. New York: Marcel Dekker; 1994:1–18.
18. Mix JM, Granger CV, LaMonte MJ, et al. Characterization of cancer patients in inpatient rehabilitation facilities: a retrospective cohort study. *Arch Phys Med Rehabil*. 2017;98(5):971–980.
19. Sliwa JA, Shahpar S, Huang ME, Spill G, Semik P. Cancer rehabilitation: do functional gains relate to 60 percent rule classification or to the presence of metastasis? *PM R*. 2016;8(2):131–137.

20. Shin KY, Guo Y, Konzen B, Fu J, Yadav R, Bruera E. Inpatient cancer rehabilitation: the experience of a national comprehensive cancer center. *Am J Phys Med Rehabil.* 2011;90(5 suppl 1):S63–S68.
21. Boake C, Meyers CA. Brain tumor rehabilitation: survey of clinical practice. *Arch Phys Med Rehabil.* 1993;74:1247 (abstract).
22. Centers for Medicare & Medicaid Services, Department of Health and Human Services. Inpatient Rehabilitation Facility Prospective Payment System. Available at: https://www.cms.gov/Outreachand-Education/Medicare-Learning-Network-MLN/MLNProducts/downloads/InpatRehabPaymtfctsht09-508.pdf.
23. Alam E, Wilson RD, Vargo MM. Inpatient cancer rehabilitation: a retrospective comparison of transfer back to acute care between patients with neoplasm and other rehabilitation patients. *Arch Phys Med Rehabil.* 2008;89(7):1284–1289.
24. Fu JB, Lee J, Shin BC, et al. Return to the primary acute care service among patients with multiple myeloma on an acute inpatient rehabilitation unit. *PM R.* 2017;9(6):571–578.
25. Fu JB, Lee J, Smith DW, Shin K, Guo Y, Bruera E. Frequency and reasons for return to the primary acute care service among patients with lymphoma undergoing inpatient rehabilitation. *PM R.* 2014;6(7):629–634.
26. Fu JB, Lee J, Smith DW, Bruera E. Frequency and reasons for return to acute care in patients with leukemia undergoing inpatient rehabilitation: a preliminary report. *Am J Phys Med Rehabil.* 2013;92(3):215–222.
27. Fu JB, Lee J, Smith DW, Guo Y, Bruera E. Return to primary service among bone marrow transplant rehabilitation inpatients: an index for predicting outcomes. *Arch Phys Med Rehabil.* 2013;94(2):356–361.
28. O'Dell MW, Barr K, Spanier D, et al. Functional outcome of inpatient rehabilitation in persons with brain tumors. *Arch Phys Med Rehabil.* 1998;79:1530–1534.
29. Fu JB, Parsons HA, Shin KY, et al. Comparison of functional outcomes in low- and high-grade astrocytoma rehabilitation inpatients. *Am J Phys Med Rehabil.* 2010;89(3): 205–212.
30. Marciniak CM, Sliwa JA, Heinemann AW, et al. Functional outcomes of persons with brain tumors after inpatient rehabilitation. *Arch Phys Med Rehabil.* 2001;82:457–463.
31. Deshpande AA, Millis SR, Zafonte RD, Hammond FM, Wood DL. Risk factors for acute care transfer among traumatic brain injury patients. *Arch Phys Med Rehabil.* 1997;78(4):350–352.
32. Stineman MG, Ross R, Maislin G, Fiedler RC, Granger CV. Risks of acute hospital transfer and mortality during stroke rehabilitation. *Arch Phys Med Rehabil.* 2003;84(5): 712–718.
33. Fu JB, Rao G, Rexer JL. Rehabilitation of patients with brain tumors. In: Stubblefield MD, ed. *Cancer Rehabilitation: Principles & Practice.* 3rd ed. Demos Medical; 2018 [In Press].
34. Fu JB, Morishita S, Yadav R. Changing paradigms in the rehabilitation of inpatients with brain tumors. *Curr Phys Med Rehabil Rep.* 2018 [In Press].
35. Guo Y, Young BL, Hainley S, Palmer JL, Bruera E. Evaluation and pharmacologic management of symptoms in cancer patients undergoing acute rehabilitation in a comprehensive cancer center. *Arch Phys Med Rehabil.* 2007;88(7):891–895.
36. Fu JB, Lee J, Tran KB, et al. Symptom burden and functional gains in a cancer rehabilitation unit. *Int J Ther Rehabil.* 2015;22(11):517–523.
37. Lovely MP, Miaskowski C, Dodd M. Relationship between fatigue and quality of life in patients with glioblastoma multiformae. *Oncol Nurs Forum.* 1999;26(5):921–925.
38. Meyers CA, Weitzner MA, Valentine AD, Levin VA. Methylphenidate therapy improves cognition, mood, and function of brain tumor patients. *J Clin Oncol.* 1998;16(7): 2522–2527.
39. Brandes AA, Scelzi E, Salmistraro G, et al. Incidence of risk of thromboembolism during treatment high-grade gliomas: a prospective study. *Eur J Cancer.* 1997;33(10): 1592–1596.
40. Benge JF, Caroselli JS, Reed K, Zgaljardic DJ. Changes in supervision needs following participation in a residential post-acute brain injury rehabilitation programme. *Brain Inj.* 2010;24(6):844–850.
41. Cope DN, Cole JR, Hall KM, Barkan H. Brain injury: analysis of outcome in a post-acute rehabilitation system. Part 1: general analysis. *Brain Inj.* 1991;5(2):111–125.
42. Stupp R, Hegi ME, Mason WP, et al. Effects of radiotherapy with concomitant and adjuvant temozolomide versus radiotherapy alone on survival in glioblastoma in a randomised phase III study: 5-year analysis of the EORTC-NCIC trial. *Lancet Oncol.* 2009;10(5):459–466.

CHAPTER 2

Safety Considerations in the Rehabilitation of Persons With Cancer of the Brain and Spinal Cord

NADIA N. ZAMAN, DO • KATHRYN GIBBS, DO • SUSAN MALTSER, DO

INTRODUCTION

Survivors of brain and spinal cord cancer often experience long-term complications secondary to the disease itself or treatment regimens, which can lead to disability and loss of function.[1] Some of the most common complications in this patient population include cognitive impairments, hemi or complete paresis, and gait and balance disturbances.[2,3] Approximately 80% of patients with primary brain tumors have an impairment in cognition at some point in the course of their disease.[1] Although variable with location of tumor and type of treatment, individuals with brain tumors have reported the rate of hemiparesis to range from 26% to 47% and gait impairment ranges from 26% to 62%.[4] Individuals with brain and spinal cord tumors also suffer from medical complications such as chemotherapy-induced cytopenia and neuropathy, osteoporosis, steroid-related myopathy and seizure.[5] Awareness of all potential disease and treatment-related complications can help the rehabilitation team to properly care for and safely direct the rehabilitation for this patient population, with the goal of preventing adverse outcomes and maximizing an individual's functional independence.

PROVIDER TRAINING

Following a multidisciplinary approach to rehabilitation, all clinicians treating those with cancer in the rehabilitation setting require knowledge of the needs specific to this patient population.

Although formal standards of competency required during residency training have yet to be established by the Accreditation Council for Graduate Medical Education (ACGME) or the American Board of Physical Medicine and Rehabilitation (ABPMR), a large number of physiatrists receive an "average" exposure to cancer rehabilitation during residency.[6] The field is also growing and Physical Medicine and Rehabilitation (PM&R) physicians recognize the vital role rehabilitation can play in the care of patients with cancer. At present time, there are five fellowship programs in cancer rehabilitation across the United States, with the hope for more in the future. The role of cancer rehabilitation has been well established and recognized by the American Physical Therapy Association and the association's work has now led to recognition by the American Board of Physical Therapy Specialties as well.[7]

The Commission on Accreditation of Rehabilitation Facilities (CARF) has outlined the requirements need for a cancer rehabilitation specialty program,[8] which focuses on an individualized, patient-centered, interdisciplinary program for those with cancer. CARF requires cancer rehabilitation programs to demonstrate "competencies and the application of evidence based practices to deliver services that address the preventative, restorative, supportive and palliative rehabilitation needs" of those which it serves.[8] With these guidelines and adequately trained physicians and therapists, a rehabilitation program is able to provide patient-centered care, specializing in the needs of this specific patient population. Communication between healthcare providers is emphasized, as is advocating to the community and legislators on behalf of patients with cancer. The goal of a cancer specialized rehabilitation program is optimizing functional independence and outcomes in an individualized manner, throughout one's course of illness, treatment, and long-term care.[8]

ENGAGING FAMILY MEMBERS IN PATIENT

Safety

Cancer patients often face seeing multiple specialists across the whole spectrum of care from acute care hospitals to rehabilitation facilities and outpatient practices. Numerous handoffs and transitions may result in miscommunication and errors. Engaging family members and educating them regarding patient's medications, precautions, and necessary follow-up will ensure patient safety through multiple transitions. In addition, patients may be engaged in learning proper techniques to assist cancer survivors with activities of daily living (ADLs) as they transition to home and community.

BRAIN AND SPINE RADIATION

Side effects of brain and spine radiation vary with the dose, duration, and amount of brain or spine treated. These side effects may present safety concerns both in the inpatient and outpatient rehabilitation setting. The timeline of common side effects can be divided into three phases: acute, early delayed, and late.[3]

Brain Radiation

Acute complications of brain radiation occur during radiation therapy (RT) and up to 6 weeks after. These effects are often due to vasogenic edema and present as an acute encephalopathy with symptoms including headache, nausea, new onset or worsening of focal neurologic deficits and seizure.[9] The acute side effects are most often seen on the inpatient rehabilitation unit and can present a safety concern, as patients may exhibit decreased safety awareness and increased risk of falls. Fortunately, RT encephalopathy is most often reversible, being easily treated or prevented with corticosteroids.[10] Although often multifactorial, RT can contribute to the fatigue a patient experiences while undergoing treatment.[11] Fatigue can hinder a patient's performance in therapy and may also increase their risk for falls on the inpatient unit.

Early delayed side effects present from 6 weeks to 6 months post RT and most commonly include persistent fatigue and focal neurologic deficits or encephalopathy, thought to be caused by demyelination of the irradiated tissue.[9,12] Similar to the complications seen in the acute phase, early delayed side effects are most often reversible when treated with corticosteroids.

Late effects occur at least 6 months to a year after completion of RT and may present several years after. Unlike the acute or early delayed side effects, these effects are usually irreversible.[9] Radiation necrosis develops with higher fractionation of radiation and is due to damage and necrosis of blood vessels, combined with demyelination of treated and surrounding brain tissue.[13] This type of necrosis leads to new focal neurologic deficits, dementia, and ataxia, all of which present safety concerns for the patient.[14] Incidence of long-term cognitive deficits varies with location of the tumor and fractionation and duration of RT, but may cause memory impairments, decreased concentration, and safety awareness.[15] Distinguishing between radiation necrosis and recurrent tumor is often difficult, as the two have similar clinical presentations. MRI imaging of the brain without a clearly defined T2 mass as well as a higher ratio of edema to enhancing lesion are more suggestive of radiation necrosis than recurrent disease.[16]

Radiation to the Spine

RT required for tumors of the spine may cause damage and fibrosis of the spinal cord itself, as well as the exiting roots and nerves and surrounding musculature. Damage to these structures may present as symptoms of myelopathy, radiculopathy, neuropathy, plexopathy, or myopathies.[17] The rehabilitation team should be aware of structures included in the irradiated field during treatment in order to properly diagnose these potential side effects.

Side effects from RT to the spinal cord presenting a safety risk include transient myelopathy, chronic progressive myelopathy, and acute paralysis. Transient myelopathy, due to demyelination, occurs in the early delayed time frame and presents as Lhermitte symptom, a shock-like sensation down the spine induced by flexion of the neck.[18] This myelopathy, although uncomfortable, resolves with time. Late radiation–induced myelopathy is most often irreversible and can be progressive in nature, leading to paralysis.[9] Demyelination and necrosis of white matter, as well as vascular necrosis all contribute to chronic radiation myelopathy.[19] Initial presentation is often with Brown-Sequard syndrome which then progresses with time to spastic paraplegia or quadriplegia with associated complications such as neurogenic bowel and bladder.[9,18] Corticosteroids may be prescribed to slow the progression. This progressive myelopathy of course increases a patient's risk for falls and skin breakdown. Lower motor neuron syndrome may occur with RT to the lower spinal cord and cauda equina, presenting as progressive lower extremity weakness.[20] Sensory impairments are rare and bowel/bladder function is usually normal with the lower motor neuron syndrome.[21] Weakness may progress very slowly, allowing patients to remain ambulatory for quite some time after initial presentation.[9] Spinal cord hemorrhage is another late complication of RT. Radiation to the spine may lead to the development of vascular malformations such as telangiectasias and cavernomas, which may rupture and bleed.

Patients present with acute onset of lower extremity weakness and back pain.[21]

Safety in Exercise with Brain and Spinal Cord Tumors

The American College of Sports Medicine (ACSM) recommends all cancer patients participate in moderate to vigorous exercise as their condition allows.[22] The ACSM also advises that a patient's physical activity level and current medical status be assessed at the time of cancer diagnosis, during treatment, and at the time of completion.[23] Assessing the patient at each interval will help to individualize exercise programs with the goal of improving overall health and function.[24] Patients participating in a supervised exercise program have shown the most significant functional improvements and for this reason it is necessary for the treating team to be aware of the patient's diagnosis, treatments, and both short- and long-term complications of the disease itself or the required treatment.[23]

Participation in a rehabilitation program for patients with brain or spinal cord tumors has shown to improve functional outcomes.[14,24] However, at present time there are no specific guidelines for the safety of exercise in patients with brain or spine cancer. Therefore, it is recommended the guidelines established by the ACSM for exercise in patients with cancer be followed. The ACSM recommends all cancer patients should avoid periods of inactivity, even when undergoing treatment, and should engage in regular aerobic, resistive, and flexibility exercises. The ACSM realizes modifications will need to be made for certain individuals, but emphasizes the goal of remaining as physically active as their condition allows.[23] A recent study found there to be no adverse outcomes when patients with high-grade glioma participated in a daily exercise program consisting of walking and resistive and balance exercises.[25]

While outlining a supervision of an individual's rehabilitation and exercise program, the following complications of medical conditions should be taken into consideration. Modifications to individualized programs should be made as needed in order to maintain patient safety.

CARDIAC AND PULMONARY SAFETY CONSIDERATIONS

Cancer survivors commonly receive cardiotoxic chemotherapeutic agents, which when combined with RT may injure cardiac muscle and coronary arteries. Awareness of cardiac compromise is warranted in order to customize the patients' rehabilitation program.[26] Cancer survivors undergoing rehabilitation should be monitored for symptoms of chest pain, dizziness fatigue, leg cramps, and claudication. Vital signs such as pulse oximetry and respiratory rate should be closely monitored during exercise.[27] Cancer survivors may experience pulmonary complications both from the cancer itself (primary and metastatic) and exposure of lungs to RT leading to pneumonitis and pulmonary fibrosis. In addition, cancer survivors are at high risk for PE and aspiration pneumonia. A high index of suspicion for dysphagia is necessary for patients with brain tumors to minimize risk of pneumonia. Cancer survivors may experience dyspnea and decreased exercise tolerance in the rehabilitation setting. It is necessary to monitor for symptoms such as shortness of breath and dizziness as well as assess oxygen saturation prior and during exercise.[28]

CYTOPENIA WHILE ON CHEMOTHERAPY

Introduction

Chemotherapy is an important part of the treatment regimen in most individuals with cancer. Temozolomide, bevacizumab, and irinotecan are commonly used in the treatment of primary brain tumors with good response rates.[29–31] Spinal cord and brain tumors resulting from metastases are generally treated with chemotherapy agents for their primary cancers. The most common cancers that metastasize to the brain are from lung, breast, melanoma, renal, and colorectal, with the incidence of metastases to the brain increasing as the survivorship of the abovementioned malignancies continue to improve.[32] All chemotherapeutic agents have short- and long-term adverse effects that can have effects on safety during rehabilitation.

Anemia

Anemia is a common complication experienced by patients undergoing chemotherapy as a part of their oncologic treatment regimen. Patients may commonly report symptoms of fatigue and dyspnea on exertion, both of which cannot only limit their activity tolerance but also affect their quality of life over time. The prevalence of anemia in adults with cancer is estimated to be as high as 39%, with numbers nearing 100% in those undergoing active chemotherapy.[33] Studies have shown greater hemoglobin concentrations are linked to better physical and functional well-being, with direct correlation between uncorrected anemia and functional disability, even increased mortality.[31,34,35] Most individuals will tolerate exercise despite having anemia, with no signs of tachycardia or dyspnea on exertion even with hemoglobin concentrations as low as 8 g/dL.[36] Cardiopulmonary functional capacity and muscular performance can be influenced by anemia, with greater functional capacity decline occurring when there is an acute drop in hemoglobin concentration rather than a gradual drop.[37] Therefore, monitoring the signs and symptoms of chemotherapy-induced anemia, as well as how rapidly the decline occurs in hemoglobin and hematocrit, is paramount to improving and maintaining a patient's physical and functional performance, as well as increasing cancer treatment tolerance.

Neutropenia

Chemotherapy-induced neutropenia is a serious adverse effect experienced by some cancer patients, and it can be associated with severe localized and systemic infections and prolonged hospitalizations.[38] The risk of serious infection increases with increasing grade and duration of neutropenia, especially neutropenia greater than 7 days' duration with neutropenic fever being considered an oncologic emergency.[39] It is important to note that these patients are most susceptible to infections that result from their own normal flora, especially those present in the gastrointestinal tract, than nosocomial infections. Therefore, it has been found that increased barrier protection, such as the use of gowns, gloves, and masks, is not useful in the prevention of infection; beneficial recommendations include proper hand hygiene among caregivers, grouping infected patients together, placing neutropenic patients in private rooms, and assigning caregivers to neutropenic patients so that their exposure to other infected patients is low.[37] In an inpatient rehabilitation setting, safety consideration should be given as to whether neutropenic patients should perform their therapies in a commonly used space or their own private rooms.[35]

Thrombocytopenia

Thrombocytopenia is the most common hematologic toxicity seen as a result of chemotherapy use and can lead to serious consequences, such as bleeding complications. It usually results from cumulative toxicity that is dose dependent and is observed 6–14 days after a treatment cycle. The predominant cause of low platelet counts secondary to chemotherapy results from decreased platelet production.[40] Temozolomide was found to be associated with the development of thrombocytopenia in 15%–20% of those undergoing treatment, with thrombocytopenia often being prolonged and possibly irreversible.[41] Aside from the changes to the chemotherapy regimen, there are only a few treatment options available for chemotherapy-induced thrombocytopenia. However, physical exercise regimens have been well tolerated in individuals undergoing active chemotherapy cycles with no signs of hemorrhage with platelets less than 10,000 cells/mm[3].[34] Therefore, the general recommendations are to limit activities to walking and ADL with platelet counts <20,000 cells/uL; light exercise with close symptom monitoring with platelet counts >20,000 cells/uL; and moderate exercise with light resistive exercises with platelet counts >30,000 cells/uL.[5] While careful consideration should be taken when evaluating thrombocytopenic patients in the rehabilitation setting, physical activities do not necessarily need to be held as long as the patient is able to tolerate the exertion.

Chemotherapy-Induced Peripheral Neuropathy

The peripheral nervous system is vulnerable to the neurotoxic effects of chemotherapy agents. Chemotherapy-induced peripheral neuropathy (CIPN) is frequently a dose-limiting adverse effect and can produce a long-standing negative impact on a patient's mobility. The nerve fibers and dorsal root ganglia of the primary sensory neurons are equally at risk of being affected, and the development of neuropathy is due to total cumulative dose and dose intensity.[42] Neuropathic changes are most often seen with platinum-based, taxane, and vinca alkaloid agents, and usually occurs in a stocking/glove distribution with sensory disturbances more common than motor disturbances. Patients will often present with decreased vibratory sensation in the toes, as well as a loss of Achilles deep tendon reflexes, with associated numbness, tingling, and paresthesia in the fingers and toes, although some patients may also experience a loss of pain and temperature sensation with taxanes.[40]

CIPN occurs during chemotherapy cycles, with symptoms decreasing after completion of treatment. However, a number of patients can continue to have altered sensation even after the cessation of the chemotherapy regimen. In a secondary data analysis of 512 female cancer survivors, 47% still reported symptoms of CIPN an average of 6 years after completion of chemotherapy, with significantly more disability and 1.8 times the risk of falls, effectively showing that those with CIPN continue to have proprioceptive and balance deficits that put them at risk for further functional disability.[43] Therefore, proper management includes baseline assessments of strength, sensation, balance, proprioception, and gait should be done prior to initiating chemotherapy, with continued screening for changes in the aforementioned clinical measures throughout the duration of the chemotherapy cycles[5,44]. Patients who have been on a chemotherapy agent known to cause CIPN should be properly monitored for fall risk throughout their rehabilitation course.

Cognitive Impairments

Changes in cognition secondary to chemotherapy, referred to colloquially as "chemo brain," can occur in a number of patients. However, cognitive impairment in this population can be multifactorial, as many of these patients not only have a brain tumor located in areas of the brain associated with memory, calculation, and executive functioning but also are on a number of medications that can cause confusion, lethargy, attention, and concentration deficits.[3] Moreover, cognitive impairment can have serious ramifications on quality of life, with reduction in learning and memory the most commonly affected. There is strong evidence that chemotherapy in cancer patients can cause a decline in short-term cognitive ability, but data regarding long-term effects still remains unclear.[45,46] For those who continue to have cognitive impairments despite stopping chemotherapy, an increase in physical activity and exercise has been shown to improve cognitive function.[47] Yoga, meditation, and Tai Chi have been indirectly linked to improving cognitive function by decreasing stress and fatigue. Pharmacologically, methylphenidate in low doses has been found to be effective in glioblastoma multiforme patients with improvement seen in memory, reasoning, and verbal fluency.[3] Donepezil, ginkgo biloba, hyperbaric oxygen, bevacizumab, and indomethacin have been studied for use in brain tumor populations as well, although the findings have been limited.[48]

Side Effects of Seizures and Anticonvulsants

Seizures are a common presenting symptom of brain tumors, occurring in 20%–80% of patients, especially those with low-grade tumors.[49,50] While some may have a seizure that leads to the diagnosis of their brain tumor, others develop seizures later in the progression of the disease. Seizures can occur with both primary brain tumors and brain metastases. Tumors involving cortical structures of the brain are more likely to produce seizures, especially those in the temporal and primary sensorimotor cortices.[51]

Traditional first-line agents for seizure management included typical anticonvulsants, such as phenytoin, carbamazepine, and valproic acid for several years. Although these medications have great efficacy for seizure control, they have the common adverse effect of cytochrome P450 enzyme induction, which leads to several drug-drug interactions, especially with chemotherapy agents and glucocorticoids. This can reduce the effective serum concentrations of chemotherapy medications; it can also reduce the efficacy of glucocorticoids in the maintenance of vasogenic edema.[48] In turn, chemotherapy metabolism by the same hepatic enzymes can cause reduction in the serum concentrations of the anticonvulsant agents, thereby increasing a patient's risk of having seizure activity, which can have devastating neurologic consequences.[49] Typical anticonvulsants also have a higher risk of causing morbilliform drug rashes when taken in conjunction with RT, with a small percentage of patients developing life-threatening reactions such as Stevens-Johnson syndrome.[52]

There have been some reports that levetiracetam can cause increased agitation or negative behavioral changes, but this was seen more often in those with baseline psychologic and behavioral derangements.[53,54] It is an otherwise well-tolerated anticonvulsant. Newer anticonvulsants, such as levetiracetam and lacosamide, have shown to be equally efficacious to the traditionally used medications, with less adverse effects experienced by the patient while undergoing treatment.[47,48,55]

Side Effects of Steroids

Glucocorticoids are an essential part of the treatment of central nervous system tumors. They are used in about 70%–100% of patients with primary central nervous system tumors and metastases and can provide transient relief of neurologic symptoms by decreasing the vasogenic edema that causes increased intracranial pressure or spinal cord compression; a marked improvement is often seen within 24 hours of administration.[56] Glucocorticoids have also been used in neuro-oncology because it can provide short-term relief of chemotherapy-induced nausea and vomiting.[57] Dexamethasone, a fluorinated steroid, is the most commonly used of these medications because of its long half-life and low mineralocorticoid effects; it is known to be beneficial in the management of mass effect secondary to tumor-associated edema and may even protect against the development of acute encephalopathic changes related to RT.[54,55,58] However, they are not without their own adverse effects (Table 2.1).

Steroid-Induced Hyperglycemia

Glucocorticoids increase serum blood sugar levels through mobilization of glucose from the liver and

TABLE 2.1
Steroid Side Effects

Side Effect of Steroid	Rehabilitation Monitoring	Treatments to Consider
Hyperglycemia	Capillary blood glucose	Insulin
Psychiatric disorders	Symptoms of depression or anxiety Insomnia	Counseling Education about diagnosis Neuroleptic medications
Gastrointestinal hemorrhage	Abdominal pain Signs of bleeding Hemoglobin and hematocrit	Administration of PPI or H2 blocker
Secondary adrenal insufficiency	Hypotension Postural dizziness/ syncope Hyponatremia Hypokalemia	Hydrocortisone Adjust activities as tolerated
Myopathy	Symmetrical proximal muscle weakness in pelvis and shoulders	Endurance and resistive exercises
Osteoporosis	Pain Falls	Calcium Vitamin D Bisphosphonates Weight-bearing exercises

TABLE 2.2
Commonly Used Chemotherapies in Primary and Metastatic CNS Tumors and Their Adverse Effects

Medication Class (Common Medication)	Adverse Effects
Alkylating agents (Temozolomide)	Cytopenia, cognitive dysfunction
Monoclonal antibodies (Bevacizumab)	Cytopenia
Topoisomerase inhibitors (Irinotecan)	Cytopenia
Taxanes (Paclitaxel)	Cytopenia, peripheral neuropathy
Platinum-based compounds (Cisplatin)	Peripheral neuropathy, ototoxicity
Vinca alkaloids (Vincristine)	Peripheral neuropathy

through induction of gluconeogenesis.[59] Elevated serum blood sugar levels was the most frequently reported adverse effect in patients with primary and metastatic brain tumors, despite no pre-existing condition of diabetes mellitus. A total of 47% of patients with brain metastases and 72% of patients with primary brain tumors reported serum blood sugar levels greater than 100 mg/dL, whereas 3.3% of patients with brain metastases and 10.6% of those with primary brain tumors reported serum blood sugar levels greater than 300 mg/dL after a mean duration of 6.9 weeks of dexamethasone treatment, although it is important to note that some brain tumor patients continued to take dexamethasone until their deaths.[54] As a result, regular monitoring of serum blood sugar levels is warranted in patients on glucocorticoids. High serum blood sugar levels should be corrected using therapeutic intervention, such as insulin, despite the patient being a nondiabetic[57] (Table 2.2).

Psychiatric Disorders

Psychiatric disorders such as anxiety, depression, and insomnia have been linked to the long-term use of glucocorticoids, although the mechanism by which this occurs is still not well understood. Anxiety, depression, and insomnia were reported in 9.9% of patients with brain metastases and 10.6% of patients with primary brain tumors.[54] Some research suggests that dexamethasone alone cannot be attributed, as many of these patients are also grappling with a terminal diagnosis and are likely experiencing psychologic changes as a result of this as well. Counseling and education are important interventions prior to initiating pharmacotherapy in these individuals, although neuroleptic medications may be required to help control the behavioral sequelae.[55] Because dexamethasone provides some neurologic benefit in these patients, it should not be withdrawn as a result of the development of these psychiatric conditions unless the patient is believed to be a danger to himself/herself or another individual.[57] Symptoms tend to resolve after stopping the steroid treatment.[55]

Risk of Gastrointestinal Hemorrhage

The development of peptic ulcer disease and gastrointestinal bleeding can be a life-threatening complication of glucocorticoid use, but this is seen very rarely today. A recent study conducted by Hempen et al. showed gastric disorders, such as a stomachache, was reported in only 3.3% of patients with brain metastases and 6.4% of patients with primary brain tumors, none of whom reported gastrointestinal hemorrhage.[54] Nevertheless, patients on glucocorticoid therapy should have prophylactic administration of H2 blockers or proton-pump inhibitors, which will likely diminish this life-threatening risk.[57]

Secondary Adrenal Insufficiency

Long-term administration of steroids at high doses can lead to secondary adrenal insufficiency through disruption of the hypothalamic-pituitary-adrenal axis, an effect that is usually temporary and reversible. Abrupt cessation or rapid tapering of steroids can cause decreased production of endogenous corticosteroids for a period of time, which can cause hypotension, postural dizziness, or syncope; these patients may also have laboratory findings of hyponatremia and hypokalemia, further exacerbating their symptoms.[57] This is particularly important in the rehabilitation setting and should be monitored by the physiatrist, with activities adjusted as the patient is able to tolerate, in order to prevent falls. Treatment often entails exogenous administration of hydrocortisone, a cortisol substitute, until the patient can recover adrenal production.[57]

Glucocorticoid-Induced Myopathy

Glucocorticoid-induced myopathy (GIM) can affect up to 60% of patients treated with glucocorticoids and occurs more frequently in those treated with fluorinated steroids.[60,55] GIM manifests as weakness that occurs due to proteolysis of myofibrils most commonly proximally and symmetrically in the pelvic girdle musculature, less commonly in the shoulder girdle and distal musculature, and usually occurs within weeks to months of the onset of glucocorticoid therapy.[57,61] This can lead to muscular atrophy and rhabdomyolysis. It is widely thought that the reduced strength in the proximal muscles can lead to decreased stability in sit-to-stand transfers and standing, both of which can lead to increased risk of falling and having fractures as well.[62] Recent studies have shown that endurance and resistance exercises can reverse muscle atrophy and weakness in those treated with glucocorticoids.[3] Therefore, there should be a focus on keeping the muscles as strong and healthy as the bones.

Osteoporosis and Bone Fragility

Glucocorticoid-induced osteoporosis is the most common form of secondary osteoporosis.[60,63] The use of glucocorticoids leads to a reduction in bone tissue integrity because of the imbalance between bone resorption and bone formation and repair, compromising the biomechanical properties of the bone.[60,64,65] A meta-analysis of previous studies showed the risk of fractures was increased at the commencement and within the first 3 months of therapy, and the increased risk was found to be dose dependent.[66] These fractures were mainly seen in the vertebrae, with hip fractures being the second most common. While the risk of fractures is high during the use of glucocorticoids, the risk of fractures decreases substantially, and often back to baseline levels, if the use of glucocorticoids is suspended.[59] Moderate-intensity weight-bearing exercise of 30 minutes per day, multiple times per week, has shown a positive impact on bone density and should be used with careful consideration in conjunction with pharmacotherapy, such as calcium and Vitamin D supplementation and bisphosphonates to further decrease the risk of fracture.[67,68]

The risk of fractures and bone fragility is also increased with bony metastases, which are commonly associated with primary cancers from the lung, breast, and prostate. The National Comprehensive Cancer Network guidelines advise cancer survivors with bony metastases to exercise with caution and ACSM follows a symptoms-based approach to exercise. For those with bony metastases, an ideal exercise program begins at low intensity and slowly progresses as the patient can tolerate.[69] Those with metastatic disease to the bone are also advised to follow modified exercise program with reduced impact, intensity and duration.[23] Studies have shown light resistive training of the paravertebral muscles in a supervised setting to be safe in patients with stable bony metastases and may help to increase bone density when concomitantly treated with bisphosphonates.[70] With bony metastases, one must be cognizant of the affected limb's functional limitations, which often requires restrictions in resistance training and off-loading weight bearing.[71] Physicians, therapists, and patients need to be aware that exercise can continue with metastatic disease to the bone, but alterations to the exercise program are required due to the increased fracture risk.

CONCLUSION

Cancer rehabilitation has the potential to offer cancer survivors improved function, mobility, and quality of life. Rehabilitation physicians need to have a thorough understanding of current treatments, subsequent complications, and precautions that patients will require.

REFERENCES

1. Kushner D, Amidei C. Rehabilitation of motor dysfunction in primary brain tumor patients. *Neuro-Oncology Pract.* 2015;2(4):185–191.
2. Mukand JA, Blackinton DD, Crincoli MG, Lee JJ, Santos BB. Incidence of neurological deficits and rehabilitation in patients with brain tumors. *Am J Phys Med Rehabilitation.* 2001;80(5):346–350.
3. Vargo M. Brain tumor rehabilitation. *Am J Phys Med Rehabil.* 2011;90(suppl):S50–S62.
4. Amidei C, Kushner D. Clinical implications of motor deficits related to brain tumors. *Neuro-Oncology Pract.* 2015; 2(4):179–184.
5. Maltser S, Cristian A, Silver JK, Morris GS, Stout NL. A focused review of safety considerations in cancer rehabilitation. *PM R.* 2017;9(9 suppl 2):S415–S428.
6. Raj VS, Balouch J, Norton JH. Cancer rehabilitation education during physical medicine and rehabilitation residency: preliminary data regarding the quality and quantity of experiences. *Am J Phys Med Rehabil.* 2014; 93(5):445–452. https://doi.org/10.1097/PHM.
7. American Physical Therapy Association. Oncology Section; 2017. www.oncologypt.org.
8. 2017 Medical Rehabilitation Program Descriptions. Carf International, Cancer Rehabilitation Speciality Program.
9. Aminoff MJ, ed. *Neurology and General Medicine.* 4th ed. Vol. 523. New York, NY: Churchill Livingstone; 2007. www.aboutcancer.com/brain_radiation_comps_aminoff.htm.
10. Correa DD, Shi W, Thaler HT, Cheung AM, DeAngelis LM, Abrey LE. Longitudinal cognitive follow-up in low grade gliomas. *J Neurooncol.* 2008;86(3):321–327.
11. Powell C, Guerrero D, Sardell S, et al. Somnolence syndrome in patients receiving radical radiotherapy for primary brain tumours: a prospective study. *Radiother Oncol.* 2011; 100(1):131.
12. Armstrong CL, Corn BW, Ruffer JE, Pruitt AA, Mollman JE, Phillips PC. Radiotherapeutic effects on brain function: double dissociation of memory systems. *Neuropsychiatry Neuropsychol Behav Neurol.* 2000;13(2):101.
13. Burger PC, Mahley Jr MS, Dudka L, Vogel FS. The morphological effects of radiation administered therapeutically for intracranial gliomas: a postmortem study of 25 cases. *Cancer.* 1979;44:1256.
14. Giordana MT, Clara E. Functional rehabilitation and brain tumour patients: a review of outcome. *Neurol Sci.* 2006;27: 240–244.
15. Dietrich J, Monje M, Wefel J, Meyers C. Clinical patterns and biological correlates of cognitive dysfunction associated with cancer therapy. *Oncologist.* 2008;13:1285.
16. Feng R, Loewenstern J, Aggarwal A, et al. Cerebral radiation necrosis: an analysis of clinical and quantitative imaging and volumetric features. *World Neurosurg.* 2018-03;111: e485–e494. https://doi.org/10.1016/j.wneu.2017.12.104.
17. O'Dell Michael, Stubblefield Michael. *Cancer Rehabilitation: Principles and Practice.* Demos Medical Publishing; 2009.
18. Fein DA1, Marcus Jr RB, Parsons JT, Mendenhall WM, Million RR. Lhermitte's sign: incidence and treatment variables influencing risk after irradiation of the cervical spinal cord. *Int J Radiat Oncol Biol Phys.* 1993;27(5): 1029–1033.
19. Okada S, Okeda R. Pathology of radiation myelopathy. *Neuropathology.* 2001;21:247.
20. Van der Sluis RW, Wolfe GI, Nations SP, et al. Post-radiation lower motor syndrome. *J Clinical Neuromuscular Disease.* 2000;2(1):10–17.
21. Agarwal A, Kanekar S, Thamburaj K, Vijay K. Radiation-induced spinal cord hemorrhage (Hematomyelia). *Neurol Int.* 2014;6(4):5553.
22. Schmitz KH, Courneya KS, Matthews C, et al. American College of Sports Medicine roundtable on exercise guidelines for cancer survivors. *Med Sci Sports Exerc.* 2010; 42(7):1409–1426. https://doi.org/10.1249/MSS.0b013e3181e0c112.
23. Stout N, Baima J, Swisher A, Winters-Stone K, Welsh J. A systematic review of exercise systematic reviews in the cancer literature (2005-2017). *PM&R.* 2017;9:S347–S384.
24. Bartolo M, Zucchella C, Pace A, et al. Early rehabilitation after surgery improves functional outcome in patients with brain tumors. *J Neuro-oncology.* 2012;107:537–544.
25. Baima J, Omer ZB, Varlotto J, Yunus S. Compliance and safety of a novel home exercise program for patients with high-grade brain tumors, a prospective, observational study. *Support Care Cancer.* 2017;25(9):2809–2814.
26. Cristian A, Tran A, Patel K. Patient safety in cancer rehabilitation. *Phys Med Rehabilitation Clin.* 2012;23(2): 441–456.
27. Bartels MN, Leight M. Cardiac complications of cancer. In: Stubblefield MD, Odell MW, eds. *Cancer Rehabilitation, Principles and Practice.* New York: Demos Medical; 2009: 349–358.
28. Bartels MN, Freeland ML. Pulmonary complications of cancer. In: Stubblefield MD, Odell MW, eds. *Cancer Rehabilitation, Pronciles and Practice.* New York: Demos Medical; 2009:331–347.
29. Stupp R, Mason WP, van der Bent MJ, et al. Radiotherapy plus concomitant and adjuvant temozolomide for glioblastoma. *N Engl J Med.* 2005;352:987–996.
30. Kreisl TN, Kim L, Moore K, et al. Phase II trial of single-agent bevacizumab followed by bevacizumab plus irinotecan at tumor progression in recurrent glioblastoma. *J Clin Oncol.* 2009;27(5):740.
31. Friedman HS, Prados MD, Wen PY, et al. Bevacizumab alone and in combination with irinotecan in recurrent glioblastoma. *J Clin Oncol.* 2009;27(28):4733.
32. Barnholtz-Sloan JS, Sloan AE, Davis FG, Vigneau FD, Lai P, Sawaya RE. Incidence proportions of brain metastases in patients diagnosed (1973 to 2001) in the Metropolitan Detroit cancer Surveillance system. *J Clin Oncol.* 2004; 22(14):2865–2872.
33. Owusu C, Cohen H, Feng T, et al. Anemia and functional disability in older adults with cancer. *J Natl Compr Canc Netw.* 2015;13(10):1233–1239.

34. Penninx BW, Pahor M, Cesari M, et al. Anemia is associated with disability and decreased physical performance and muscle strength in the elderly. *J Am Geriatr Soc.* 2004;52(5):719–724.
35. Denny SD, Kuchibhatla MN, Cohen HJ. Impact of anemia on mortality, cognition, and function in community-dwelling elderly. *Am J Med.* 2006;119(4):327–334.
36. Elter T, Stipanov M, Heuser E, et al. Is physical exercise possible in patients with critical cytopenia undergoing intensive chemotherapy for acute leukaemia or aggressive lymphoma? *Int J Hematol.* 2009;90:199–204.
37. Paul KL. Rehabilitation and exercise considerations in hematologic malignancies. *Am J Phys Med Rehabil.* 2011; 90(suppl):S76–S82.
38. Khan S, Dhadda A, Fyfe D, et al. Impact of neutropenia on delivering planned chemotherapy for solid tumours. *Eur J Cancer Care.* 2008;17:19–25.
39. Shelton BK. Evidence-based care for the neutropenic patient with leukemia. *Semin Oncol Nurs.* 2003;19(2):133–141.
40. Vadhan-Raj S. Management of chemotherapy-induced thrombocytopenia: current status of thrombopoietic agents. *Semin Hematol.* 2009;46(1 suppl 2):S26–S32.
41. Gerber DE, Grossman SA, Zeltzman M, Parisi MA, Kleinberg L. The impact of thrombocytopenia from temozolomide and radiation in newly diagnosed adults with high-grade gliomas. *Neuro Oncol.* 2007;9(1):47–52.
42. Argyriou AA, Bruna J, Marmiroli P, Cavaletti G. Chemotherapy-induced peripheral neurotoxicity (CIPN): an update. *Crit Rev Oncol Hematol.* 2012;82(1):51–77.
43. Winters-Stone KM, Horak F, Jacobs PG, et al. Falls, functioning, and disability among women with persistent symptoms of chemotherapy-induced peripheral neuropathy. *J Clin Oncol.* 2017;35(23):2604–2612.
44. Stubblefield MD, Burstein HJ, Burton AW, et al. NCCN task force report: management of neuropathy in cancer. *J Natl Comp Cancer Netw.* 2009;7:S1–S26.
45. Hess LM, Huang HQ, Hanlon AL, et al. Cognitive function during and six months following chemotherapy for front line treatment of ovarian, primary peritoneal or fallopian tube cancer: an NRG oncology/gynaecologic oncologic group study. *Gynecol Oncol.* 2015;139: 541–545.
46. Cruzado JA, López-Santiago S, Martínez-Marín V, José-Moreno G, Custodio AB, Feliu J. Longitudinal study of cognitive dysfunctions induced by adjuvant chemotherapy in colon cancer patients. *Support Care Cancer.* 2014;22:1815–1823.
47. Zimmer P, Baumann FT, Oberste M, et al. Effects of exercise interventions and physical activity behavior on cancer related cognitive impairments: a systematic review. *Biomed Res Int.* 2016;2016:1820954. https://doi.org/10.1155/2016/1820954.
48. Gehring K, Sitskoorn MM, Aaronson NK, et al. Interventions for cognitive deficits in adults with brain tumours. *Lancet Neurol.* 2008;7:548–560.
49. Rosati A, Buttolo L, Stefini R, Todeschini A, Cenzato M, Padovani A. Efficacy and safety of levetiracetam in patients with glioma. *Arch Neurol.* 2010;67(3):343–346.
50. Usery JB, Michael M, Sills AK, Finch CK. A prospective evaluation and literature review of levetiracetam use in patients with brain tumors and seizures. *J Neurooncol.* 2010; 99:251–260.
51. Vecht CJ, van Breemen M. Optimizing therapy of seizures in patients with brain tumors. *Neurology.* 2006;67(suppl): S10–S13.
52. Błaszczyk B, Lasoń W, Czuczwar SJ. Antiepileptic drugs and adverse skin reactions: an update. *Pharmacol Rep.* 2015;67(3):426–434.
53. Hurtado B, Koepp MJ, Sander JW, Thompson PJ. The impact of levetiracetam on challenging behavior. *Epilepsy Behav.* 2006;8(3):588.
54. Helmstaedter C, Fritz NE, Kockelmann E, Kosanetzky N, Elger CE. Positive and negative psychotropic effects of levetiracetam. *Epilepsy Behav.* 2008;13(3):535.
55. Milligan TA, Hurwitz S, Bromfield EB. Efficacy and tolerability of levetiracetam versus phenytoin after supratentorial neurosurgery. *Neurology.* 2008;71:665–669.
56. Hempen C, Weiss E, Hess CF. Dexamethasone treatment in patients with brain metastases and primary brain tumors: do the benefits outweigh the side-effects? *Support Care Cancer.* 2002;10(4):322–328.
57. Roth P, Happold C, Weller M. Corticosteroid use in neuro-oncology: an update. *Neurooncol Pract.* 2015;2(1):6–12.
58. Piette C, Munuat C, Foidart JM, Deprez M. Treating gliomas with glucocorticoids: from bedside to bench. *Acta Neuropathol Berl.* 2006;112:651–664.
59. Roth P, Wick W, Weller M. Steroids in neurooncology: actions, indications, side effects. *Curr Opin Neurol.* 2010; 23(6):597–602.
60. Canalis E, Mazziotti G, Giustina A, Bilezikian JP. Glucocorticoid-induced osteoporosis: pathophysiology and therapy. *Osteoporos Int.* 2007;18:1319–1328.
61. van Staa TP. The pathogenesis, epidemiology and management of glucocorticoid-induced osteoporosis. *Calcif Tissue Int.* 2006;79(3):129–137.
62. Canalis E, Bilezikian JP, Angeli A, Giustina A. Perspectives on glucocorticoid-induced osteoporosis. *Bone.* 2004;34: 593–598.
63. Mazziotti G, Angeli A, Bilezikian JP, Canalis E, Giustina A. Glucocorticoid-induced osteoporosis: an update. *Trends Endocrinol Metab.* 2006;17(4):144–149.
64. Jia D, O'Brien CA, Stewart SA, Manolagas SC, Weinstein RS. Glucocorticoids act directly on osteoclasts to increase their life span and reduce bone density. *Endocrinology.* 2006;147(12):5592–5599.
65. O'Brien CA, Jia D, Plotkin LI, et al. Glucocorticoids act directly on osteoblasts and osteocytes to induce their apoptosis and reduce bone formation and strength. *Endocrinology.* 2004;145(4):1835–1841.
66. van Staa TP, Leufkens HG, Abenhaim L, Zhang B, Cooper C. Oral corticosteroids and fracture risk: relationship to daily and cumulative doses. *Rheumatol Oxf.* 2000; 39(12):1383–1389.
67. Silver JK, Baima J, Mayer RS. Impairment-driven cancer rehabilitation: an essential component of quality care and survivorship. *CA Cancer J Clin.* 2013;63:295–317.

68. Stubblefield M, Schmitz KH, Ness KK. Physical functioning and rehabilitation for the cancer survivor. *Semin Oncol.* 2013;40:784–795.
69. Wolin K, Schwartz A, Matthews C, Courneya K, Schmitz K. Implementing the exercise guidelines for cancer survivors. *The J Support Oncol.* 2012;10(5):171–177.
70. Rief H, Petersen L, Omlor G, et al. German Bone Research Group. The effect of resistance training during radiotherapy on spinal bone metastases in cancer patients - a randomized trial. *Radiotherapy Oncol.* 2014;112:133–139.
71. O'Toole GBP, Herklotz M. Bone metastases. In: Stubblefield M, O'Dell M, eds. *Cancer Rehabilitation: Principles and Practice.* New York: Demos Publishing; 2009: 773–785.

CHAPTER 3

Inpatient Rehabilitation Outcome Measures in Persons With Brain and Spinal Cord Cancer

VERONICA J. CHEHATA, BSBIOLOGY, MD • MATTHEW SHATZER, DO • ADRIAN CRISTIAN, MD, MHCM

INTRODUCTION

Inpatient rehabilitation of individuals with brain and spinal cord tumors plays a distinctive role in their cancer care continuums. This chapter focuses on inpatient rehabilitation outcomes in such patients with respect to function, length of stay (LOS), discharge to community, acute transfers, quality of life (QoL), and survivorship. The management and treatment of brain and spinal cord tumors as well as impairments and complications commonly affecting these patients are covered elsewhere in this book.

Rehabilitation of patients with brain and spinal cord tumors undoubtedly presents a unique challenge, as a result of the medical and therapeutic complexities associated with these cancer diagnoses. There are a broad range of associated impairments which include but are not limited to cognitive and/or communication deficits, dysphagia, aphasia, hemiplegia, paraplegia, tetraplegia, spasticity, contractures, pressure ulcers, and neurogenic bowel and bladder.[1,2]

Inpatient rehabilitation of noncancer patients with stroke, traumatic brain injury (TBI), or spinal cord injury (SCI), who may present with some of the abovementioned impairments, has been well established. Intuitively, the same rehabilitation principles should be applied to patients with brain and spinal cord tumors. However, the key differences between patients with brain and spinal cord tumors and their noncancer counterparts are the uncertainties associated with cancer, which include prognosis, progressive functional decline, medical complexity, and concomitant chemotherapy or radiation, to name a few.[1] These, in addition to financial considerations, likely explain why such cancer patients may be less likely to be admitted to acute inpatient rehabilitation.[3]

In order to assess the value of inpatient rehabilitation for patients with brain and spinal cord tumors, as well as their candidacy for it, it is pivotal to evaluate the functional improvements made in inpatient rehabilitation as well as other outcomes such as LOS, discharge to community, acute transfer rate, QoL, and survivorship. It has been suggested that selection of patients for inpatient rehabilitation is often based on prognosis for survival and anticipated functional outcome on discharge.[4]

Evidently, patients with brain and spinal cord tumors do benefit from inpatient rehabilitation. Patients with brain tumors show improved functional scores that are maintained after discharge. These improvements are achieved regardless of tumor type, lesion, and presence of metastasis.[5] Additionally, patients with brain tumors make similar functional gains to stroke and TBI patients, despite shorter LOSs. Similarly, patients with spinal cord tumors have been found to have improved Functional Independence Measure (FIM) scores, as well as improved mood, QoL, and survival after inpatient rehabilitation.[6] Such promising results warrant the attention of providers to admitting and selecting brain and spinal cord cancer patients to acute inpatient rehabilitation when appropriate.

DESCRIPTION OF OUTCOME MEASURES

Functional Independence Measure (FIM): The FIM is an 18-item, clinician-reported scale that assesses function in six areas including self-care, continence, mobility, transfers, communication, and cognition. Each of the 18 items is graded on a scale of 1–7 based on level of independence in that item (1 = total assistance required, 7 = complete independence).[7,8] FIM scores can be measured at admission to and discharge from inpatient rehabilitation. The difference between the admission and discharge scores constitutes the FIM change or FIM gain. FIM efficiency refers to the rate of FIM change with time.

Karnofsky Performance Status (KPS): A clinician-reported scale that rates patients' global performance status on a scale of 0–100, scored in intervals of 10. A score of 0 signifies death, while a score of 100 indicates normal function with no evidence of disease.[7,8]

Eastern Cooperative Oncology Group (ECOG) Performance Status: A clinician-reported scale comparable to the KPS, scored from 0 to 5, with 0 indicating "Fully active, able to carry on all predisease performance without restriction," and 5 indicating death.[8,9]

Spinal Cord Independence Measure (SCIM): A validated and sensitive tool used to detect functional improvements in traumatic and nontraumatic SCI. It has been suggested as a more optimal tool to assess functional outcomes in patients with spinal cord tumors as opposed to the FIM.[10]

Functional Assessment of Cancer Therapy-Brain (FACT: BR): A 54-item scale used to assess QoL in patient with brain tumor using Likert scales. The tool assesses QoL components, including physical, social, emotional, and functional well being, in addition to other considerations.[7]

OUTCOMES: BRAIN TUMOR

Functional Outcomes

Several studies have shown improvement in functional status in patients with brain tumors who undergo inpatient rehabilitation. Marciniak et al. showed that patients with both primary and metastatic tumor types improved functionally after inpatient rehabilitation, with comparable *total* FIM change (motor and cognitive) and equivalent FIM efficiencies across all tumor groups.[11] Similarly, Tang et al. showed that patients with brain metastasis, glioblastoma multiforme, and other brain tumors made functional gains from inpatient rehabilitation admission to discharge.[12]

In a study that prospectively evaluated 10 patients with brain tumors, Huang et al. showed significant functional gains as measured by the FIM, the disability rating scale (DRS), and the KPS score.[7] FIM and DRS scores improved from admission to discharge to 3-month follow-up, whereas KPS scores only showed significant improvement from admission to 3-month follow-up. Their study shows that functional gains are sustained at 3 months and suggests that the KPS may not be useful in detecting more subtle changes.[7]

A more recent, larger study examined the effect of inpatient rehabilitation on functional outcomes in 100 patients who underwent surgical resection after newly diagnosed glioblastoma multiforme. The study showed that 93.7% of patients had improvement in functional status from admission to discharge, with the largest gains in mobility, self-care, communication/social cognition, and sphincter control. Additionally, 22% of the patients were deemed to be "high responders" who improved a minimum of two levels of independence based on FIM scores from admission to discharge.[13]

Comparing Functional Outcomes in Relationship to Other Factors

Several studies have attempted to further characterize the functional gains made by patients with brain tumors in inpatient rehabilitation with regard to tumor type, tumor recurrence, and concomitant therapy.

Marciniak et al. did note a difference in *motor* FIM gains across tumor types (lowest gains in meningioma and astrocytoma compared with metastasis and "other"); however, such differences were deemed secondary to differing LOSs.[11] Similarly, a retrospective review of charts comparing 21 patients with low-grade astrocytoma with 21 patients with high-grade astrocytoma by Fu et al. showed that while both groups made functional gains, the patients with high-grade astrocytoma had higher total FIM gains (21.7 vs. 13), but again likely secondary to longer LOS (13 vs. 9 days).[14] FIM efficiencies were comparable in the two groups.[14] Thus it appears that patients with more advanced tumors such as metastatic tumors and high-grade astrocytomas had higher FIM gains, but likely due to longer LOS.

With regard to tumor recurrence, Marciniak et al. showed that patients with recurrence had lower FIM motor gains and FIM efficiencies compared with those patients undergoing rehabilitation after initial tumor diagnosis.[11]

With respect to concomitant treatment, Marciniak et al. also found that patients receiving concomitant radiotherapy had greater motor FIM efficiency scores, thought likely due to tumor shrinkage. However, the authors also note that patients who received radiotherapy tended to not have tumor recurrence.[11] In contrast, Tang et al. showed that concomitant treatment with chemotherapy or radiation was not a predictor of FIM gain.[3,12]

Length of Stay

Several studies between 1998 and 2006 show that brain tumor patients undergoing inpatient rehabilitation have LOSs between 18 and 25 days.[2,7,11,15–17] A later study by Fu et al. showed even shorter LOS in high- and low-grade astrocytoma patients (13 days vs. 9 days, respectively).[14]

Discharge Home

Patients with brain tumors show relatively high rates of discharge home after inpatient rehabilitation, with most studies reporting rates between 80% and 92%.[2,7,11,14–17] Tang et al. showed slightly lower rates of 76%, 72%, and 70% in glioblastoma, metastatic tumors, and other tumors, respectively.[3,12]

Acute Transfer

While most studies have not measured the rate of acute transfers as a primary outcome, several have reported it. Marciniak et al. showed an acute transfer rate of 25%.[11] Several have compared such rates with that of the rate of acute transfer in TBI and stroke patients as in the following sections.

Quality of Life

Poor functional status has been linked to poor QoL in cancer survivors, including patients with brain tumors. To date, few studies have specifically examined the correlation between inpatient rehabilitation functional and QoL outcomes in patients with brain tumors. In one study, Huang et al. used the FACT-BR measure to assess QoL in a prospective study of 10 patients with brain tumors. They found insignificant improvement in scores from admission to discharge, with significant improvement between admission and 1-month follow-up and admission and 3-month follow-up.[7] This was deemed likely to the fact that patients only perceived improvement in QoL when they were able to reintegrate back into their home and community environments. Of note, functional levels on the three scales measured (FIM, DRS, KPS) did not correlate with FACT-BR scores, which the authors note is similar to the results in three prior studies.[7] Similarly, Kim et al. found insignificant improvements in QoL (using the European Organization for Research and Treatment of Cancer Quality of Life Questionnaire-Core 30) in 25 brain tumor patients undergoing inpatient rehabilitation. As in Huang's study,[7] the authors felt that longer follow-up was necessary to evaluate the effect of inpatient rehabilitation on QoL.[18]

Survival

Inherent to cancer rehabilitation as a whole is the question of survival and prognosis as it pertains to function. The study by Tang et al. showed that positive prognosis was associated with high FIM gain, low dexamethasone dose, and lack of organ metastasis in patients with brain metastasis. In patients with glioblastoma, low admission dexamethasone dose and high FIM gain indicated better survival prognosis.[3,12]

Roberts et al. also examined survival time in their study of patients with glioblastoma multiforme who underwent inpatient rehabilitation. They reported a median survival time of 14.3 months in patients who underwent inpatient rehabilitation versus 17.9 months in patients who did not undergo inpatient rehabilitation; however, this was not statistically significant after adjustment for confounders (age, extent of resection, and KPS score). They concluded that the lack of survival difference in the two groups may be clinically relevant in the sense that the patients admitted to inpatient rehabilitation had lower KPS scores than those who did not require inpatient rehabilitation, presumably due to worse overall clinical condition and potentially worse prognosis. They thus argue that inpatient rehabilitation may have "level[ed] the survival prognosis" for these patients with initial lower function. Namely, inpatient rehabilitation provided a survival benefit to these patients. Additionally, this study noted that "mobility responders" or patients with FIM mobility gains trended toward longer survival.[13]

Comparison to TBI and Stroke

As the neurologic impairments in patients with brain tumors are similar to those in stroke and TBI, several studies have compared outcomes in patients with brain tumors to those in patients with TBI and stroke, as inpatient rehabilitation in these groups is well established.

O'Dell et al. retrospectively compared outcomes after inpatient rehabilitation in patients with brain tumors with those in a group of case-matched patients with TBI.[2] They found that although the absolute FIM gains were higher in the TBI group, FIM efficiencies were comparable, likely due to the shorter LOS in the brain tumor group (18 days vs. 22 days). Also, there was a trend toward higher gains in patients with diagnosis of meningioma, lesions in the left hemisphere (thought due to generally poorer outcomes in right-sided lesions, due to neglect), and those not receiving concomitant radiotherapy. Discharge home rates were comparable in the two groups (82.5% in the brain tumor group vs. 92.5% in the

TBI group). The rate of acute transfer in the brain tumor group was 7.5% versus 0% in the TBI group.[2]

Huang et al. also compared patients with brain tumor to those with TBI and found no significant difference with regard to total admission and discharge FIMs or FIM efficiencies.[16] Admission cognitive FIM was lower in the TBI group. As in O'Dell's study,[2] FIM change was higher in the TBI group. The tumor group had lower LOSs and greater discharge to the community—TBI patients were more likely to be discharged to institutionalized settings (26% vs. 13.4%). It is thought that patients with brain tumors may have better family support hence increased rates of discharge home. In contrast to O'Dell's study,[2] side of lesion did not result in differences in the rehabilitation LOS.[16] Bilgin et al. more recently performed a similar study comparing patients with TBI and brain tumor, using lesion side and gender as matching criteria.[19] They found that patients with TBI had initial lower functional status but displayed better functional recovery than patients with brain tumor. As in Huang's study,[16] lesion side had no effect on functional outcome in either group.[19]

Similarly Huang et al. retrospectively compared outcomes in patients with brain tumors to those in stroke patients admitted to inpatient rehabilitation.[15] They reported no significant difference between the two groups with regard to total admission FIM, total discharge FIM, total FIM change, or FIM efficiency. However, stroke patients did experience greater change in ADL-FIM scores from admission to discharge as compared with their counterparts with brain tumors. On the other hand, patients with brain tumors had higher motor FIM scores. There were no significant differences in cognitive FIM between the two groups. With regard to LOS, the brain tumor group had significantly shorter LOS than the stroke group (25 days vs. 34 days). Discharge to the community was greater than 85% in both groups. Additionally, LOS for patients with right-sided stroke was an average of 10 days longer than in patients with right-sided tumor. Also, the right-sided stroke group experienced higher rates of ADL-FIM change than their right-sided tumor counterparts.[15]

In another study, Greenberg et al. compared rehabilitation outcomes in patients with brain tumors (meningiomas and gliomas) who survived craniotomy to those with stroke. They found similar functional outcomes in all groups tested, with shorter LOS in patients with brain tumor (24 days for the meningioma group, 23 days for the glioma group, 75.4 days for the stroke group). FIM efficiency was found to be lower (although not statistically significant) in the stroke group likely secondary to increased LOS.[17]

Finally, Bartolo et al. compared 75 patients with brain tumor (meningioma and glioblastoma) status post neurosurgery (rehabilitation started within 2 weeks of surgery) with a control group of 75 matched stroke patients.[20] They found improvement in function across both groups. Subgroup analysis showed that patients with meningioma had significantly higher FIM motor and ADL gains as compared with patients with glioblastoma or stroke. These differences were thought to be secondary to the benign nature of meningiomas as compared with glioblastomas. With regard to the stroke group, the differences were thought to be due to the ischemic or hemorrhagic nature of brain damage as opposed to the "space-occupying" nature of meningiomas. Overall they show that early rehabilitation after surgery is key.[20]

OUTCOMES: SPINAL CORD TUMOR

Functional Outcomes

Studies evaluating patients with spinal cord tumors undergoing inpatient rehabilitation show functional benefits. An early study by Murray et al. in 27 patients with spinal cord tumors showed improved function after inpatient rehabilitation, which was maintained at 1-year follow-up in patients with incomplete SCIs (Frankel 2, 3, and 4).[21] Another study in patients with both primary and secondary spinal cord tumors specifically showed improvement in upper and lower extremity dressing, wheelchair use and transfers, ambulation, and stair climbing. These improvements were sustained at 3 months post discharge.[22] In a later study by Tan et al., comparing patients with primary versus secondary spinal cord tumor, FIM gain was significantly greater in patients with primary tumors.[23]

Thus patients with metastatic spinal cord tumors show improvement after inpatient rehabilitation. In a study by Parsch et al., patients with metastatic spinal cord compression showed improvements in their FIM scores from 62 to 84.[24] FIM efficiency in this study was 0.33, which the authors noted was within the reported range for non traumatic complete paraplegic patients, but lower than expected for traumatic SCI patients.[24] Similarly, a study by Tang et al. showed improvements in FIM score from 83 to 102 from admission to discharge, with a similar FIM efficiency to the Parsch study, of 0.38.[25] Overall, a review of several studies on functional outcome in patients with metastatic spinal cord tumors after inpatient rehabilitation showed FIM gain to be at least 15, with FIM efficiencies between 0.33 and 0.42.[26]

Length of Stay

LOS for patients with spinal cord tumors undergoing inpatient rehabilitation is mostly in the range of 15–50 days[26] with the exception of an early study by Hacking et al. (LOS 111 days)[4] and a study in the Netherlands (LOS of 104 days; the authors noted that inpatient rehabilitation LOS in the Netherlands is generally longer than in other countries).[27] With regard to factors that affect LOS, one study in patients with metastatic tumors found LOS to vary with the incidence of pressure ulcers. Namely, patients without pressure ulcers had LOS of 42 days, whereas patients with pressure ulcers had significantly longer LOS of 123 days.[24] With regard to primary tumors compared with secondary tumors, a retrospective 12-year study in Australia showed a median LOS of 47.5 days, with a trend toward shorter LOS in patients with primary tumors.[28]

Discharge to Community

The vast majority of patients with spinal cord tumors undergoing inpatient rehabilitation are discharged home. In one study, 84% of patients were discharged home.[22] In a study of patients with metastatic tumors, the rate of discharge home was 82%.[29] In a retrospective study by Tan et al., 62% were discharged home, with a noticeable trend of more patients with secondary tumors being discharged to nursing or palliative care.[23,28] Also, patients with complete SCIs were more likely to be discharged to palliative care.[23]

In the only prospective study of patients with metastatic spinal cord tumors who received 2 weeks of inpatient rehabilitation (compared with a group who did not receive rehabilitation), 75% of the rehabilitation group were discharged home versus 20% of the "No Rehab" group.[30]

Acute Transfers

While the rate of acute transfers has not been measured as a primary outcome in most studies, several have reported it. A study of metastatic spinal cord tumors reported a rate of approximately 16% (11 of 68 patients), in addition to 6 of 68 patients who died on the ward.[24] Another study of both primary and secondary tumors showed a lower rate of 11%.[28] In a general study of inpatient cancer rehabilitation, Alam et al. showed that patients with spinal cord neoplasms had a significantly higher rate of transfer to acute care compared with controls (23% vs. 10%).[31] Overall, patients with spinal cord tumor resulting in malignant spinal cord compression are more likely to have their rehabilitation interrupted by transfer to the acute care hospital as compared with patients with other nontraumatic etiologies of spinal cord injury.[10]

Quality of Life

While QoL is certainly recognized as a key aspect of cancer survivorship, as in brain tumor, few studies have evaluated the effect of inpatient rehabilitation and functional outcomes on QoL outcomes. Of these two rare studies by Ruff et al., measured level of pain, self-reported depression, and satisfaction of life as secondary outcomes (amid others) in patients with spinal epidural metastasis undergoing inpatient rehabilitation. Their initial study showed that such patients had lower prevalence of clinical depression, lower pain scores, and higher satisfaction with life. Their follow-up study showed that such benefits with regard to pain, depression, and QoL persisted until end of life.[30,32]

For sure, QoL is related to pain, and this has certainly been noted in several studies.[22,33,34] McKinley reported that 64%–90% of patients had disabling pain.[33] Similarly, Tan et al. showed that patients with pain had worse FIM efficiencies and longer median LOS.[23] More studies are needed to evaluate the interplay of pain, QoL, and functional outcomes in inpatient spinal cord tumor rehabilitation.

Survival

Much of the research focused on functional outcomes in inpatient rehabilitation of patients with spinal cord tumors has also focused on survival and prognostication. An early study by Hacking et al. noted six factors associated with prolonged survival greater than 1 year after discharge and improved functional level. These included tumor biology, SCI as the presenting symptom of malignancy, slow progression of neurologic symptoms (>1 week), tumor treated with a combination of surgery and radiotherapy, (partial) bowel control at admission, and (partial) independence regarding transfer activities at admission.[1,4]

Some studies have noted that the most significant and reliable factor for functional prognosis and survival was higher FIM score on admission, or pretreatment motor function.[24,33] However, Tang et al. did not find admission FIM score to be a significant prognostic factor, but rather FIM gain or improvement in function during inpatient rehabilitation.[25] Other studies found improved survival and functional outcome in less severely injured patients,[21,24] but with conflicting results on whether there is a correlation between completeness of injury and survival.[3] Tumor type and level of lesion were deemed less predictive in the sense of survival outcomes on one study[24] and did not reach significance at all in another.[25]

In the prospective study by Ruff et al., the difference in survival between the Rehab and "No Rehab" groups was 20 weeks (26 weeks vs. 6 weeks, respectively). The shorter survival in the "No Rehab" group was deemed secondary to complications of myelopathy and increased rates of depression.[30]

Comparing Spinal Cord Tumors to Traumatic Spinal Cord Injury

McKinley et al. compared patients with spinal cord tumors (neoplastic group) with traumatic SCI patients. Motor FIM scores were higher in the neoplastic group, but discharge FIM scores and FIM change were lower. FIM efficiencies were similar in both groups. LOS was shorter in the neoplastic group, but discharge rates to home were similar in both groups. Overall they noted the difficulties inherent in comparing these two groups in light of the differences in the two study populations with regard to gender, age, and impairment.[33] The study by McKinley in 2000 showed similar results.[35] Shorter LOS may be in part secondary to the incomplete nature of injury and the predominance of paraplegia. Shorter life expectancy and overall prognosis likely also play a role. Patients and families may prefer earlier discharge to allow for maximal time at home and improved QoL.[35]

Comparing Spinal Cord Tumors to Other Nontraumatic Spinal Cord Injury

Fortin et al. compared malignant spinal cord compression to other forms of nontraumatic SCI and found significant improvement in FIM scores from admission to discharge in the malignant spinal cord compression group. However the other nontraumatic SCI group demonstrated higher FIM gain and higher motor FIM subscores on discharge.[10]

CONCLUSIONS

Taken together, the current literature demonstrates that patients with brain and spinal cord cancer do make functional progress in inpatient rehabilitation with high rates of discharge home. As compared with their noncancer counterparts (patients with TBI, stroke, or SCI), they have comparable functional outcomes, shorter LOSs, and higher rates of acute transfer. The few available studies on functional outcomes as they pertain to QoL certainly show a positive association. Similarly, those studies that evaluate the effect of inpatient rehabilitation and functional gain on survival also show a positive correlation.

Several difficulties are apparent in the literature overall. First and foremost is the heterogeneous nature of the cohorts across studies. This includes differences in tumor histology, location, and recurrence, as well as different scales used for functional assessment. In addition, most studies have small samples sizes and are retrospective in nature.[36] Further prospective, large sample size studies are necessary, with a focus on maintenance of gains in the long term. Further studies are needed to evaluate the effect of inpatient rehabilitation on survival and QoL.

The complex interplay between function and survival superimposed on the medical complexity inherent to patients with brain and spinal cord cancer warrants further clarity on the expected functional benefits of inpatient rehabilitation, as they relate to the overall cancer care continuum. Thus clearer criteria for the appropriate selection and admission of such patients to inpatient rehabilitation may be established.

REFERENCES

1. Kirshblum S, O'Dell MW, Ho C, Barr K. Rehabilitation of persons with central nervous system tumors. *Cancer.* 2001;92(Suppl 4):1029–1038.
2. O'Dell MW, Barr K, Spanier D, Warnick RE. Functional outcome of inpatient rehabilitation in persons with brain tumors. *Arch Phys Med Rehabil.* 1998;79:1530–1534.
3. Huang ME, Silwa JA. Inpatient rehabilitation of patients with cancer: efficacy and treatment considerations. *PM R.* 2011;3:746–757.
4. Hacking HG, Van As HH, Lankhorst GJ. Factors related to the outcome of inpatient rehabilitation in patients with neoplastic epidural spinal cord compression. *Paraplegia.* 1993;31:367–374.
5. Shahpar S, Mhatre PV, Huang ME. Update on brain tumors: new developments in neuro-oncologic diagnosis and treatment, and impact on rehabilitation strategies. *PM R.* 2016;8(7):678–689.
6. Raj VS, Lofton L. Rehabilitation and treatment of spinal cord tumors. *J Spinal Cord Med.* 2013;36(1):4–11.
7. Huang ME, Wartella JE, Kreutzer JS. Functional outcomes and quality of life in patients with brain tumors: a preliminary report. *Arch Phys Med Rehabil.* 2001;82:1540–1546.
8. Chevile AL. Metrics in cancer rehabilitation. In: Stubblefield MD, Michael OW, eds. *Cancer Rehabilitation: Principles and Practice*. New York: Demos Medical Publishing; 2009:1025–1034.
9. Oken M, Creech R, Tormey D, et al. Toxicity and response criteria of the Eastern Cooperative Oncology Group. *Am J Clin Oncol.* 1982;5:649–655.
10. Fortin CD, Voth J, Jaglal SB, Craven BC. Inpatient rehabilitation outcomes in patients with malignant spinal cord compression compared to other non-traumatic spinal cord injury: a population based study. *J Spinal Cord Med.* 2015;38(6):754–764.
11. Marciniak CM, Sliwa JA, Heinemann AW, Semik PE. Functional outcomes of persons with brain tumors after inpatient rehabilitation. *Arch Phys Med Rehabil.* 2001;82:457–463.

12. Tang V, Rathbone M, Park Dorsay J, Jiang S, Harvey D. Rehabilitation in primary and metastatic brain tumours: impact of functional outcomes on survival. *J Neurol.* 2008;255:820–827.
13. Roberts PS, Nuño M, Sherman D, et al. The impact of inpatient rehabilitation on function and survival of newly diagnosed patients with glioblastoma. *PM R.* 2014;6(6): 514–521.
14. Fu JB, Parsons HA, Shin KY, et al. Comparison of functional outcomes in low- and high-grade astrocytoma rehabilitation inpatients. *Am J Phys Med Rehabil.* 2010;89(3): 205–212.
15. Huang ME, Cifu DX, Keyser-Marcus L. Functional outcome after brain tumor and acute stroke: a comparative analysis. *Arch Phys Med Rehabil.* 1998;79:1386–1390.
16. Huang ME, Cifu DX, Keyser-Marcus L. Functional outcomes in patients with brain tumor after inpatient rehabilitation: comparison with traumatic brain injury. *Am J Phys Med Rehabil.* 2000;79:327–335.
17. Greenberg E, Treger I, Ring H. Rehabilitation outcomes in patients with brain tumors and acute stroke: comparative study of inpatient rehabilitation. *Am J Phys Med Rehabil.* 2006;85:568–573.
18. Kim BR, Chun MH, Han EY, Kim DK. Fatigue assessment and rehabilitation outcomes in patients with brain tumors. *Support Care Cancer.* 2012;20(4):805–812.
19. Bilgin S, Kose N, Karakaya J, Mut M. Traumatic brain injury shows better functional recovery than brain tumor: a rehabilitative perspective. *Eur J Phys Rehabil Med.* 2014;50(1): 17–23.
20. Bartolo M, Zucchella C, Pace A, et al. Early rehabilitation after surgery improves functional outcome in inpatients with brain tumours. *J Neurooncol.* 2012;107(3):537–544.
21. Murray PK. Functional outcome and survival in spinal cord injury secondary to neoplasia. *Cancer.* 1985;55: 197–201.
22. McKinley WO, Conti-Wyneken AR, Vokac CW, Cifu DX. Rehabilitative functional outcome of patients with neoplastic spinal cord compressions. *Arch Phys Med Rehabil.* 1996;77:892–895.
23. Tan M, New PW. Retrospective study of rehabilitation outcomes following spinal cord injury due to tumour. *Spinal Cord.* 2012;50:127–131.
24. Parsch D, Mikut R, Abel R. Postacute management of patients with spinal cord injury due to metastatic tumour disease: survival and efficacy of rehabilitation. *Spinal Cord.* 2003;41:205–210.
25. Tang V, Harvey D, Park Dorsay J, Jiang S, Rathbone MP. Prognostic indicators in metastatic spinal cord compression: using functional independence measure and Tokuhashi scale to optimize rehabilitation planning. *Spinal Cord.* 2007;45:671–677.
26. Fattal C, Fabbro M, Rouays-Mabit H, Verollet C, Bauchet L. Metastatic paraplegia and functional outcomes: perspectives and limitations for rehabilitation care. Part 2. *Arch Phys Med Rehabil.* 2011;92(1):134–145.
27. Eriks IE, Angenot EL, Lankhorst GJ. Epidural metastatic spinal cord compression: functional outcome and survival after inpatient rehabilitation. *Spinal Cord.* 2004;42: 235–239.
28. Tan M, New P. Survival after rehabilitation for spinal cord injury due to tumor: a 12-year retrospective study. *J Neurooncol.* 2011;104(1):233–238.
29. Guo Y, Young B, Palmer JL, Mun Y, Bruera E. Prognostic factors for survival in metastatic spinal cord compression: a retrospective study in a rehabilitation setting. *Am J Phys Med Rehabil.* 2003;82:665–668.
30. Ruff RL, Adamson VW, Ruff SS, Wang X. Directed rehabilitation reduces pain and depression while increasing independence and satisfaction with life for patients with paraplegia due to epidural metastatic spinal cord compression. *J Rehabil Res Dev.* 2007;44(1):1–10.
31. Alam E, Wilson RD, Vargo MM. Inpatient cancer rehabilitation: a retrospective comparison of transfer back to acute care between patients with neoplasm and other rehabilitation patients. *Arch Phys Med Rehabil.* 2008;89(7):1284–1289.
32. Ruff RL, Ruff SS, Wang X. Persistent benefits of rehabilitation on pain and life quality for nonambulatory patients with spinal epidural metastasis. *J Rehabil Res Dev.* 2007; 44(2):271–278.
33. McKinley WO, Huang ME, Brunsvold KT. Neoplastic versus traumatic spinal cord injury: an outcome comparison after inpatient rehabilitation. *Arch Phys Med Rehabil.* 1999;80:1253–1257.
34. Fattal C1, Gault D, Leblond C, et al. Metastatic paraplegia: care management characteristics within a rehabilitation center. *Spinal Cord.* 2009;47(2):115–121.
35. McKinley WO, Huang ME, Tewksbury MA. Neoplastic vs. traumatic spinal cord injury: an inpatient rehabilitation comparison. *Am J Phys Med Rehabil.* 2000;79:138–144.
36. Formica V, Del Monte G, Giacchetti I, et al. Rehabilitation in neuro-oncology: a meta-analysis of published data and a mono-institutional experience. *Integr Cancer Ther.* 2011; 10(2):119–126.

CHAPTER 4

Tumors of the Brain

SEONG-JIN MOON, MD • DANIEL T. GINAT, MD, MS •
R. SHANE TUBBS, MS, PA-C, PHD • MARC D. MOISI, MD, MS

BACKGROUND

Tumors of the brain present a special challenge for both patients and physicians. Every year, a new brain tumor is discovered in 6.4 cases per 100,000 persons with an overall 5-year survival rate of approximately 33.4%.[1] Nearly 700,000 Americans live with a primary brain tumor. Brain tumors can occur at any age, but the greatest incidence is with ages 65 years and older, and there is a slightly higher predominance in men than in women.[2,3] Over a person's lifetime, there is an approximately 0.6% risk of being diagnosed with a central nervous system cancer. The impact that a diagnosis of brain tumor has on a patient cannot be overstated: some brain tumors can cause significant disability and drastically worsen quality of life, whereas others do not. New treatments offer opportunities to extend life and minimize disability.

CLASSIFICATION

Intracranial tumors are generally classified into either malignant or benign tumors. Furthermore, malignant tumors can be either primary or metastatic. Metastatic lesions are more common than primary tumors.[4] Generally, the proportion of adults with brain tumors increases with age, given that metastatic lesions are more prone to develop over time. The most prevalent brain tumor types in adults are meningiomas, which make up nearly 33.8% of all primary brain tumors[5]; gliomas (i.e., glioblastomas, ependymomas, astrocytomas, oligodendrogliomas) make up almost 80% of malignant brain tumors.[6] Intracranial tumors are often divided into World Health Organization (WHO) classification scale, which can provide patients and clinicians with further information regarding prognosis and management.[7] The WHO scale divides brain tumors into four different classes, from 1 through 4. WHO grade 1 tumors are generally nonmalignant, slower growing, better prognostic lesions. WHO grade 2 tumors are generally nonmalignant but can also be malignant and have a higher propensity for recurrence than grade 1 tumors. WHO grade 3 tumors are aggressive malignant lesions and often recur as higher grade lesions. WHO grade 4 tumors exhibit the most aggressive of lesions and generally exhibit a very high recurrence rate—they demonstrate the poorest prognosis for patients.

CLINICAL PRESENTATION

The clinical presentation of intracranial tumors can vary widely and run the spectrum from a patient who presents with clinical obtundation to an asymptomatic presentation. The location of an intracranial tumor along with its size and mass effect dictates its clinical presentation. Many patients present with clinical signs and symptoms of increased intracranial pressure: headache, nausea/vomiting, ocular palsies, altered mental status, loss of balance, seizures, or papilledema.[8] Some patients can present solely with one clinical symptom, whereas others present with no symptoms at all. For lesions within the frontal lobe, memory, reasoning, personality, and thought processing can be affected. For lesions within the temporal lobe, behavior, memory, hearing, vision, emotion, and speech can be affected. For lesions within the parietal lobe, sensory perception and spatial relations can be affected. For lesions within the occipital lobe, vision can be affected. For lesions within the brainstem or cerebellum, balance and coordination can be affected. A pituitary tumor can compress the optic nerve and cause a bitemporal hemianopsia. A tumor within Broca's area can present with expressive aphasia, whereas a tumor within Wernicke's area can present with fluent aphasia. Meningiomas are dural-based lesions; they are found alongside the dural meninges, and their clinical effects are often related to local mass effect on surrounding tissue. Glioblastomas are very aggressive WHO grade 4 neoplasms with a poor prognosis for recovery. Primary cerebellar lesions that are not metastatic in origin are often hemangioblastomas.[9] Often, such lesions can cause considerable mass effect on surrounding tissue and structures and also have significant surrounding edema as well.

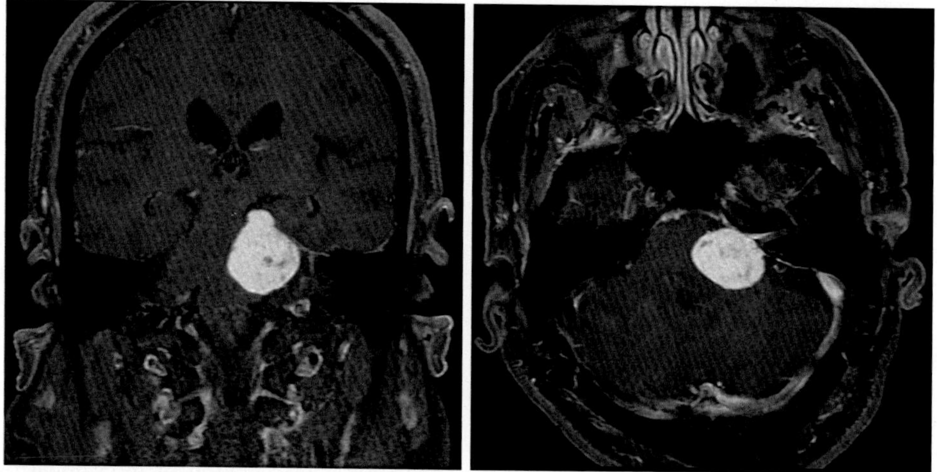

Meningioma. Axial postcontrast T1 MR images show a dural-based mass along the inferior aspect of the left tentorium cerebellum, with a dural tail that extends to the left internal auditory canal.

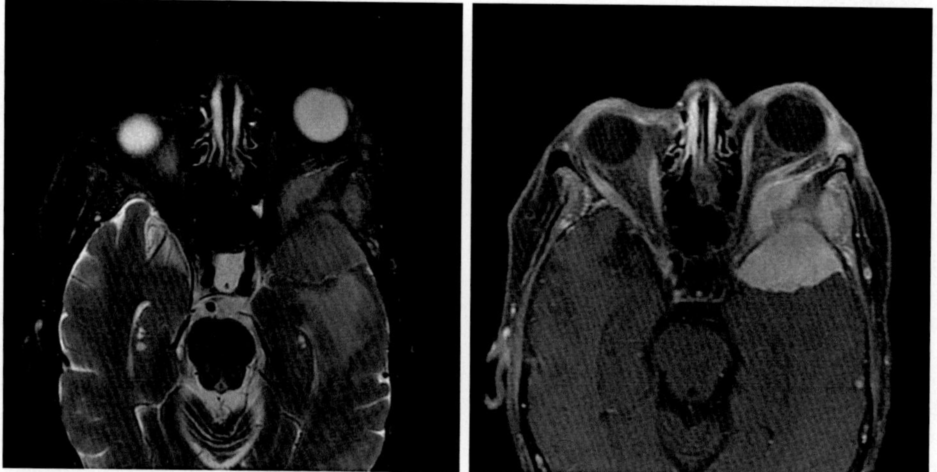

Meningioma. Axial T2 and postcontrast T1 MR images show an enhancing mass centered in the left sphenoid triangle with associated vasogenic edema in the left temporal lobe and extension into the left orbit.

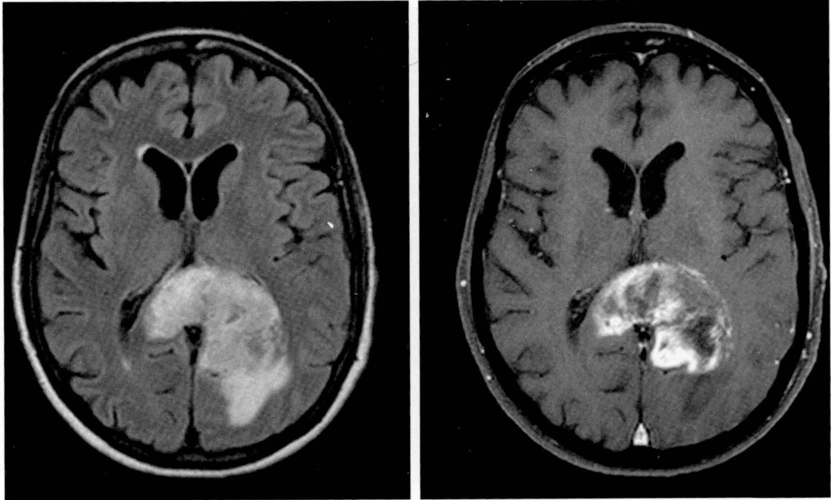

Glioblastoma. FLAIR and postcontrast T1 MR images show a heterogeneously enhancing mass that spans posterior corpus callosum.

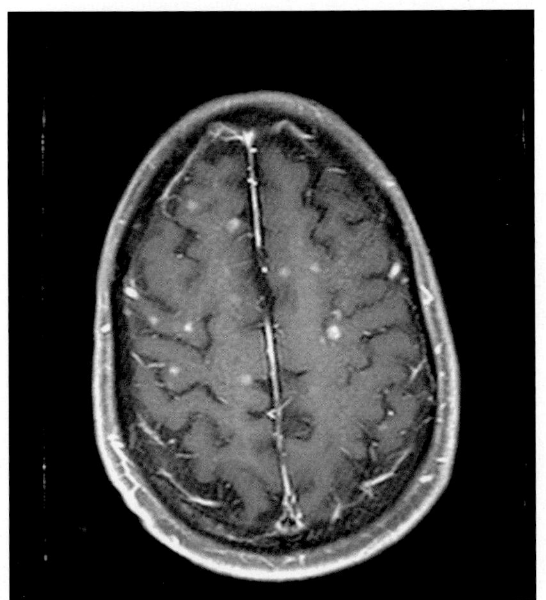

Lung cancer metastases. Axial postcontrast T1 MRI shows multiple enhancing nodules in the bilateral cerebral hemispheres.

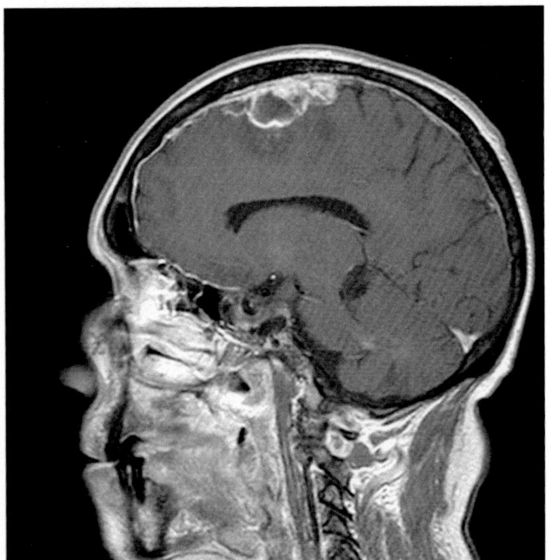

Breast cancer metastasis. Sagittal postcontrast T1 MRI shows a heterogeneously enhancing dural-based mass along the frontal convexity.

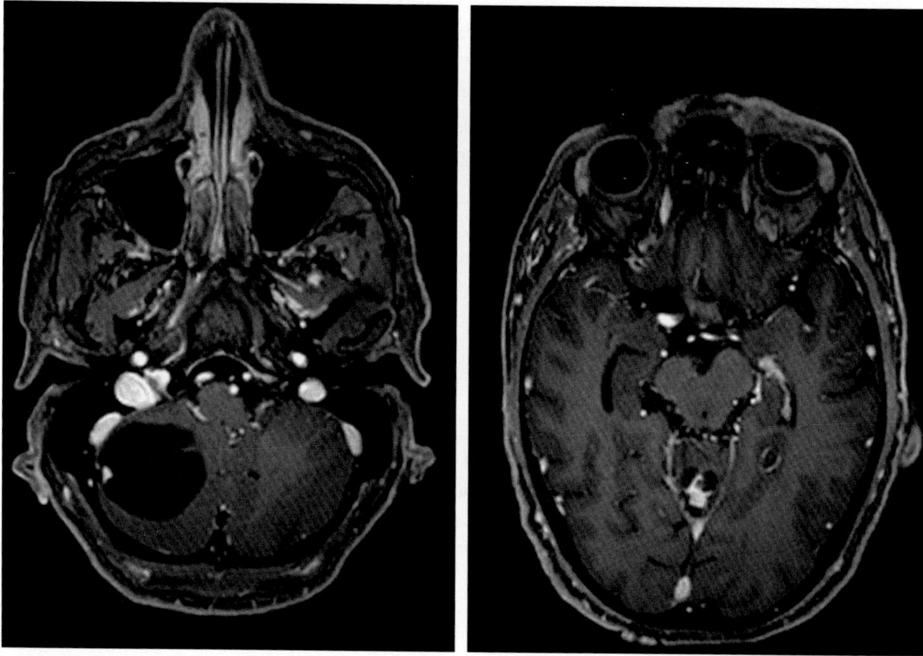

Hemangioblastoma. Axial postcontrast T1 MR images show cystic tumors in the cerebellum with enhancing nodules.

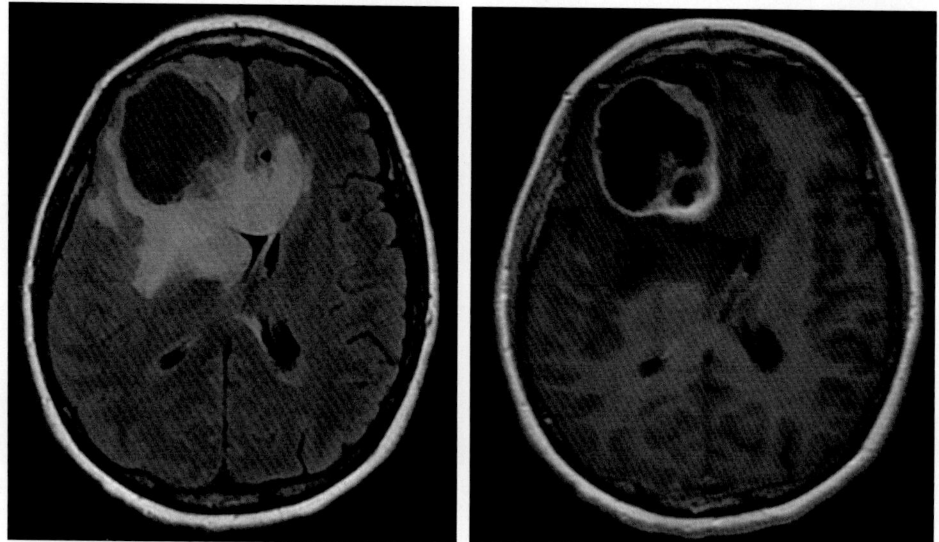

Primitive Neuroectodermal Tumor (PNET). Axial FLAIR and postcontrast T1 MR images show a mass in the right frontal lobe with irregular peripheral enhancement and surrounding edema with midline shift.

PHYSICAL EXAMINATION

A thorough physical and neurologic examination should be performed on all patients with intracranial tumors. Neurologic examination consists of a mental status examination with a complete cranial nerve assessment, along with motor/sensory testing, reflex testing, and cerebellar testing. Elements of complex motor system testing and speech and memory testing should also be assessed. As stated previously, the location of an intracranial tumor dictates its presentation. For example, a patient with a tumor present within the motor strip may present with profound contralateral motor weakness, whereas a patient with a pituitary tumor may complain of visual blurriness or generalized hormone discrepancy. A cerebellar tumor may present in a patient with primary gait imbalance, or a patient with hearing difficulty may present with a vestibular schwannoma. A thorough cranial nerve assessment can also provide further clues for the astute clinician in localizing the location and most likely differential diagnoses of intracranial tumors.

DIAGNOSIS

Diagnosis of adult intracranial lesions is generally through a combination of history and physical examination findings, corroborated by imaging support. A clinician approaching a patient with either known or suspected concern for intracranial tumors should collect a thorough history, which often provides clues to the location, duration, and classification of intracranial tumors. In general, a physician will order a computed tomography (CT) scan of the head or a magnetic resonance imaging scan of the brain to better evaluate intracranial tumors. The aforementioned imaging sequences provide structural and anatomic characteristics of the intracranial tumors in question, which aids clinicians in generating a differential diagnosis as well as in further management. MR spectroscopy and PET scans offer further clues into the nature of such intracranial tumors, which in turn can aid in making an accurate diagnosis.[10]

For some intracranial tumors, identification of the vascular supply is critical to the subsequent management. These intracranial tumors warrant further vascular imaging, in the form of CT angiography/ magnetic resonance angiography (CTA/MRA), as well as venous modalities as well i.e., CT venography/ magnetic resonance venography (CTV/MRV). For intracranial tumors that warrant critical vascular findings and close affinity with vascular structures, a diagnostic cerebral angiogram may be necessary.[11]

MANAGEMENT

Adult intracranial tumors are best managed by a multidisciplinary team of clinicians. Management options include observation surveillance, surgical resection, chemotherapy, radiation therapy, or a combination thereof. No two intracranial tumors are the same, which means that no two intracranial tumors are managed the same.

A variety of scales may aid the patient and clinician in determining the baseline functional status of a patient, which aids in the patient's decision-making. In neuro-oncology, some notable examples include the Karnofsky performance status scale[12] (outlined in the following section) and the Eastern Cooperative Oncology Group (ECOG)[13] performance status. Such scales assist the patient and clinician in making the most informed decision regarding further therapies and different treatment modalities.

Karnofsky Performance Status Scale Definitions	**Rating (%)**	**Criteria**
Able to carry on normal activity and to work; no special care needed.	100	Normal no complaints; no evidence of disease.
	90	Able to carry on normal activity; minor signs or symptoms of disease.
	80	Normal activity with effort; some signs or symptoms of disease.
Unable to work; able to live at home and care for most personal needs; varying amount of assistance needed.	70	Cares for self; unable to carry on normal activity or to do active work.
	60	Requires occasional assistance, but is able to care for most of his/her personal needs.
	50	Requires considerable assistance and frequent medical care.
Unable to care for self; requires equivalent of institutional or hospital care; disease may be progressing rapidly.	40	Disabled; requires special care and assistance.
	30	Severely disabled; hospital admission is indicated although death not imminent.
	20	Very sick; hospital admission necessary; active supportive treatment necessary.
	10	Moribund; fatal processes progressing rapidly.
	0	Dead

Eastern Cooperative Oncology Group (ECOG) Performance Status*

Grade	ECOG
0	Fully active, able to carry on all predisease performance without restriction
1	Restricted in physically strenuous activity but ambulatory and able to carry out work of a light or sedentary nature, e.g., light house work, office work
2	Ambulatory and capable of all self-care but unable to carry out any work activities. Up and about more than 50% of waking hours
3	Capable of only limited self-care, confined to bed or chair more than 50% of waking hours
4	Completely disabled. Cannot carry on any self-care. Totally confined to bed or chair
5	Dead

*Published in Oken MM, Creech RH, Tormey DC, Horton J, Davis TE, McFadden ET, Carbone PP. Toxicity And response criteria of the Eastern Cooperative Oncology Group. Am J Clin Oncol 1982; 5: 649–655.

Management of the patient with an intracranial tumor requires addressing the tumor itself as well as its neurologic sequelae. For example, a patient who is acutely obtunded from a large brain tumor should have his/her airway evaluated and stabilized first. Seizures should be controlled either with medication or, if sometimes required, deep sedation. Hydrocephalus due to obstruction caused by an intracranial tumor can be managed in the acute setting with an external ventricular drain versus emergent decompressive surgery for resection of said lesion. If hydrocephalus persists, the patient may require cerebrospinal fluid diversion, likely in the form of a ventriculoperitoneal shunt.[14]

If surgical resection is a possibility, a consultation with a neurosurgeon should be made so that the details and feasibility of such a surgery, as well as risks and benefits, could be explained to the patient and his/her family. Some intracranial lesions are more amenable to gross total resection, whereas other tumors will require a surgical biopsy first, which in turn will dictate further management. The neurosurgeon may discuss with the patient which surgical approach and operative management would be best to treat the patient's intracranial tumor. For example, a neurosurgeon may discuss with the patient the possibility of approaching a pituitary tumor via a transsphenoidal approach or by a pterional craniotomy. How the neurosurgeon delivers such medical information is often as important as the medical information itself.[15] Different surgical approaches that are specific to the individual characteristics and location of the tumor may be utilized; however, the basic operative principle is to provide the neurosurgeon the maximal exposure through the operative corridor, without any or minimal damage to the surrounding normal tissue. Supratentorial tumors are often approached with a standard pterional craniotomy, whereas infratentorial tumors are often approached with a retrosigmoid craniotomy.[16]

Some intracranial tumors are not amenable to surgical resection, or the characteristics of such a lesion make it more appropriate to be managed with radiation therapy instead. For example, if a lesion is small, or present in several parts of the brain, or within an area of the brain where surgical resection may potentially cause more harm than benefit, radiation therapy is a consideration. A consultation with a radiation oncologist can provide the patient with a variety of radiotherapy treatment options to target the tumor(s). For example, a patient with diffuse multiple metastases that are too many for surgical resection may benefit from whole brain radiation therapy, whereas a patient with a single small lesion that is radiosensitive may benefit from stereotactic radiosurgery. Patients who also undergo surgical resection of their intracranial tumors often receive radiation therapy to the surgical resection bed.[17]

Chemotherapy is also utilized as an adjunct for some tumors. A consultation with a neuro-oncologist should be made, and the variety of chemotherapeutic regimens should be discussed. Traditionally, the utilization of chemotherapy within the brain was limited, as the unique nature of the blood-brain barrier limited the efficacy of the medication traveling across the barrier.[18] Recent studies and research have paved the way for new chemotherapeutic drugs, however, and some patients receive a combination of surgery, radiation therapy, and chemotherapy as a result. Taxol is a well-known example.[19]

While chemotherapy and radiation regimens have evolved, some guidelines have proven successful in changing the standard of care. One prominent example is the advent of the Stupp protocol in 2005. The Stupp regimen tackled the most aggressive of primary intracranial neoplasms, glioblastoma multiforme (GBM). For newly diagnosed GBM, the Stupp regimen called for maximal surgical resection, followed by radiation therapy, in conjunction with either simultaneous or adjuvant chemotherapy, specifically temozolomide.[20] Temozolomide is an alkylating/methylating drug, where its mechanism is to alkylate usually the N-7 or

O-6 positions of guanine residues in DNA. The Stupp regimen compared those patients undergoing surgery with chemotherapy and radiation to those patients undergoing external beam radiation alone: the study demonstrated a median survival of 14.6 months in the former group compared with 12.1 months in the latter group. Other agents such as PCV (procarbazine, lomustine, vincristine) have found success in the treatment of recurrent low-grade oligodendrogliomas/astrocytomas, whereas other patients have benefitted from carmustine (Gliadel) wafers which are implanted in the surgical resection cavity after craniotomy.[21]

Preoperative embolization to reduce the vascular supply to a tumor and potentially aid in surgical resection is also a consideration.[22]

POSTMANAGEMENT COURSE

Postoperative management is equally as important as the surgical resection of the tumor itself. For intracranial tumors that undergo surgical resection, postoperative management is critical, with close neurologic monitoring and strict blood pressure control, generally provided in the ICU. One of the most common issues that patients with resection of their intracranial tumors experience is an acute hypertensive episode, which can generally be managed with careful neurologic checks in the ICU.[23] Patients can sometimes have a weaning steroid protocol as well, and there are a variety of tools that the neurosurgeon or neurointensivist can utilize in the immediate perioperative setting to enable a smooth transition to recovery. Postoperative seizures remain a major concern as well.[24,] Some studies have suggested that the prevalence of seizures can be as much as 30%–40% of patients with supratentorial brain tumors.[24–26] One study compared the efficacy of levetiracetam versus phenytoin and found that the levetiracetam group experienced a lower frequency of postoperative seizures.[27] Many patients who undergo surgical resection then undergo a phase of radiation therapy to the surgical resection bed.

For patients who have undergone their initial treatment phase, it is often the case that patients will have to follow through generally every 2–4 months to make sure there are no recurrent signs. This is generally managed with serial imaging and close follow-up with their neuro-oncologist, neurosurgeon, and radiation oncologist. The primary purpose of such follow-up is to ensure that the patient does not have any further recurrence of the intracranial tumor and to have the patient and patient's family involved in all aspects of recovery, as well.

Family support and social needs is also an important factor in the general recovery and the total care of the patient with an intracranial tumor. For many patients and their families, a revelation that their loved one has an intracranial tumor is often met with much consternation and sometimes outright fear. It is therefore critical to guide the patient and their family through this trying time and to not only address the patient's medical concerns but also social needs, as well.[28]

CONCLUSION

Intracranial tumors in the adult patient present a challenging clinical problem for physicians and often require a general management combination of surgical resection, radiation therapy, and chemotherapy. Patients who undergo such a combination require strict follow-up and close postoperative care, including overarching rehabilitation needs and social support. Such attention to a multifaceted approach for patients with intracranial tumors allows the clinician to provide the best overall care for the patient, in some of their most trying moments.

REFERENCES

1. Ostrom QT, Gittleman H, Liao P, et al. CBTRUS statistical report: primary brain and other central nervous system tumors diagnosed in the United States in 2010–2014. *Neuro Oncol.* 2017;19(suppl_5):v1–v88. https://doi.org/10.1093/neuonc/nox158.
2. Howlader N, Noone AM, Krapcho M, et al., eds. *SEER Cancer Statistics Review, 1975–2014*. Bethesda, MD: National Cancer Institute; April 2017. https://seer.cancer.gov/archive/csr/1975_2014/results_merged/sect_01_overview.pdf. based on November 2016 SEER data submission, posted to the SEER web site.
3. Sun T, Plutynski A, Ward S, Rubin JB. An integrative view on sex differences in brain tumors. *Cell Mol Life Sci.* 2015; 72(17):3323–3342. https://doi.org/10.1007/s00018-015-1930-2.
4. Owonikoko TK, Arbiser J, Zelnak A, et al. Current approaches to the treatment of metastatic brain tumours. *Nat Rev Clin Oncol.* 2014;11(4):203–222. https://doi.org/10.1038/nrclinonc.2014.25.
5. Wiemels J, Wrensch M, Claus EB. Epidemiology and etiology of meningioma. *J Neurooncol.* 2010;99(3):307–314. https://doi.org/10.1007/s11060-010-0386-3.
6. Ostrom QT, Bauchet L, Davis FG, et al. The epidemiology of glioma in adults: a "state of the science" review. *Neuro Oncol.* 2014;16(7):896–913. https://doi.org/10.1093/neuonc/nou087.
7. Louis DN, Perry A, Reifenberger G, et al. *Acta Neuropathol.* 2016;131:803. https://doi.org/10.1007/s00401-016-1545-1.

8. Comelli I, Lippi G, Campana V, Servadei F, Cervellin G. Clinical presentation and epidemiology of brain tumors firstly diagnosed in adults in the Emergency Department: a 10-year, single center retrospective study. *Ann Transl Med.* 2017;5(13):269. https://doi.org/10.21037/atm.2017.06.12.
9. Hussein MR. Central nervous system capillary haemangioblastoma: the pathologist's viewpoint. *Int J Exp Pathol.* 2007;88(5):311–324. https://doi.org/10.1111/j.1365-2613.2007.00535.x.
10. Bruzzone MG, D'incerti L, Farina LL, Cuccarini V, Finocchiaro G. CT and MRI of brain tumors. *Q J Nucl Med Mol Imaging.* 2012;56(2):112–137.
11. Wetzel SG, Cha S, Law M, et al. Preoperative assessment of intracranial tumors with perfusion MR and a volumetric interpolated examination: a comparative study with DSA. *AJNR Am J Neuroradiol.* 2002;23(10):1767–1774.
12. Karnofsky DA, Abelmann WH, Craver LF, Burchenal JH. The use of the nitrogen mustards in the palliative treatment of carcinoma – with particular reference to bronchogenic carcinoma. *Cancer.* 1948;1(4):634–656.
13. Oken MM, Creech RH, Tormey DC, et al. Toxicity and response criteria of the Eastern Cooperative Oncology Group. *Am J Clin Oncol.* 1982;5(6):649–655.
14. Reddy GK, Bollam P, Caldito G, et al. *J Neurooncol.* 2011; 103:333. https://doi.org/10.1007/s11060-010-0393-4.
15. Jagadeesh H, Bernstein M. Patients' anxiety around incidental brain tumors: a qualitative study. *Acta Neurochir.* 2014;156(2):375–381. https://doi.org/10.1007/s00701-013-1935-2.
16. Schödel P, Schebesch K-M, Brawanski A, Proescholdt MA. Surgical resection of brain metastases—impact on neurological outcome. *Int J Mol Sci.* 2013;14(5):8708–8718. https://doi.org/10.3390/ijms14058708.
17. Chan MD, Tatter SB, Lesser G, Shaw EG. Radiation oncology in brain tumors: current approaches and clinical trials in progress. *Neuroimaging Clin N Am.* 2010;20(3):401–408.
18. Vick NA, Khandekar JD, Bigner DD. Chemotherapy of brain tumors. The "Blood-Brain barrier" is not a factor. *Arch Neurol.* 1977;34(9):523–526. https://doi.org/10.1001/archneur.1977.00500210025002.
19. Joo KM, Park K, Kong DS, et al. Oral paclitaxel chemotherapy for brain tumors: ideal combination treatment of paclitaxel and P-glycoprotein inhibitor. *Oncol Rep.* 2008; 19(1):17–23.
20. Stupp R, Mason WP, Van den bent MJ, et al. Radiotherapy plus concomitant and adjuvant temozolomide for glioblastoma. *N Engl J Med.* 2005;352(10):987–996.
21. Ewend MG, Brem S, Gilbert M, et al. Treatment of single brain metastasis with resection, intracavity carmustine polymer wafers, and radiation therapy is safe and provides excellent local control. *Clin Cancer Res.* 2007;13(12): 3637–3641.
22. Kuroiwa T, Tanaka H, Ohta T, Tsutsumi A. Preoperative embolization of highly vascular brain tumors: clinical and histopathological findings. *Noshuyo Byori.* 1996; 13(1):27–36.
23. Hanak BW, Walcott BP, Nahed BV, et al. Post-operative intensive care unit requirements following elective craniotomy. *World Neurosurg.* 2014;81(1):165–172. https://doi.org/10.1016/j.wneu.2012.11.068.
24. Gokhale S, Khan SA, Agrawal A, Friedman AH, McDonagh DL. Levetiracetam seizure prophylaxis in craniotomy patients at high risk for postoperative seizures. *Asian J Neurosurg.* 2013;8(4):169–173. https://doi.org/10.4103/1793-5482.125658.
25. Glantz MJ, Cole BF, Forsyth PA, et al. Practice parameter: anticonvulsant prophylaxis in patients with newly diagnosed brain tumors. Report of the Quality Standards Subcommittee of the American Academy of Neurology. *Neurology.* 2000;54(10):1886–1893.
26. Van breemen MS, Rijsman RM, Taphoorn MJ, Walchenbach R, Zwinkels H, Vecht CJ. Efficacy of anti-epileptic drugs in patients with gliomas and seizures. *J Neurol.* 2009;256(9):1519–1526.
27. Iuchi T, Kuwabara K, Matsumoto M, Kawasaki K, Hasegawa Y, Sakaida T. Levetiracetam versus phenytoin for seizure prophylaxis during and early after craniotomy for brain tumours: a phase II prospective, randomised study. *J Neurol Neurosurg Psychiatr.* 2015;86(10):1158–1162.
28. Ownsworth T, Goadby E, Chambers SK. Support after brain tumor means different things: family caregivers' experiences of support and relationship changes. *Front Oncol.* 2015;5:33. https://doi.org/10.3389/fonc.2015.00033.

FURTHER READING

1. Pekmezci M, Perry A. Neuropathology of brain metastases. *Surg Neurol Int.* 2013;4(suppl 4):S245–S255. https://doi.org/10.4103/2152-7806.111302.
2. Vargo M. Brain tumor rehabilitation. *Am J Phys Med Rehabil.* 2011;90(5 suppl 1):S50–S62.
3. Pace A, Parisi C, Di lelio M, et al. Home rehabilitation for brain tumor patients. *J Exp Clin Cancer Res.* 2007;26(3): 297–300.
4. Greenberg E, Treger I, Ring H. Rehabilitation outcomes in patients with brain tumors and acute stroke: comparative study of inpatient rehabilitation. *Am J Phys Med Rehabil.* 2006;85(7):568–573.

CHAPTER 5

Brain Tumor Rehabilitation

TERRENCE MACARTHUR PUGH, MD • JOANNA EDEKER, DPT • BRITTANY LORDEN, OT • VISHWA S. RAJ, MD

EPIDEMIOLOGY

There are 700,000 people living in the United States with a primary brain tumor. Approximately 80,000 new cases of primary brain tumors are expected to be diagnosed in 2017, with 26,000 of these expected to be malignant.[1] There are an expected 16,700 deaths in 2017 from primary brain tumors accounting for 2.8% of all cancer deaths.[2] The median age for diagnosis of primary brain tumors is 59 years old; however, these are the most common cancer in those aged 0–14 years.[1]

TUMOR TYPES

As of 2016, the World Health Organization (WHO) updated the brain tumor staging recommendations to include not only microscopic histology but also by incorporating molecular parameters into the classification of central nervous system (CNS) tumors. Tumors are staged from I to IV, with stage I tumors classified the most benign and stage IV being the most malignant (Table 5.1).[3,4] The most common type of brain tumor is a meningioma, which represents nearly 37% (27,110 in 2017) of all primary brain tumors. Gliomas account for 24.7% of all brain tumors and 74.6% of all malignant tumors.[1] Tumors included within the glioma category are astrocytomas (which include glioblastomas), oligodendrogliomas, and ependymomas.[5] Gliomas carry the highest mortality rate among brain tumors, with a median survival rate of approximately 12–15 months despite many advances in treatment.[6] Glioblastomas account for 14.9% of all primary brain tumors and 55.4% of all gliomas, with an estimated 12,390 new diagnoses in 2017. Pituitary tumors a typically benign and there are an anticipated 14,230 new tumors in 2017 (16% of all primary brain tumors). Lymphomas and oligodendrogliomas account for 2% of primary brain tumors, whereas medulloblastomas represent 1%.[1] Within an inpatient rehabilitation population, 20%–30% of brain tumor admissions are glioblastomas and approximately 20% are meningiomas.[7]

The exact incidence of metastatic brain tumors is not known; however, metastatic disease to the brain is diagnosed in between 200,000 and 300,000 patients per year. These are diagnosed with computed tomography (CT) or magnetic resonance imaging (MRI) when neurologic symptoms manifest. Lung, breast, melanoma, colon, and renal carcinomas are the most common primary sites for metastatic spread to the brain.[8] The majority (approximately 80%) of metastatic brain lesions present as multiple tumors, whereas only 15%–20% present as a single lesion. A total of 85% of metastatic lesions are located within the cerebrum, whereas 15% present within the cerebellum. The probability of cerebellar metastases is highest in lung and breast cancers; however, the majority of brain metastases are located within the watershed areas of the brain such as the gray-white matter junction.[9] The location of the lesion corresponds to the symptoms that manifest within the patient (Fig. 5.1).[8] A total of 25% –30% of brain tumors admitted to inpatient rehabilitation facilities are due to metastatic disease.[7]

DIAGNOSIS

Presenting Symptoms

Patients with brain tumors may present with a variety of symptoms that may be nonspecific or are more closely correlated to intracranial pathology. The most common presenting symptom of a tumor is a headache, with 40%–80% being tension type and migraine in approximately 10%.[10] Epileptic seizures may also be a functionally limiting complication of patients with metastatic and primary brain malignancy. Approximately 50% of patients with an intracranial malignancy will have an epileptic episode during their disease.[11] As previously stated, focal neurologic deficits as presenting

TABLE 5.1
World Health Organization Grades of Select Central Nervous System (CNS) Tumors

Diffuse astrocytic and oligodendroglial tumors		Desmoplastic infantile astrocytoma and ganglioglioma	I
Diffuse astrocytoma, IDH-mutant	II	Papillary glioneuronal tumor	I
Anaplastic astrocytoma, IDH-mutant	III	Rosette-forming glioneuronal tumor	I
Glioblastoma, IDH-wild type	IV	Central neurocytoma	II
Glioblastoma, IDH-mutant	IV	Extraventricular neurocytoma	II
Diffuse midline glioma, H3 K27M-mutant	IV	Cerebellar liponeurocytoma	II
Oligodendroglioma, IDH-mutant and 1p/19q codeleted	II	**Tumors of the pineal region**	
Anaplastic oligodendroglioma, IDH-mutant and 1p/19q-codeleted	III	Pineocytoma	I
Other astrocytic tumors		Pineal parenchymal tumor of intermediate differentiation	II or III
Pilocytic astrocytoma	I	Pineoblastoma	IV
Subependymal giant cell astrocytoma	I	Papillary tumor of the pineal region	II or III
Pleomorphic xanthoastrocytoma	II	**Embryonal tumors**	
Anaplastic pleomorphic xanthoastrocytoma	III	Medulloblastoma (all subtypes)	IV
Ependymal tumors		Embryonal tumor with multilayered rosettes. C 19MC-altered	IV
Subependymoma	I	Medulloepithelioma	IV
Myxopapillary ependymoma	I	CNS embryonal tumor. NOS	IV
Ependymoma	II	Atypical teratoid/rhabdoid tumor	IV
Ependymoma. *RELA* fusion-positive	II or III	CNS embryonal tumor with rhabdoid features	IV
Anaplastic ependymoma	III	**Tumors of the cranial and paraspinal nerves**	
Other gliomas		Schwannoma	I
Angiocentric glioma	I	Neurofibroma	I
Chordoid glioma of third ventricle	II	Perineurioma	I
Choroid plexus tumors		Malignant peripheral nerve sheath tumor (MPNST)	II, III, or IV
Choroid plexus papilloma	I	**Meningiomas**	
Atypical choroid plexus papilloma	II	Meningioma	I
Choroid plexus carcinoma	III	Atypical meningioma	II
Neuronal and mixed neuronal-glial tumors		Anaplastic (malignant) meningioma	III
Dysembryoplastic neuroepithelial tumor	I	**Mesenchymal, nonmeningothelial tumors**	
Gangliocytoma	I	Solitary fibrous tumor / hemangiopericytoma	I, II, or III
Ganglioglioma	I	Hemangioblastoma	I
Anaplastic ganglioglioma	III	**Tumors of the sellar region**	
Dysplastic gangliocytoma of cerebellum (Lhermitte-Duclos)	I	Craniopharyngioma	I
		Granular cell tumor	I
		Pituicytoma	I
		Spindle cell oncocytoma	I

WHO Classification of CNS tumors

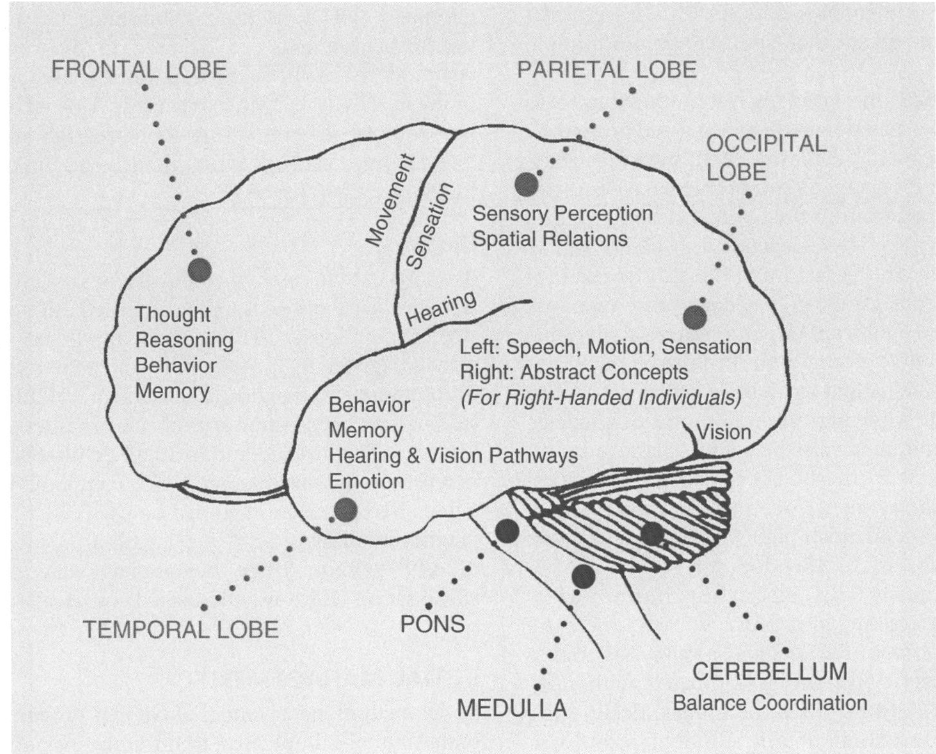

FIG. 5.1

symptoms of malignancy are dependent on the location of the tumor. Physical examination, including fundoscopic examination which could signal increase in intracerebral pressure, is key to finding a diagnosis.

Imaging

Structural MRI remains the standard of care for diagnosis and in management of intracranial neoplasms. The primary role of structural MRI is to determine the location of the tumor, extent of involvement, and the effect of compression due to edema on the brain parenchyma, vessels, or other structures. Standardized protocols exist and the recommended imaging sequence involves a three-dimensional (3D) T1, axial fluid-attenuated inversion recovery (FLAIR), axial diffusion-weighted imaging (DWI), axial gadolinium contrast–enhanced T2, and 3D gadolinium contrast–enhanced T1 obtained on a 1.5 T MRI system. Two-dimensional sequences can be substituted if time is limited or if there are other contraindications. Structural sequences, which include T2-weighted, FLAIR, and T1-weighted images with and without contrast, are the basis for MRI examinations. For presurgical examinations, 3D T2-weighted images and 3D T1-weighted images may be useful in planning.[12]

MRI offers superior views of the soft tissues of the brain as opposed to other neuroimaging techniques. Intravenous contrast shows enhancement of areas that have had disruption of the blood-brain barrier (BBB). Degree of contrast enhancement is highly correlated with tumor grade; however, some lower grade gliomas, i.e., WHO grade I tumors such as pilocytic astrocytoma and ganglioglioma, have intense enhancement signals.[12,13] Hyperintense signals on T2 and FLAIR imaging is identified as peritumoral edema and can be vasogenic or infiltrative edema. Vasogenic edema is due to increase in extracellular fluid and plasma due to poorly formed capillaries feeding into the tumor. It can also be seen in metastatic disease or noninfiltrating tumors such as meningiomas. Infiltrative edema associated with gliomas is due to a combination of vasogenic edema and tumor cells that penetrate white matter tracts within the brain. This enhancement may be difficult to differentiate from the actual primary mass lesion.[12] Contrast-enhanced MRI is more sensitive that nonenhanced MRI or CT in detecting intracranial lesions, either primary or metastases.[14,15] However, CT may be used in patients that have a contraindication to MRI.

There has been increased interest in functional MRI (fMRI) and its utilization in diagnosing and prognostic value in intracranial neoplasms. fMRI measures activity of neurons by giving a ratio of the deoxyhemoglobin to oxyhemoglobin in the brain and is reported as the blood oxygen level dependent (BOLD) signal. The interest lies in the fact that fMRI can be used for mapping of sensorimotor, language, and memory, which can have significant impact on surgical planning and intraoperative evaluation. Task-based fMRI involves asking the patient to oscillate between a resting and active state while performing a motor or language task. This technique can also be used to characterize tumors. A decrease in the BOLD signal in the affected brain tissue shows alterations in blood flow, which can be used to distinguish high- v. low-grade tumors. Resting state fMRI (rs-fMRI) does not require the patient to perform any tasks and can be performed while the patient is receiving anesthesia. At times there are small fluctuations in BOLD signals known as resting state networks (RSNs). When compared with task-based fMRI, rs-MRI can map the brain quickly using RSN in a shorter amount of time. Although promising, rs-fMRI needs further investigation before it has more clinical utility.[12]

As previously stated, MRI is the gold standard for imaging in regard to diagnosis of gliomas; however, MRI is not without its limitations. MRI alone oftentimes gives limited information when grading a tumor or delineation of the tumor. There is also difficulty in distinguishing between necrotic tissue and recurrent tumor. A rapidly enlarging, contrast-enhanced tumor is usually considered a progressive lesion, even in the absence of worsening neurologic dysfunction, as opposed to a treatment side effect such as radiation necrosis.[16]

Recent studies have shown that positron emission tomography (PET) scanning has utility in the diagnosis of gliomas. Owing to improved ability to radioactively label amino acids, PET scans can be used to aid in therapy planning and monitoring in glioblastomas. PET scanning can also be used in noninvasive grading of gliomas. There is also better delineation of tumor invasion, more precision with surgical or radiation planning, and improved posttreatment monitoring and prognostic evaluations. ^{18}F-2-fluoro-2-deoxy-D-glucose (^{18}F-FDG) is the most well-studied and validated radiotracer available in nuclear medicine literature. It has also been proven to be cost effective. In lower grade gliomas, ^{18}F-FDG is used to monitor for anaplastic transformation and can be used in prognosis. This technique is useful because it can be used to assess biologic activity in living organisms. This technique is not without its limitations though. High uptake of ^{18}F-FDG in normal, healthy brain tissue limits its use in cerebral brain tissue.[16]

Biopsy

Biopsy is used in cases when the diagnosis with imaging is inconclusive or needs to be confirmed. Intraoperative stereotactic biopsy (STB) showed correlation with the actual diagnosis 90% of the time, and a 96% sensitivity in obtaining a diagnostic specimen.[17] More recent studies have been examining other techniques to obtain biopsies when needed and in a more cost-effective and in a time conscious manner. When compared with CT-guided STB, ultrasound-guided biopsy (USGB) showed diagnostic utility of 93%–91% with a procedure time of 149–94 min. Three hematomas were seen the USGB group which were managed conservatively.[18]

INITIAL MANAGEMENT

Initial medical management of patients presenting with brain tumors is imperative to minimize risk of complications and irreversible brain damage associated with delay. The following section discusses some of these early interventions.

Steroids

Nearly all patients with an intracranial neoplasm receive steroids during their disease. However, there is not a standardized method of dosing or weaning.[19] Steroids help minimize symptom burden due to associated vasogenic edema. Dexamethasone has been the steroid of choice due to its low mineralocorticoid activity, but methylprednisolone and prednisone have also been used. Dexamethasone has a half-life of 36–54 hours which provides extended coverage after dosing. Standard starting dose is 16 mg divided into four daily doses.[20] The goal of steroid management is to taper to the minimum effective dose once the patient is symptomatically stable. This dose will minimize symptom burden and maximize functional benefit while minimizing risk of the long-term side effects associated with prolonged steroid use. One study showed 29% of patients were able to be weaned off steroid therapy within 3 months of completion of radiation[21]; however, 55%–58% of patients had to have steroid dosage increased during radiation therapy (RT).[22] Steroid-induced myopathy is a potential complication of long-term steroid usage and manifests as proximal muscle weakness most notably in the lower extremities, but in more severe cases, it can be seen in the neck extensor muscles and respiratory muscles.[23] Other more common side effects include anxiety, insomnia, psychosis, and delirium. Hiccups may also be seen and can be treated with baclofen among other medications.[23] Despite a lack of definitive evidence showing gastrointestinal (GI) bleeding in patients on corticosteroids are often prescribed a proton pump inhibitor or an H_2 receptor antagonist. Associated endocrine side effects including Cushing's syndrome and steroid-induced hyperglycemia usually resolve upon discontinuation of therapy. Corticosteroids also have detrimental effects on bone. Fractures of the spine and hip can also occur, with impaired calcium absorption being the proposed mechanism. Supplementation of calcium and vitamin D should be considered. Avascular necrosis of the hip can also occur.[23] There are also other potential benefits of dexamethasone in brain tumor patients. A recent case report showed potential antineoplastic effects in glioblastoma multiforme (GBM) with dexamethasone and levetiracetam; however, this would need to be further proven by randomized control trials.[24] Affronti et al. also showed that dexamethasone in combination with palonosetron was effective in preventing chemotherapy-induced nausea and vomiting (CINV) in patients receiving treatment for gliomas while maintaining quality of life (QoL).[25] Palonosetron, dexamethasone, and aprepitant were also effective in improving CINV in patients receiving temozolomide.[26]

Seizure Management

Seizures are among the most common presenting symptoms in patients with brain tumors. Surgical resection of the malignancy has been shown to effectively control the seizure.[27] Location of the tumor is an important determinant in the likelihood of having seizures during the illness. Seizures are more common in oligodendrogliomas that are located in the cortex[28] and in lesions of the insula and temporal lobe.[29] White matter and posterior fossa tumors do not often cause seizures, although multifocal deep tumors can be the cause of epileptic episodes.[23] Metastatic disease causes seizures in 20%–40% of patients when they are hemorrhagic, multiple, and/or involve the temporal lobe.[30] There is conflicting evidence about the use of chemoradiation therapy in brain tumor treatment and its effectiveness in managing seizure activity, and further randomized control trials are recommended.[23]

Administration of antiepileptic drugs (AEDs) is standard of care in patients with intracranial malignancy who present with seizure activity,[31] and a 1996 survey found that 55% of practitioners administered prophylactic AEDs to brain tumor patients.[32] Although the use of prophylactic AEDs seems to becoming more of a routine practice, this has not been proven to statistically significantly reduce the risk of seizures.[23] Further clinical trials are recommended. The use of AEDs is often limited by side effect profiles and drug interactions; however, newer AEDs such as levetiracetam, lamotrigine, lacosamide, and pregabalin are better tolerated.[23] Levetiracetam has no known drug interactions and has become a favorite among clinicians as a prophylactic AED. Lacosamide has been proven to be an effective second-line therapy in conjunction with other AEDs or as monotherapy in reducing seizures associated with brain tumors.[11] Valproic acid has also been shown to be effective; however, as it is a CYP450 inhibitor, it may increase toxicity associated with certain chemotherapeutic medications.[23]

Venous Thromboembolism Risk Management

Patients with brain tumors are at high risk for developing deep venous thrombosis (DVT) or pulmonary embolism (PE). DVT or PE has been shown to occur in glioma patients 3%–20% of the time[33] and in up to 60% of GBM patients.[34] This alone should give providers a low threshold for investigation of potential VTE if needed; however, treatment of these is contingent on whether the patient has a hemorrhagic lesion or if there is an increased risk for hemorrhage. Metastatic disease from lung and breast cancer has a lower incidence of hemorrhage when compared with patients with melanoma or renal cell carcinoma.[23] If there are contraindications to chemoprophylaxis in patients with a known DVT, consideration can be made for placement of an inferior vena cava filter. These should be restricted to patients with absolute contraindications to chemoprophylaxis. Low-molecular weight heparin products, such as enoxaparin, can be used for prophylactic and treatment dosing in patients with VTE. Unfractionated heparin products are generally used in patients with renal insufficiency or at higher risk for bleeding due to its ability to be reversed.[35] More recently, direct Xa inhibitors, such as rivaroxaban, have been used in treating VTE in oncology patients. Rivaroxaban received approval in 2012 after the EINSTEIN trials for treatment of VTE; however, these data could not be reliably extrapolated to an oncology population as only 5% of the population studied had active cancer and the study did not account for complications that arise during cancer treatment such as drug interactions, bleeding, and thrombocytopenia.[36] Mantha et al. explored this in a 2017 study in patients who had a cancer-related VTE with similar rates of bleeding risk and recurrent VTE as other published studies. However, this study did not include patients with a primary brain tumor, only those with metastatic disease.[36] A recent case report showed that severe postoperative bleeding was found in a patient with a DVT started on rivaroxaban after thoracic surgery for lung cancer[37] indicating that caution should be used when initiating any anticoagulant.

TREATMENT

Chemotherapy

The treatment of a brain tumor involves a combination of surgery, chemotherapy, and RT. The first-line chemotherapy for GBM is temozolomide, which is an oral alkylating agent. The effectiveness of this chemotherapy is determined by the methylation status of the O^6-methylguanine methyltransferase (MGMT) genes. MGMT functions to displace alkyl groups from compounds and works within the DNA direct reversal repair pathway. Loss or silencing of this gene by methylation may increase the likelihood of developing malignancy with exposure to other alkylating agents. High levels of MGMT within malignant cells create temozolomide resistance by blocking the effectiveness of the medicine. Therefore, methylation of MGMT increases the efficacy of temozolomide.[38] Temozolomide has also been shown to improve long-term survival in patients with anaplastic gliomas with leptomeningeal spread.[39] More recent studies suggest that the addition of the vascular endothelial growth factor (VEGF) receptor inhibitor cediranib to the standard GBM treatment of radiation and temozolomide may improve overall survival.[40] Neutropenia and myelosuppression are rare with temozolomide alone; however, the risk doubles with the addition of bevacizumab.[23] If thrombocytopenia occurs, platelet transfusions are recommended for platelet counts less than 10,000 or less than 20,000 if the patient is febrile, has an active hemorrhage, or is demonstrating signs of sepsis.[23]

Bevacizumab is a human-derived monoclonal antibody against VEGF that has shown improvement in 6-month survival in previous trials. It is commonly used in treatment of recurrent GBM. It is known that high-grade gliomas produce large quantities of VEGF which promotes endothelial proliferation, and overexpression of this growth factor is directly proportional to blood vessel density, grade of tumor, and patient outcome. VEGF promotes angiogenesis; however, these vessels are often disorganized, which causes an increase in leakiness of the BBB. Bevacizumab functions to help the vessels function more normally, which in turn improves oxygenation and drug delivery. An intact BBB decreases vasogenic edema, which can improve symptoms by reducing mass effect.[41] Although the effectiveness of bevacizumab is apparent, negative side effects can occur. It has been shown to increase the risk of cancer-associated hypercoagulability while also increasing the risk of hemorrhage.[23] Other less common side effects include posterior reversible encephalopathy syndrome, GI perforation, and impaired wound healing.[23]

Chemotherapy intervention for metastatic disease depends on the type of cancer. A recent case report showed 25 months of disease-free progression in a patient with intracranial non–small cell lung cancer (NSCLC) with crizotinib then ceritinib. Targeted therapy against the ALK oncogene has been proven effective in patients with NSCLC.[42]

Radiation Therapy

Whole brain radiation therapy (WBRT) is becoming less favorable in managing metastatic disease due to the concern of neurocognitive toxicity. In patients that are candidates for WBRT with extensive intracranial metastatic disease, the standard doses are 3000 cGy in 10 daily fractions or 2000 cGy in 5 daily fractions. The addition of radiosensitizers does not improve overall survival when compared with WBRT alone.[43] In a randomized control trial of patients with metastatic NSCLC, patients who received WBRT and optimum supportive care, defined as dexamethasone and a proton pump inhibitor for GI prophylaxis, had no statistically significant improvement in quality-adjusted life years or median survival when compared with those who received optimum supportive care alone.[44] Stereotactic radiosurgery (SRS) alone is the treatment of choice in patients with one to three brain metastases. In younger patients with limited extracranial disease and four or more intracranial disease, there have also been positive results. SRS has been shown to have local control rates at 1 year of approximately 90% with minimal toxicity in patients with prior surgery or with SRS alone. Radionecrosis rates are approximately 20% after initial SRS.[45] In 2014 the American Society for Radiation Oncology (ASTRO) released the following statement to help clinicians choose appropriate radiation techniques in patients with limited metastatic disease:

> *Don't routinely add adjuvant whole brain radiation therapy to stereotactic radiosurgery for limited brain metastases.*
>
> *Randomized studies have demonstrated no overall survival benefit from the addition of adjuvant whole brain radiation therapy (WBRT) to stereotactic radiosurgery (SRS) in the management of selected patients with good performance status and brain metastases from solid tumors. The addition of WBRT to SRS is associated with diminished cognitive function and worse patient-reported fatigue and QoL. These results are consistent with the worsened, self-reported cognitive function and diminished verbal skills observed in randomized studies of prophylactic cranial irradiation for small cell or non–small cell lung cancer. Patients treated with radiosurgery for brain metastases can develop metastases elsewhere in the brain. Careful surveillance and the judicious use of salvage therapy at the time of brain relapse allow appropriate patients to enjoy the highest QoL without a detriment in overall survival. Patients should discuss these options with their radiation oncologist.*
>
> TSAO.[43]

Discussions between healthcare providers and the patients regarding prognosis and goals of therapy should be a routine part of the communication prior to initiating any intervention.

Surgical Resection

Surgical resection of brain tumors may also be considered for patients that have significant disease burden and to minimize symptoms. Several randomized trials have recommended the use of surgery for single brain metastatic disease to increase survival.[43] Gamma knife radiosurgery (GKRS) is a good treatment option for small meningiomas, and a study shows that 97.9% showed 5-year tumor control.[46] A recent study showed that the 5-year recurrence rate of grade I meningiomas to be 10% after complete resection and as high as 45% with subtotal resection. RT and GKRS are good for preventing recurrence in lower and higher grade meningiomas. However, further surgery could not be reliably recommended due to high rates of recurrence and complication rates.[47] In a study of patients with stage II and III ependymomas, adult patients with a gross total resection saw a statistically significant increase in progression-free survival as compared with those with subtotal resection. This finding was independent of those who received postoperative adjuvant RT.[48]

REHABILITATION INTERVENTIONS

Brain tumors, as well as the treatment of the lesions, can cause a multitude of medical and functional impairments for the survivor. The impairments that manifest within the patient are often correlated to baseline functional status. Brain tumor–related impairments include headaches, seizures, neurocognitive dysfunction, varying levels of paresis, and dysphagia.[49] The benefits of rehabilitation for brain tumor survivors includes improved mobility, pain management, improvement of fatigue, improved QoL, preserved dignity, and establishment of resources and supportive services.[50] The healthcare team develops rehabilitation goals within the limitations of the patient's illness, environment, and social support. Goals are objective, realistic, attainable, and involve the patient and caregivers. A collaborative effort with professional members of the team, the patient, and the patient's support network provide services to patients throughout the course of illness. Treatment plans are individualized to meet each survivor's unique and specific needs.[51] The purpose of rehabilitation, for those with brain tumors, is similar to that for patients with other intracranial disease processes; however, the pathology of the tumor, the anticipated progression of disease, and any associated cancer treatments must be considered and play a role in goal setting.[52] If tumor progression and treatment causes a functional decline or a fluctuation in abilities, rehabilitation assumes a supportive role and goals are adjusted to accommodate the patient's limitations.[53] It is imperative to remember that survivors who participate in rehabilitation programs have been shown to make functional gains, even though they have significant medical comorbidities.[53] Health-related quality of life (HRQoL) is commonly used as an outcome measure for brain tumor patients.[54,55] Improvements in HRQoL is related to longer survival in high-grade glioma patients, including those with recurrent tumors. Not only did these survivors make HRQoL gains, they were also able to improve functionality with rehabilitation interventions.[56] Higher functionality is directly correlated with better survival outcomes for patients with brain cancer.[57,58] Despite the prognosis, a survivor can benefit from rehabilitation services to maximize QoL and function.[52]

Neurocognitive Stimulants

Neurocognitive functional impairment has been seen in as many as 75% of glioma patients with left or right temporal lobe tumors,[59] with reports of impairments in up to 90% of patients who receive WBRT.[60] The mechanism associated with radiotherapy-induced cognitive dysfunction is thought to be related to neuronal inflammation and degeneration of the hippocampus.[61] Temozolomide can also impair cognition through some of the same mechanisms.[62] Multiple agents have been hypothesized to help with neurocognitive functioning in brain tumor patients. Memantine was the drug of choice in a recent randomized control trial in patients receiving WBRT; however, it was underpowered and did not show statistical significance, but there were still incremental cognitive benefits.[23] Donepezil, in irradiated patients, was proven to be beneficial in brain tumor patients and improved neurocognitive functioning, mood, and HRQoL.[63] Modafinil and methylphenidate are also reasonable medications to try due to their favorable side effect profiles.[23]

Aphasia

Broca's and Brodmann's areas, near the inferior frontal gyrus in the dominant hemisphere, control complex speech, and insults to this area can cause an expressive aphasia.[64] Patients with this type of aphasia have difficulty with the motor coordination of speech. Other types of aphasias that patients may experience include fluent aphasias such as Wernicke's aphasia or a conductive aphasia. Global aphasia affects all aspects of language, whereas anomic aphasia manifests as difficulties with recalling words, names, or numbers.[65] Approximately 30%–50% of patients with primary brain tumors will experience aphasia, which is a higher rate than patients with a stroke affecting the dominant hemisphere.[64] There are multiple techniques to help treat aphasia which are used by a speech and language pathologist in order to maximize communication and limit social barriers experienced by brain tumor survivors.[66]

Dysphagia

Treatment of dysphagia should be treated similarly to swallowing deficits following CVA and can achieve similar functional outcomes. A retrospective study found that 63% of brain tumor patients and 73% of stroke patients admitted to acute rehabilitation were identified as having dysphagia.[67] When stroke and brain tumor patients with dysphagia were matched, both had similar statistically significant functional gains in swallowing, with 50% of patients consuming a regular diet by time of discharge home. Dysphagia has been described in 85% of brain tumor patients at end of life.[67]

Cognitive Rehabilitation

Cognitive deficits that are present in brain tumor patients may be due to not only the pathology but also the treatment. Historic data indicate that cognitive impairments are present in at least 30% of patients following surgical intervention and extending to 90% long term. The impact of oncologic treatments may induce progressive deterioration over time, unlike deficits occurring following other brain pathologies.[68] Chemotherapy-related cognitive dysfunction, more commonly known as "chemo brain" is a possible side effect of chemotherapy drugs. Chemotherapy is thought to cause an alteration in cytokines which subsequently causes changes in epigenetic factors that impairs brain metabolism leading to cognitive dysfunction.[69] Other risk factors for developing chemo brain include older age, lower education level, other medical comorbidities, and living alone.[70] Symptoms include forgetfulness, difficulty concentrating, difficulty with multitasking, feeling disorganized, and difficulty with learning new skills. Chemo brain is not a new phenomenon; however, research has focused more attention on examining this impairment in more recent years. The onset, length, and extent of chemo brain varies.[71]

Typically, cognitive rehabilitation interventions can be adaptive or restorative in approach with most rehabilitation programs combining both approaches. Successful cognitive programs focus on the individual's ability to function within their daily activities, not simply on practiced therapy tasks. Thus, it is crucial in cognitive therapy to individualize interventions to processes that are relevant to the patient's daily environments. Cognitive therapy should also include educational and metacognitive strategies for the patient to understand and demonstrate insight regarding their deficits to apply to their own life and environment. Although limited studies have been conducted, the results of the studies addressing cognitive rehabilitation in patients with brain tumors confirm improved cognitive function in survivors receiving structured cognitive rehabilitation.[68] Consideration must also be made to patients with brain tumors as decision-making capacity may also be affected. Caregivers should be involved in medical decision-making whenever possible.[72]

Activities of Daily Living

Activities of daily living (ADL) give an objective measure of a patient's functional status. These can be divided in basic activities of daily living (BADL) and instrumental activities of daily living (IADL).[73] BADL include bathing, dressing, and toileting, which are necessary for self-maintenance,[74] whereas IADL include more complex tasks such as finances, shopping, and using electronics.[75] Oncologists commonly use the

Karnofsky Performance Scale (KPS), which only accounts for BADL.[76] Occupational therapists help develop plans of care that help the patient reach maximum functional independence. The functional independence measure (FIM) is an objective scale used to document functional gains in brain tumor patients, and the patients have similar FIM change as TBI patients after undergoing rehabilitation.[77] Although these scales are routinely used, they have limitations, and current research is exploring if they can effectively be utilized in the brain tumor population.[73]

Transfer Training

In various rehabilitation settings, the therapists assess the safest technique for a person with a tumor to perform transfers with family assistance if needed. Therapists help determine the type of transfer and other equipment needed to ensure a safe discharge. Considerations of the patient's strength, tone, balance, midline orientation, size, cognition, and prognosis should be accounted for in the management of cancer patients.[52] The treating therapy team provides education to the cancer survivor and caregivers to ensure safety throughout the process. Transfer training includes bed mobility, transfers into and out of bed or a wheelchair, toilet transfers, shower transfers, car transfers, and floor transfers.[52] An oncology patient may experience fluctuating fatigue levels or a progressively worsening disease process that can influence the level of assistance or equipment needed. A mechanical lift is used when a patient is dependent or unable to assist and other transfer techniques are unsafe. A transfer board is an assistive device used to bridge the gap from the wheelchair to the bed when a patient is too weak or too imbalanced to transfer by unloading through lower extremities.[52,78,79]

Gait Training

If the brain tumor affects motor control or planning, the patient may present with gait impairments such as ataxia. Ataxia, which may occur with cerebellar lesions, can cause a lack of coordination within the patient. Treatments to address impaired motor control and motor planning may include aquatic therapy to utilize buoyancy, applying weights to the limbs or trunk, vibratory stimulation, and neuromuscular electrical stimulation (NMES).[80] Gait speed and Timed Up and Go (TUG) are tests that can be performed in various settings. Gait speed is considered among some as the "sixth vital sign" and is a reliable measure of functional capacity with well-documented predictive value for major health-related outcomes.[81] TUG correlates with the patient's fall risk[82] and can be useful in goal setting.

Exercise

The value of exercise for the cancer survivor continues to be researched and not only approved but encouraged throughout the continuum of cancer care. Exercise not only addresses functional decline but also addresses fatigue, cognitive impairments, anxiety, and depression.[83] The amount of time performing aerobic exercise has shown an inverse relationship with mortality in brain tumor survivors, compared with the counterparts who exercised less.[84] Ongoing research attempts to answer the question if exercise can prevent disease progression.[85]

Neuromuscular Electrical Stimulation/ Functional Electrical Stimulation

NMES is a low level electrical current applied to affected muscles to facilitate muscle contractions to create repetitive movements with a hemiparetic limb. NMES enables neuromuscular reeducation or motor relearning.[86] NMES can be used to address hemiparesis and impaired motor control secondary to brain tumors for the upper extremity and the lower extremity. The application of NMES to a hemiparetic limb encourages neural plasticity with the goal of long-term functional improvement of treated limb.[87] Functional electrical stimulation (FES), also known as a neuroprosthesis, is stimulation provided to specific muscles while the user is performing a functional mobility task. FES is specifically programmed for the user, which makes it customizable. If a user chooses to purchase a system for home use, FES for foot drop could replace an ankle foot orthosis.[88] Although modalities such as NMES and FES have been proven to be effective, these modalities may be contraindicated in patients with unmanaged tumor or active disease.[89]

Equipment

A therapist recommends the appropriate durable medical equipment (DME) for the survivor and properly educates on safely using the DME. The appropriate DME will be determined based on the impairments present while simultaneously considering the prognosis of the patient. The goal is to allow as much independence as possible while maintaining safety. DME includes, but is not limited to, bedside commodes, shower chairs, tub transfer benches, canes, walkers, wheelchairs, hospital beds, transfer boards, gait belts, and mechanical lifts.[52] The therapist should account for rapid changes in function associated with malignancy. For example, the patient may currently be ambulating, but with small functional declines, the patient may require transition to a wheelchair for mobility. Insurance justification for custom DME might be more challenging for the oncology population, but if it is medically necessary and appropriate, then it is worth the fight to facilitate function and safety for the survivor.[79]

Spasticity

Both transcutaneous electrical nerve stimulation (TENS) and NMES have been researched to address spasticity, but as of now, neither have provided long-term lasting effects on spasticity.[88] Serial casting is commonly used to address spasticity and furthermore, prevent contractures via prolonged stretching.[90,91] Positioning can also be beneficial for spasticity, including use of splints for optimal positioning; however, limited evidence demonstrates the impact on function with use of splints. A multitargeted approach (botulinum toxin in addition to casting) is most likely more beneficial than a single treatment for spasticity management.[92] Providers may prescribe systemic pharmacologic therapy including baclofen, dantrolene, or tizanidine. Patients can also be evaluated for intrathecal baclofen in more severe cases.[104]

Pain

Pain is a common symptom experienced in the oncology population, with greater than 60% of survivors reporting pain.[93] It can not only negatively affect HRQoL but also impair function. The cause of pain may be directly or indirectly related to the cancer, i.e., a result of the cancer itself or side effects of cancer treatments, immobility, and/or psychologic factors. Pain in patients with an intracranial malignancy may be neuropathic or nociceptive. Central neuropathic pain is caused by a direct insult to the CNS from vascular dysfunction, infection, demyelination, trauma, or a tumor.[94] Headache is the most common type of pain in brain tumor patients, occurring in 23%–90% of patients and is likely attributable to tumor growth or surrounding edema. Somatic or nociceptive pain is more common in other systemic cancers, but only occurs in 10%–30% of brain tumor patients.[95]

Depending on the type and degree of pain, a combination of pharmacologic and nonpharmacologic options may provide the best results of managing oncologic pain. Treatment of somatic pain may necessitate the use of opioid and nonopioid analgesics, but while treating neuropathic pain, a provider may use neuropathic pain medications such as tricyclic antidepressants, carbamazepine, and gabapentin. For chronic pain management, behavioral modification techniques may also prove beneficial.[104]

Use of nonpharmacologic pain management techniques including therapeutic modalities and manual therapy can be beneficial in pain management. According to Cheville et al., therapeutic modalities used to manage pain can be grouped into four categories as follows: those that modulate nociception, stabilize or unload painful structures, influence physiologic processes that indirectly influence nociception, or alleviate pain arising from the overloading of muscles and connective tissues that often occurs after surgery or with sarcopenia in late-stage cancer.[96]

Therapeutic modalities utilized to address pain management may include heat therapy, cryotherapy, ultrasound, TENS, NMES,[86] fluidotherapy, light or laser therapy.[97]

Desensitization can be incorporated to address neuropathic pain with therapeutic exercises or with fluidotherapy.[97] TENS is a commonly used therapeutic modality used for pain management. It is postulated to work via the gate theory, which uses a noxious stimulus to block pain signals.[98,99] In the past, therapeutic modalities have listed malignancies as a contraindication due to the insufficient research around changes in blood flow and movement of cells, and in turn, the potential detriment on the body.[86] However, views on the use of therapeutic modalities with the oncology population are evolving and may be used with caution by weighing the risks and benefits of the treatment. It was once thought that most therapeutic modalities are free of adverse effects for the oncologic population[96]; however, more recent studies show that caution should be used with any modality.[89]

Manual therapy pain management techniques to address myofascial pain includes soft tissue mobilization, myofascial release, manual traction, therapeutic massage, trigger point dry needling. Therapeutic exercises can be utilized to strengthen and stabilize muscles and stretching to address impaired range of motion. Repositioning and pressure reliefs, whether sitting or in supine, may also assist with pain management from immobility.[96]

Complementary and Alternative Medicine

Complementary and alternative medicine (CAM) therapies can be integrated into a comprehensive pain management program. CAM techniques have been shown to improve QOL in patients with glioma.[100] Acupuncture and support groups have been shown to be efficacious in managing cancer-related pain.[101,102] Psychologic factors such as emotional distress, depression, anxiety, and feelings of loss of control can negatively influence pain and impair mobility. Cotreatment with a psychologist who can help implement behavioral strategies to help with pain including use of coping skills, hypnosis, relaxation, and imagery.[103] Other types of CAM include reflexology, meditation, art, dietary supplements, aromatherapy, massage, healing touch, and Reiki.

Bowel and Bladder

Bowel management is important for maintaining continence and QoL. Most tumors cause an upper motor neuron bowel and can be managed with a combination of stool softeners, colonic irritants, colonic stimulants, and suppositories.[104] Bowel incontinence can also be improved with a toileting schedule.[105] Neurogenic bladder can present in patients with brain tumors as a hypotonic (flaccid) or a spastic bladder. Bladder balance is imperative to limit vesicoureteral reflux and decrease risk of urinary tract infection and renal disease.[104] Intermittent catheterization, which can be taught to the patient or caregiver, is preferred to Foley catheter placement to minimize infectious risk. As with bowel management, improved bladder continence helps protect the skin and helps the patient avoid embarrassment.[104]

CONCLUSION

Brain tumor rehabilitation is an important aspect of cancer rehabilitation. Patients who have been diagnosed with intracranial malignancy have many physical, cognitive, and psychologic impairments that can be improved through rehabilitation interventions. Grade of tumor or stage of the malignancy should be considered when developing the rehabilitation plan. A multidisciplinary team approach is often needed to obtain maximal functional benefit for the patient. Communication of the physiatry team with medical oncology, radiation oncology, and surgical oncology can be beneficial in making sure that goals of care and treatment strategies are aligned. This will help ensure the best outcome for the patient.

REFERENCES

1. American Brain Tumor Association: Brain Tumor Statistics. http://www.abta.org/about-us/news/brain-tumor-statistics/.
2. National Cancer Institute SEER Database. https://seer.cancer.gov/statfacts/html/brain.html.
3. Louis DN, Perry A, Reifenberger G, et al. The 2016 World Health Organization classification of tumors of the central nervous system: a summary. *Acta Neuropathol*. 2016; 131:803. https://doi.org/10.1007/s00401-016-1545-1.
4. Gupta A, Dwivedi T. A simplified overview of World Health Organization classification update of central nervous system tumors 2016. *J Neurosci Rural Pract*. 2017; 8(4):629–641. https://doi.org/10.4103/jnrp.jnrp_168_17.
5. American Cancer Society: Types of Brain and Spinal Cord Tumors in Adults. https://www.cancer.org/cancer/brain-spinal-cord-tumors-adults/about/types-of-brain-tumors.html.
6. Lucena-Cacace A, Otero-Albiol D, Jimenez-Garcia MP, et al. NAMPT overexpression induces cancer stemness and defines a novel tumor signature for glioma prognosis. *Oncotarget*. 2017;8(59):99514–99530. https://doi.org/10.18632/oncotarget.20577.
7. Stubblefield MD, O'Dell MW. *Cancer Rehabilitation: Principles and Practice*. New York: Demos Medical; 2009 [Chapter 43].
8. American Brain Tumor Association: Metastatic Brain Tumors. http://www.abta.org/secure/metastatic-brain-tumor.pdf.
9. Kyeong S, Cha YJ, Ahn SG, et al. Subtypes of breast cancer show different spatial distributions of brain metastases. *PLoS One*. 2017;12(11):e0188542. https://doi.org/10.1371/journal.pone.0188542.
10. Forsyth PA, Posner JB. Headaches in patients with brain tumors: a study of 111 patients. *Neurology*. 1993;43(9): 1678–1683.
11. Sepulveda-Sanchez JM, Conde-Moreno A, Baron M, et al. Erratum: efficacy and tolerability of lacosamide for secondary epileptic seizures in patients with brain tumor: a multicenter, observational retrospective study. *Oncol Lett*. 2017;14(4):4410. https://doi.org/10.3892/ol.2017.6689.
12. Villaneuva-Meyer JE, Mabray MC, Cha S. Current clinical brain tumor imaging. *Neurosurgery*. 2017;81(3): 397–415. https://doi.org/10.1093/neuros/nyx103.
13. Smirniotopoulos JG, Murphy FM, Rushing EJ, et al. Patterns of contrast enhancement in the brain and meninges. *Radiographics*. 2007;27(2):525–551.
14. Davis PC, Huddgins PA, Peterman SB, et al. Diagnosis of cerebral metastases: double-dose delayed CT vs contrast-enhanced MR imaging. *AJNR Am J Neuroradiol*. 1991; 12(2):293–300.
15. Schaefer PW, Budzik Jr RF, Gonzalez RG. Imaging of cerebral metastases. *Neurosurg Clin N Am*. 1996;7(3): 393–423.
16. Verger A, Langen KJ. PET imaging in glioblastoma: use in clinical practice. In: De Vleeschouwer, ed. *Glioblastoma*. Brisbane (AU): Codon Publications; September 2017 (Chapter 9).
17. Firlik KS, Martinez AJ, Lunsford LD. Use of cytological preparations for the intraoperative diagnosis of stereotactically obtained brain biopsies: a 19-year experience and survey of neuropathologists. *J Neurosurg*. 1999;91(3):454–458.
18. Satyarthee GD, Chandra PS, Sharma BS, et al. Comparison of stereotactic and ultrasound-guided biopsy of solid supratentorial tumor: a preliminary report. *Asian J Neurosurg*. 2017;12(4):664–669. https://doi.org/10.4103/1793-5482.215765.

19. Schwarzrock C. Collaboration in the presence of cerebral edema: the complications of steroids. *Surg Neurol Int.* 2016;7(suppl 7):S185–S189. https://doi.org/10.4103/2152-7806.179228.
20. Ryan R, Booth S, Price S. Corticosteroid-use in primary and secondary brain tumour patients: a review. *J Neurooncol.* 2012;106(3):449–459.
21. Marantidou A, Levy C, Duquesne A, et al. Steroid requirements during radiotherapy for malignant gliomas. *J Neurooncol.* 2010;100(1):89–94.
22. Deutsch MB, Panageas KS, Lassman AB, et al. Steroid management in newly diagnosed glioblastoma. *J Neurooncol.* 2013;113(1):111–116.
23. Schiff D, Lee EQ, Nayak L, et al. Medical management of brain tumors and the sequelae of treatment. *Neuro Oncol.* 2015;17(4):488–504. https://doi.org/10.1093/neuonc/nou304.
24. Peddi P, Ajit NE, Burton GV, et al. Regression of a glioblastoma multiforme: spontaneous versus a potential antineoplastic effect of dexamethasone and levetiracetam. *BMJ Case Rep.* December 23, 2016. pii: bcr2016217393. https://doi.org/10.1136/bcr-2016-217393.
25. Affronti ML, Woodring S, Peters KB, et al. A Phase II single-arm trial of palonosetron for the prevention of acute and delayed chemotherapy-induced nausea and vomiting in malignant glioma patients receiving multidose irinotecan in combination with bevacizumab. *Clin Risk Manag.* 2016;13:33–40. https://doi.org/10.2147/TCRM.S122480.
26. Matsuda M, Yamamoto T, Ishikawa E, et al. Combination of palonosetron, aprepitant, and dexamethasone effectively controls chemotherapy-induced nausea and vomiting in patients treated with concomitant temozolomide and radiotherapy: results of a prospective study. *Neurol Med Chir (Tokyo).* 2016;56(11):698–703.
27. Alexiou GA, Varela M, Sfakianos G, et al. Benign lesions accompanied by intractable epilepsy in children. *J Child Neurol.* 2009;24(6):697–700.
28. You G, Sha ZY, Yan W, et al. Seizure characteristics and outcomes in 508 Chinese adult patients undergoing primary resection of low-grade gliomas: a clinicopathological study. *Neuro Oncol.* 2012;14(2):230–241.
29. Lee JW, Wen PY, Hurwitz S, et al. Morphological characteristics of brain tumors causing seizures. *Arch Neurol.* 2010;67(3):336–342.
30. Maschio M. Brain tumor-related epilepsy. *Curr Neuropharmacol.* 2012;10(2):124–133.
31. Weller M, Stupp R, Wick W. Epilepsy meets cancer: when, why, and what to do about it? *Lancet Oncol.* 2012;13(9):e375–e382.
32. Glantz MJ, Cole BF, Friedberg MH, et al. A randomized, blinded, placebo-controlled trial of divalproex sodium prophylaxis in adults with newly diagnosed brain tumors. *Neurology.* 1996;46(4):985–991.
33. Perry JR. Thromboembolic disease in patients with high-grade glioma. *Neuro Oncol.* 2012;14(suppl 4):iv73–iv80.
34. Sawaya R, Zuccarello M, Elkalliny M, et al. Postoperative venous thromboembolism and brain tumors: Part I. Clinical profile. *J Neurooncol.* 1992;14(2):119–125.
35. Jo JT, Schiff D, Perry JR. Thrombosis in brain tumors. *Semin Thromb Hemost.* 2014;40(3):325–331.
36. Martha S, Laube E, Miao Y, et al. Safe and effective use of rivaroxaban for treatment of cancer-associated venous thromboembolic disease: a prospective cohort study. *J Thromb Thrombolysis.* 2017;43(2):166–171. https://doi.org/10.1007/s11239-016-1429-1.
37. Kuwata T, Kanayama M, Hirai A, et al. Postoperative thoracic hemorrhage after right upper lobectomy with thoracic wall resection during rivaroxaban anticoagulant therapy for deep leg vein thrombosis: a case report. *Int J Surg Case Rep.* 2017;41:340–342. https://doi.org/10.1016/j.ijscr.2017.11.015.
38. Han L, Kamdar MR. MRI to MGMT: predicting methylation status in glioblastoma patients using convolutional recurrent neural networks. *Pac Symp Biocomput.* 2018;23:331–342.
39. Bae JW, Hong EK, Gwak HS. Response of leptomeningeal dissemination of anaplastic glioma to temozolomide: experience of two cases. *Brain Tumor Res Treat.* 2017;5(2):99–104. https://doi.org/10.14791/btrt.2017.5.2.99.
40. Andronesi OC, Esmaeili M, Bora RJH, et al. Early changes in glioblastoma metabolism measured by MR spectroscopic imaging during combination of anti-angiogenic cediranib and chemoradiation therapy are associated with survival. *NPJ Precis Oncol.* 2017;1. pii: 20. https://doi.org/10.1038/s41698-017-0020-3.
41. Li Y, Ali S, Clarke J, et al. Bevacizumab in recurrent glioma: patterns of treatment failure and implications. *Brain Tumor Res Treat.* 2017;5(1):1–9. https://doi.org/10.14791/btrt.2017.5.1.1.
42. Zhu Z, Chai Y. Crizotinib resistance overcome by ceritinib in an ALK-positive non-small cell lung cancer patient with brain metastases: a case report. *Med Baltim.* 2017;96(45):e8652. https://doi.org/10.1097/MD.0000000000008652.
43. Tsao MN. Brain metastases: advances over the decades. *Ann Palliat Med.* 2015;4(4):225–232. https://doi.org/10.3978/j.issn.2224-5820.2015.09.01.
44. Mulvenna P, Nankivell M, Baron R, et al. Dexamethasone and supportive care with or without whole brain radiotherapy in treating patients with non-small cell lung cancer with brain metastases unsuitable for resection or stereotactic radiotherapy (QUARTZ): results from a phase 3, non-inferiority, randomised trial. *Lancet.* 2016;388(10055):2004–2014. https://doi.org/10.1016/S0140-6736(16)30825-X.
45. Rana N, Pendyala P, Cleary RK, et al. Long-term outcomes after salvage stereotactic radiosurgery (SRS) following in-field failure of initial SRS for brain metastases. *Front Oncol.* 2017;7:279. https://doi.org/10.3389/fonc.2017.00279.
46. Kollová A, Liscák R, Novotný Jr J, et al. Gamma knife surgery for benign meningioma. *J Neurosurg.* 2007;107:325–336.

47. Ryu HS, Moon KS, Lee KH, et al. Recurred intracranial meningioma: a retrospective analysis for treatment outcome and prognostic factor. *Brain Tumor Res Treat*. 2017;5(2):54–63. https://doi.org/10.14791/btrt.2017.5.2.54.
48. Chai YH, Jung S, Lee JK, et al. Ependymomas: prognostic factors and outcome analysis in a retrospective series of 33 patients. *Brain Tumor Res Treat*. 2017;5(2):70–76. https://doi.org/10.14791/btrt.2017.5.2.70.
49. Khan F, Amatya B, Drummond K, et al. Effectiveness of integrated multidisciplinary rehabilitation in primary brain cancer survivors in an Australian community cohort: a controlled clinical trial. *J Rehabil Med*. 2014;46(8):754–760. https://doi.org/10.2340/16501977-1840.
50. Cromes GF. Implementation of interdisciplinary cancer rehabilitation. *Rehabil Couns Bull*. 1978;21:230–237.
51. Silver JK, Baima J, Mayer RS. Impairment-driven cancer rehabilitation: an essential component of quality care and survivorship. *CA Cancer J Clin*. 2013;63(5):295–317.
52. Cheville A. Rehabilitation of patients with advanced cancer. *Cancer*. 2001;92:1039–1048. https://doi.org/10.1002/1097-0142(20010815)92:4+<1039::AID-CNCR1417>3.0.CO;2-L.
53. Yoshioka H. Rehabilitation for the terminal cancer patients. *Am Phys Med Rehabil*. 1994;73:199–206.
54. Taphoorn MJ, Sizoo EM, Bottomley A. Review on quality of life issues in patients with primary brain tumors. *Oncologist*. 2010;15:618–626.
55. Bunevicius A, Tamasauskas S, Deltuva V, et al. Predictors of health-related quality of life in neurosurgical brain tumor patients: focus on patient-centered perspective. *Acta Neurochir*. 2014;156:367–374.
56. Bosma I, Reijneveld JC, Douw L, et al. Health-related quality of life of long-term high-grade glioma survivors. *Neuro Oncol*. 2009;11:51–58.
57. Carson KA, Grossman SA, Fisher JD, Shaw EG. Prognostic factors for survival in adult patients with recurrent glioma enrolled on to the new approaches to brain tumor therapy CNS consortium phase I and II clinical trials. *J Clin Oncol*. 2007;25(18):2601–2606.
58. Tang V, Rathbone M, Park Dorsay J, et al. Rehabilitation in primary and metastatic brain tumours: impact of functional outcomes on survival. *J Neurol*. 2008;255(6):820–827.
59. Noll KR, Ziu M, Weinber JS, et al. Neurocognitive functioning in patients with glioma of the left and right temporal lobes. *J Neurooncol*. 2016;128(2):323–331. https://doi.org/10.1007/s11060-016-2114-0.
60. Crossen JR, Garwood D, Glatstein E, et al. Neurobehavioral sequelae of cranial irradiation in adults: a review of radiation-induced encephalopathy. *J Clin Oncol*. 1994;12(3):627–642.
61. Monje ML, Toda H, Palmer TD. Inflammatory blockade restores adult hippocampal neurogenesis. *Science*. 2003;302(5651):1760–1765.
62. Dietrich J, Han R, Yang Y, et al. CNS progenitor cells and oligodendrocytes are targets of chemotherapeutic agents in vitro and in vivo. *J Biol*. 2006;5(7):22.
63. Shaw EG, Rosdhal R, D'Agostino Jr RB, et al. Phase II study of donepezil in irradiated brain tumor patients: effect on cognitive function, mood, and quality of life. *J Clin Oncol*. 2006;24(9):1415–1420.
64. Prater S, Anand N, Wei L, et al. Crossed aphasia in a patient with anaplastic astrocytoma of the non-dominant hemisphere. *J Radiol Case Rep*. 2017;11(9):1–9. https://doi.org/10.3941/jrcr.v11i9.3154.
65. Hillis AE. Aphasia: progress in the last quarter of a century. *Neurology*. 2007;69:200.
66. Cicerone KD, Langenbahn DM, Braden C, et al. Evidence-based cognitive rehabilitation: updated review of the literature from 2003 through 2008. *Arch Phys Med Rehabil*. 2011;92:519–530.
67. *Am J Phys Med Rehabil*. 2011;90(5 suppl 1):S50–S62.
68. Back M, Back E, Kastelan M, et al. Cognitive deficits in primary brain tumours: a framework for management and rehabilitation. *J Cancer Ther*. 2014;5(1):74–81. https://doi.org/10.4236/jct.2014.51010.
69. Wang XM, Walitt B, Saligan L, et al. Chemobrain: a critical review and causal hypothesis of link between cytokines and epigenetic reprogramming associated with chemotherapy. *Cytokine*. 2015;72(1):86–96. https://doi.org/10.1016/j.cyto.2014.12.006.
70. Vitali M, Ripamonti CI, Roila F, et al. Cognitive impairment and chemotherapy: a brief overview. *Crit Rev Oncol Hematol*. 2017;118:7–14. https://doi.org/10.1016/j.critrevonc.2017.08.001.
71. Boykoff N, Moieni M, Subramanian S. Confronting chemobrain: an in-depth look at survivors' reports of impact on work, social networks, and health care response. *J Cancer Surviv*. 2009;3(4):223–232.
72. Veretennikoff K, Walker D, Biggs V, et al. Changes in cognition and decision making capacity following brain tumor resection: illustrated with two cases. *Brain Sci*. 2017;7(10). pii: E122. https://doi.org/10.3390/brainsci7100122.
73. Oort Q, Dirven L, Meijer W, et al. Development of a questionnaire measuring instrumental activities of daily living (IADL) in patients with brain tumors: a pilot study. *J Neurooncol*. 2017;132(1):145–153. https://doi.org/10.1007/s11060-016-2352-1.
74. Lawton MP, Brody EM. Assessment of older people: self-maintaining and instrumental activities of daily living. *Gerontologist*. 1969;9(3):179–186. https://doi.org/10.1093/geront/9.3_Part_1.179.
75. Overdorp EJ. The combined effect of neuropsychological and neuropathological deficits on instrumental activities of daily living in older adults: a systematic review. *Neuropsychol Rev*. 2016;26(1):92–106. https://doi.org/10.1007/s11065-015-9312-y.
76. Mackworth N, Fobair P, Prados MD. Quality of life self-reports from 200 brain tumor patients: comparisons with Karnofsky performance scores. *J Neurooncol*. 1992;14(3):243–253. https://doi.org/10.1007/BF00172600.
77. O'Dell MW. Functional outcome of inpatient rehabilitation in persons with brain tumors. *Arch Phys Med Rehabil*. 1998;79(12):1530–1534. https://doi.org/10.1016/S0003-9993(98)90414-2.

78. Avin KG, Hanke TA, Kirk-Sanchez N, et al. Management of falls in community-dwelling older adults: clinical guidance statement from the academy of geriatric physical therapy of the American Physical Therapy Association. *Phys Ther.* 2015;95(6):815–834.
79. Umphred DA. *Neurological Rehabilitation.* 5th ed. St. Louis: Mosby Elsevier; 2007 [Chapter 23].
80. Umphred DA. *Neurological Rehabilitation.* 5th ed. St. Louis: Mosby Elsevier; 2007 [Chapter 25].
81. Peel NM, Kuys SS, Klein K. Gait speed as a measure in geriatric assessment in clinical settings: a systematic review. *J Gerontol.* 2013;68(1):39–46.
82. Hurria A, Gupta S, Zauderer M, et al. Developing a cancer-specific geriatric assessment. *Cancer.* 2005;104: 1998–2005.
83. Cormie P, Nowak AK, Chambers SK, et al. The potential role of exercise in neuro-oncology. *Front Oncol.* 2015;5:1–6.
84. Ruden E, Reardon DA, Coan AD, et al. Exercise behavior, functional capacity, and survival in adults with malignant recurrent glioma. *J Clin Oncol.* 2011;29(21):2918–2923.
85. Betof AS, Dewhirst MW, Jones LW. Effects and potential mechanisms of exercise training on cancer progression: a translational perspective. *Brain Behav Immun.* 2013;30: 75–87.
86. Pope G, Mockett S, Wright J. A survey of electrotherapeutic modalities. *Physiotherapy.* 1995;81:82–91.
87. Nudo RJ, Plautz EJ, Frost SB. Role of adaptive plasticity in recovery of function after damage to motor cortex. *Muscle Nerve.* 2001;24:1000–1019.
88. Frontera W, DeLisa J, Gans BM, et al. *DeLisa's Physical Medicine and Rehabilitation: Principles and Practice.* 5th ed. Philadelphia: Lippincott Williams & Wilkins; 2010 [Chapter 71].
89. Maltser S, Cristian A, Silver JK, et al. A focused review of safety considerations in cancer rehabilitation. *PMR Contemp Issues Cancer Rehabil.* 2017;9:S415–S428.
90. Tyson S, Kent R. The effect of upper limb orthotics after stroke: a systematic review. *NeuroRehabilitation.* 2011; 28:29–36.
91. Logan LR. Rehabilitation techniques to maximize spasticity management. *Top Stroke Rehabil.* 2011;18(3):203–211.
92. Farina S, Migliorini C, Gandolfi M, et al. Combined effects of botulinum toxin and casting treatments on lower limb spasticity after stroke. *Funct Neurol.* 2008;23:87–91.
93. Davis MP, Lasheen W, Gamier P. Practical guide to opioids and their complications in managing cancer pain: what oncologists need to know. *Oncology.* 2007;21(10): 1229–1238.
94. Watson JC, Sandroni P. Central neuropathic pain syndromes. *Mayo Clin Proc.* 2016;91:372–385.
95. Pace A, Dirven L, Koekkoek JAF, et al. European Association for Neuro-Oncology (EANO) guidelines for palliative care in adults with glioma. *Lancet Oncol.* 2017; 18(6):e330–e340. https://doi.org/10.1016/S1470-2045(17)30345-5.
96. Cheville AL, Basford JR. The role of rehabilitation medicine and the physical agents in the treatment of cancer-associated pain. *J Clin Oncol.* 2014;32:1691–1702.
97. Goodwin PJ. Pain in patients with cancer. *J Clin Oncol.* 2014;32(16):1637–1639.
98. Melzack R, Wall PD. Pain mechanism: a new theory. *Science.* 1965;150(3699):971–979.
99. Keskin EA, Onur O, Keskin HL, et al. Transcutaneous electrical nerve stimulation improves low back pain during pregnancy. *Gynecol Obstet Invest.* 2012;74:76–83.
100. Mobed K, Liu R, Stewart S, et al. Quality of life and patterns of use of complementary and alternative medicines among glioma patients. *J Support Oncol.* 2009;7(6): W23–W31.
101. Alimi D, Rubino C, Leandri EP, et al. Analgesic effect of auricular acupuncture for cancer pain: a randomized, controlled, blinded trial. *J Clin Oncol.* 2003;21: 4120–4126.
102. Goodwin PJ, Leszcz M, Ennis M, et al. The effect of group psychosocial support on survival in metastatic breast cancer. *N Engl J Med.* 2001;345:1719–1726.
103. Syrjala KL, Jensen MP, Mendoza ME, et al. Psychological and behavioral approaches to cancer pain management. *J Clin Oncol.* 2014;32:1703–1711.
104. Kirshblum S, O'Dell MW, Ho C, et al. Rehabilitation of persons with central nervous system tumors. *Cancer.* 2001;92:1029–1038. https://doi.org/10.1002/1097-0142(20010815)92:4+<1029::AID-CNCR1416> 3.0.CO;2-P.
105. Mukand JA, Blackinton DD, Crincoli MG, Lee JJ, Santos BB. Incidence of neurologic deficits and rehabilitation of patients with brain tumors. *Am J Phys Med Rehabil.* 2001;80:346–350.

CHAPTER 6

Cognitive Deficits in Brain Cancer

SARAH KHAN, DO • KOMAL PATEL, MD • GONZALO A. VAZQUEZ-CASALS, PHD

INTRODUCTION

The average annual mortality in the United States between the years 2010–2014 was 4.33 per 100,000, with over 75,000 deaths being attributed to primary malignant brain or other CNS tumors.[1] Gliomas are the most common primary brain tumor, making up between 70% and 81% of all malignant intracranial primary tumors.[2–4] The cause is largely unknown. They are classified according to the World Health Organization (WHO) grades 1–4, based on increasing severity of malignancy. Males are more commonly affected than women in a 3:2 ratio.

A grade 4 glioma is known as a glioblastoma and is the most aggressive and accounts for 50%–70% of diffuse gliomas. The average age of diagnosis is 60 years. Anaplastic gliomas are grade 3 lesions including astrocytomas, oligodendrogliomas, or mixed gliomas. They make up 15%–25% of primary brain tumors and usually present around 45 years of age.[2,4] These higher grade gliomas have been found to present with focal neurologic deficits and cognitive changes of up to 3 months duration and in some cases, headaches of up to 1 month duration.[4]

The remaining 15%–25% of gliomas are low grade—grade 2 and grade 1 gliomas. Grade 2 gliomas include oligodendrogliomas and oligoastrocytomas. Astrocytomas can be grade 1 or grade 2 lesions. These tumors typically present with seizures between 30–45 years of age.[2,4] Oligodendrogliomas tend to have a median survival of 10–15 years from diagnosis, and astrocytomas and oligoastrocytomas have a median survival of 6 years[5] (Table 6.1).

Patients suspected of intracranial lesions should be assessed with MRI, including T1-weighted spin echo, T2 fluid-attenuated inversion recovery (FLAIR), and gadolinium. Lesions suggestive of tumor will have hyposignal on T1 and hypersignal on T2. Lesion biopsy will allow for definitive diagnosis.

Prognosis is based on phenotype and tumor grading. Favorable prognostic factors include younger age, complete surgical resection of tumor, good functional performance status, and good cognition.[2,3] Management includes steroid treatment in a tapering dose for edema control and antiepileptics for seizure management or prophylaxis. Levetiracetam is usually the antiepileptic of choice as it has a low likelihood to have drug interactions with chemotherapy medications, good tolerability, relatively rapid titration, and intravenous availability.[6] Usually surgical resection of tumor is followed by radiation therapy typically starting 3–4 weeks post operation, once the surgical bed has healed adequately to prevent necrosis from radiation. Ideally, chemotherapy is started shortly after radiation therapy in patients who can tolerate both. The ability to tolerate concurrent chemotherapy and radiation predicts a more favorable prognosis.

Meningiomas, or tumors of CNS dural coverings, have long been the most common nonglial intracranial tumor, accounting for a little over 36% of all such tumors, with an incidence of about 8.3 per 100,000.[1,7,8] First described in 1922 by Harvey Cushing, meningiomas have, as a majority, been found to be benign (WHO grade 1) but are typically diagnosed at an older age, with the median age of diagnosis being 66 years old.[1,7,8] Furthermore, meningiomas tend to occur with greater frequency in those with certain conditions, such as neurofibromatosis type 2 and multiple endocrine neoplasia type 1.[7] Currently, the WHO criteria has three grades for meningiomas: grade 1 meningiomas are benign, grade 2 meningiomas are atypical, and grade 3 meningiomas are malignant[7,8] (Table 6.2).

Surgery is necessary for establishing a definitive diagnosis and removal of the tumor, but gross total resection (GTR) is only achieved about 50% of the time.[7,8] Depending on the extent of resection of the meningioma, the Simpson criteria has been able to better predict the risk of tumor recurrence. But there still remains some uncertainty, and hence there is some variability in treatment options. Available treatments include surgical resection with recurrence being based on the Simpson classification Table 6.3, single-session

TABLE 6.1
World Health Organization (WHO) Grading, Classification, and Survival Rates Among Gliomas[3, 4]

WHO Grading	Histologic Classification	Average Age of Presentation	5-year Survival Rate (%)
I	Pilocytic astrocytoma	20–30	95
II	Diffuse astrocytoma	30–45	50
	Oligoastrocytoma		60
	Oligodendroglioma		70
III	Anaplastic astrocytoma	45	50–60
	Anaplastic oligodendroglioma		
	Oligoastrocytoma		
IV	Glioblastoma	60	5

TABLE 6.2
World Health Organization (WHO) Classification of Meningiomas and the 15 Variations Based on Microscopic Cell Analysis

WHO grade 1—Benign	WHO Grade 2—Atypical	WHO Grade 3—Malignant
Meningothelial	Chordoid	Papillary
Fibrous	Clear cell	Rhabdoid
Transitional/Mixed	Atypical	Anaplastic
Psammomatous		
Angiomatous		
Microcystic		
Secretory		
Lymphoplasmacyte-rich		
Metaplastic		

Found on American Association of Neurological Surgeons website, http://www.aans.org/Patients/Neurosurgical-Conditions-and-Treatments/Meningiomas.

TABLE 6.3
Simpson Grades of Resection[9]

Grade	Definition	Recurrence Rate
1	Gross total resection (GTR) of tumor, dural attachments, and abnormal bone	9
2	GTR of tumor, coagulation of dural attachments	19
3	GTR of tumor without resection or coagulation of dural attachments or extradural extensions	29
4	Partial tumor resection	44
5	Simple decompression (biopsy)	

stereotactic radiosurgery, hypofractionated stereotactic radiation therapy, and conventionally fractionated external beam radiation therapy.

The primary objective of surgery for meningiomas is that which is classified as Simpson grades 1–3.[7,10] In benign meningiomas, GTR is considered definite therapy. Simpson grades 4 and 5 or subtotal resections, on the other hand, carry a substantially higher rate of progression, even with benign meningiomas.[7,10] Moreover, other treatment options such as radiation therapy are typically used as an adjunct therapy to subtotal resection, treatment for tumor recurrence, for tumors in surgically inaccessible areas, or tumors of high-grade histology.[7] On the other hand, chemotherapy has a limited role in meningiomas and hence is rarely used.

Clinical presentation in brain tumors can be very diverse, involving any conceivable neurologic or neuropsychologic sign or symptom by virtue of their localization, tumor type, and growth characteristics. In turn, the clinical presentation interacts with different patient characteristics including age, cerebral lateralization, premorbid abilities and skills, and environmental demands. Slowly growing tumors are often associated with an insidious onset, and subtle progression of symptoms not unlike it is observed in neurodegenerative disorders such as dementia. If cognitive symptoms are the earliest signs of a tumor, the impairments are usually severe enough to interfere with the patient's daily activities. Unawareness, which may accompany the impairments resulting from a brain tumor, may also delay its identification. While relatives and friends may misattribute the cognitive, emotional, and personality changes to other benign causes, it is common for them to retrospectively identify subtle tumor signs that were present before the condition was suspected. Initial presentation may involve a single breakthrough event such as a seizure or an episode of altered mental status or aphasic/dysphasic speech. At times, prior to the emergence of cognitive symptoms, focal, noncognitive neurologic signs such as numbness or tingling, or signs of increased intracranial pressure—headaches, nausea, vomiting, drowsiness, and visual abnormalities—may be present.[11]

Inpatient and outpatient rehabilitation therapy to address functional impairments as a result of weakness, mobility, and ADL impairment and cognitive deficits due to the effects of the tumor itself or the side effects of cancer treatment is of benefit. Patients and their families should also be referred to psychologic counseling and support to address coping strategies to address the psychologic stress and social impact of this progressive disease.

TUMOR-RELATED COGNITIVE DECLINE

Early in the course of diagnosis, patients with gliomas, meningiomas, and cerebral metastasis often exhibit neurocognitive deficits that impact general functioning and overall quality of life. In general, for all of these tumor types, deficits have been noted in multiple cognitive domains. Even patients considered to be in good neurologic status at diagnosis were shown to have significant deficits in neuropsychologic assessments of processing speed, executive functioning, and memory. Larger tumor volume, tumors affecting the frontal lobe, and left cortical lesions seem to be associated with greater neurocognitive dysfunction.[12] It appears that in patients with gliomas, executive functioning tends to be the most commonly affected. Attention and memory have also been noted to be frequently impaired. These cognitive deficits have been observed both prior to and after surgical resection. Meningioma tumors tend to more frequently affect frontal lobe functions of attention, executive functioning, and memory. Patients with cerebral metastatic lesions are most commonly affected by memory deficits.

Gliomas

There are a handful of studies addressing cognitive deficits in glioma early in diagnosis. In a neuropsychologic assessment of patients with both low- and high-grade gliomas prior to the initiation of any treatment, deficits were found in multiple cognitive domains, most commonly executive functioning. Greater than 60% of patients had impairment in at least one cognitive domain of executive functioning, attention, memory, language, visuospatial functioning, and processing speed. Patients with high-grade glioma are affected with a greater degree of cognitive impairment compared with patients with low-grade glioma.[13]

Neuropsychologic evaluation of a group of patients with low-grade gliomas found 60% of these patients had cognitive deficits, mainly in executive functioning but also in domains of attention and memory. Two-third had subjective complaints of fatigue or attentional disturbances that had been progressively increasing over the past 6–12 months. There was a positive correlation between subjective complaints and impairments on neuropsychologic testing.[14]

Another study showed 1/3 of patients with high-grade glioma exhibited cognitive decline after treatment with chemotherapy and radiation. However, the overwhelming majority of these patients had progression of their tumor within 4 months. This finding suggests that cognitive decline often appears to be related to tumor progression rather than treatment.[15] It has also been shown that there is a significant correlation between deficits on the neuropsychologic tests of the Controlled Oral Word Association (COWA), which assesses executive functioning, and Trails Making Test B, which measures attention, with increased mortality. A significant, but less prominent, correlation was also observed in deficits on the executive task of similarities and the attention task of digit span on chance of survival.[16] There was no association between tumor laterality and survival.

It is noteworthy to mention that much of the literature on this topic is limited by small study sample sizes and heterogeneity of assessment measures used. Almost all patients had cortical lesions. Overall, a sizable percentage of these patients exhibited some degree of cognitive impairment on neuropsychologic evaluation.

Meningioma

Most patients with meningioma demonstrate cognitive deficits in several domains, particularly frontal lobe functions. A systematic review assessing cognitive deficits in patients with meningioma (mostly affecting the cortex) before and/or just after treatment found that in general, patients with meningioma have cognitive deficits mainly in attention, memory, and executive functioning. Typically post resection most studies found improvement in cognition, but patients still had deficits compared with healthy controls. Most studies did not find significant association of tumor laterality and cognitive impairment. A couple studies suggested that right-sided lesions tend to improve more post resection compared with left-sided lesions.[17]

Skull base meningioma tumors can also affect cognition. A prospective study assessing neuropsychologic measures in patients with skull base meningioma prior to and at 3–5 months and 9–12 month periods after surgical resection showed about 10%–15% of patients showed decline in long-term verbal memory, working memory, and processing speed within 3 months after surgical resection, but only 5%–10% of patients showed long-term impairments persisting at 12 months. No significant effect was noted for measures of anxiety and depression. Authors did not speculate or comment on factors associated with a decline in neurocognitive status.[18] Anterior skull base meningiomas affecting the ventromedial prefrontal cortex exhibited significant decline in behavioral adaptive functioning, but do not affect basic cognitive functioning.[19]

Brain Metastasis

Common primary tumors with metastasis to the brain include lung, breast, melanoma, and colon cancer. Compared with glioma and meningioma, there is limited literature regarding cognitive deficits related to brain metastasis. Overall, patients with brain metastasis were significantly impaired in most cognitive domains compared with controls. Memory deficits were found to be the most prominent. Language, executive functioning, and fine motor dexterity were also found to be significantly impacted in a number of patients. Attention was found to be the least affected.[20] Cognitive deficits would be expected based on the region of brain affected and the extent and size of metastatic lesions in the brain.

TREATMENT-RELATED COGNITIVE IMPAIRMENTS

Overall, the treatments for malignancies have improved, allowing for individuals with cancer to better fight off their disease process. With increased survivorship among patients with malignancies comes the long-term sequelae of the treatments we provide them. In particular, individuals with brain malignancies experience cognitive impairments related to treatments such as radiation therapy, chemotherapy, and surgery.[21] Much of the improvement in treating brain tumors has come from this increased aggressiveness in attacking the tumor, combining multiple treatment options.[22] The cognitive impairments as a result of these treatments, however, are a feature that may limit a patient's functional recovery, as they typically affect the processes of learning, concentration, memory, spatial information processing, reasoning, attention, and processing speed.[21–25] There has been some variability in the literature as to the effect that tumor size and grade actually have on cognitive impairments. It is therefore important to identify and address other potential causes of these impairments, helping to minimize these effects, especially since cognitive function has been shown to be a sensitive independent predictor of survival.[22,26,27]

Neurosurgery

The choice of surgical procedures (i.e., craniotomy, stereotactic biopsy, image-guided biopsies) and the location of the tumor will determine the impact on cognition. Also, the extent of surgical intervention will determine the risk of cognitive deficit. Many intracranial tumors are susceptible to be treated by means of neurosurgical resection. Even large meningiomas can frequently be excised completely. Surgery for metastatic tumors is continuously evolving and has benefitted from improved neuroimaging resulting in improvement in intraoperative targeting, anesthetic techniques, and survival rates.

Complete surgical removal of an intracranial tumor typically results in a relatively stable and focal chronic postsurgical neuropsychologic profile during the recovery period. In the case of space-occupying tumors from the cranium, their removal frequently results in neuropsychologic improvement compared with the patient's presurgical status.[17,28]

Radiation Therapy

Radiation therapy has proven to be a curative therapeutic tool in the treatment of cancer, but it has also been shown to have a negative impact on quality of life as well as neurocognitive function.[21,29] The effect of a brain tumor itself on a patient's function and cognitive status is dependent on location, but radiation-induced brain injury is a dynamic process affecting all cell types: endothelial and oligodendroglial cells, astrocytes, microglia, neurons, and neuronal stem cells.[29] The effects of radiation therapy are divided into acute, early, delayed, and late delayed processes, with late delayed effects believed to be the cause of neurologic consequences.[21] Delayed effects may present up to 20 years after treatment. Characteristics of radiation therapy that contribute to the risk of radiation-induced brain injury include total dose, dose per fraction (higher risk with greater than 2 Gy dose per fraction), total time and volume, radiation quality and volume, hyperfractionated schedules, shorter overall treatment time, presence of comorbid vascular risk factors, and adjunctive therapy.[22,29,30,31] Radiation therapy causes both demyelinating and axonal damage, which are hallmarks of brain white matter damage. The proposed mechanism is believed to be by damaging oligodendrocytes and disrupting cerebral vascular endothelial cells leading to coagulative necrosis, vessel wall thickening, and focal mineralization, affecting brain white matter more than brain gray matter.[21,22] Radiation to larger volumes of brain and higher doses have also been shown to produce higher grade lesions on magnetic resonance imaging,[32] and the amount of demyelination and damage to the white matter track integrity correlates with the extent of cognitive impairment.[21,23] Additionally, radiation therapy is generally not given as a monotherapy, rather combined with chemotherapy targeted against the tumor as well.

Partial brain radiotherapy results in variable effects across patients, with prevalent impairment of memory and processing speed. Extent of impairment of verbal versus visual memory may vary from the early to the last postradiation phases. However, the initial neuropsychologic profiles do not appear to accurately predict profiles after 3 years.

Limited field radiation appears to have less delayed consequences than those seen in whole brain radiation. Most patients appear to have minimal or no cognitive deterioration during the first several years, with some variability among cases.[33–35] Increasingly more used in the treatment of several types of brain tumors, stereotactic radiosurgery, has a more focused effect and therefore limits the amount of radiation delivered to normal tissue and the contingent neurocognitive deficits.[36]

Chemotherapy

Typically speaking, radiation therapy is localized to a certain region of the body; however, chemotherapy has a more systemic effect. There are a vast number of chemotherapeutic agents available for cancer treatment, each affecting an individual's body differently but also carrying their own side effect profile. White matter in the brain is significantly vulnerable to effects of chemotherapy, with onset of identifiable changes possibly delayed for months. A wide range of incidence for cognitive impairments in those receiving chemotherapy has been reported, but of more recent it is believed to be greater than 70% and typically manifesting as concentration impairments, memory loss, reasoning, and attention deficits.[23–25,37–40] These deficits are typically referred to as "chemobrain." This is not to say that the high incidence of cognitive impairments in those being treated with chemotherapy is solely due to the medications themselves, but may be a contributing factor in addition to the tumor itself.

Most chemotherapeutic agents used do not even cross the blood-brain barrier, with the exception of 5-Fluorouracil, methotrexate,[23] and a few others which were found in low levels including cisplatin,[41] carmustine,[42] and paclitaxel.[43] Even so these chemotherapeutic agents are believed to increase overall oxidative stress resulting in cognitive impairments.[23,37] Chemotherapy produces a wide variety of cognitive impairments, most of which are dose dependent.[24] Furthermore, as many cancer treatment plans are multifaceted, it has been shown that the toxicity of radiation, as mentioned earlier, is likely to be synergistic with the toxicity of chemotherapies, further exacerbating these symptoms.[23,30] Historically, it was believed that these cognitive impairments were related to psychologic factors such as depression, anxiety, or other cancer-related side effects such as fatigue.[24,40] Furthermore, prophylactic medications such as antiepileptic medications may exacerbate fatigue and lethargy. Steroids are used to reduce edema and may cause insomnia, anxiety, or emotional lability. Both of these types of medications may exacerbate cognitive impairments. As we, medical professionals, look to be more aggressive in treating an individual's cancer, we must remember the potential for side effects related to the treatments we are providing.

ASSESSMENT OF COGNITIVE DEFICITS IN BRAIN TUMOR

Patients with intracranial tumors, whether they are primary brain tumors, meningiomas, lymphomas, or brain metastases, will eventually present with some degree of cognitive impairment or deficits. In the following section some considerations are presented largely based on Anderson and Ryken's lucid presentation about the neuropsychologic assessment of the direct effects of intracranial tumors as well as those resulting from their treatment[11]; some basic assessment protocols will be discussed as well.

In contemporary practice, patients are diagnosed with intracranial brain tumors by means of neuroimaging techniques. Thus, the purpose of a cognitive or neuropsychologic evaluation consists of the description of a patient's profile of cognitive strengths and weakness in order to inform in management. Other possible reasons for pursuing neuropsychologic evaluation prior to formal diagnosis may include (1) collecting objective evidence supporting a patient's complaints of cognitive difficulties before more expensive procedures are ordered; (2) ruling out psychogenic and/or unusual cognitive complaints; and (3) addressing personality and emotional factors if the previous point is demonstrated.

Neuropsychologic assessment has the advantage of covering a broad range of cognitive domains, thus being susceptible of detecting the usually circumscribed cognitive dysfunction resulting from a brain tumor, so the location of a tumor determines the associated neuropsychologic signs and symptoms observed. However, there is considerable variability in the neuropsychologic sequelae of brain tumors similarly located by neuroimaging means,[44] which means that typical principles of dysfunction localization may not necessarily apply. Plastic compensatory processes may be facilitated by gradual tumor growth. Similarly, space-occupying tumors may result in neuropsychologic deficits not expected from lesion location alone. Therefore, there is no specific or particular cognitive profile indicative or suggestive of a brain tumor.

Generally, neuropsychologic evaluations occur after some kind of treatment has started. Such evaluations are helpful to (1) monitor beneficial versus neurotoxic effects of treatment, (2) evaluate for evidence indicating tumor growth, (3) monitor pace recovery, (4) assess residual competencies, and (5) guide rehabilitation efforts. Current treatment alternatives for brain tumor can result in beneficial and detrimental effects on cognition; actually, it is not infrequent for patients to concurrently receive multiple treatment modalities. Timing of the evaluation is also critical, as differences exist between long-term versus short-term cognitive sequelae of radiation therapy and chemotherapy. Therefore, developing sensitive and practical methods of monitoring for tumor recurrence in at-risk patients is crucial.

Neuropsychologic assessment, compared with other laboratory tests (e.g., neuroimaging, EEG), has the advantage of being easily repeatable, noninvasive, and relatively inexpensive. Evidence about the sensitivity of neuropsychologic evaluations in this area has increased over the years. For example, measures of memory and attention shifting have demonstrated predictive power for tumor recurrence in glioblastoma multiforme patients.[45]

An initial neuropsychologic evaluation of a patient with a suspected or known brain tumor has to minimally include a screening of all the classical domains of cognition, as well as of his/her emotional state and relevant personality traits. The latter is necessary due to the fact that the psychologic reaction to such a life-threatening diagnosis may range widely from nonreality-based optimism to absolute despair and pessimism. Identification of individuals who might benefit from psychosocial interventions, including psychotherapy/counseling, and/or pharmacologic approaches for depression and anxiety, is another important aspect of the neuropsychologic evaluation.

Assessment

Assessing cognitive deficits in patients being treated for brain tumors is not essentially different than when conducted with patients with other conditions such as traumatic brain injury (TBI) or cerebrovascular accidents. However, cognitive difficulties tend to be more diffuse in adults and reflect the contribution of current brain tumor treatment in dysfunction in the frontal-subcortical brain systems, as well as psychologic symptoms such as depression and anxiety.

The strategy and focus of the assessment is closely related to the referral questions. More often than not, the evaluation focuses on attention, executive functions, language, memory and learning, visuospatial skills, and psychologic adjustment.

In the acute rehabilitation setting, most patients with intracranial tumors have undergone some kind of tumor resection or biopsy, likely resulting in some degree of diffuse and focal cognitive deficits. Typically, these deficits may include decreased awareness and impairment in attention, executive functions, short-term memory, visuospatial skills, and aspects of language. Given their relatively short length of stay, neuropsychologic evaluations will typically make use of screening instruments to efficiently identify areas of deficit in need of interventions. Also, a hierarchical strategy may be used, matching the screening instrument to the patient examined, based on the observed level of functioning (i.e., the more apparently impaired the patient, the simpler screener will be used). Cognitive measures such as the Mini Mental State Examination (MMSE[46]), the Montreal Cognitive Assessment MoCA[47]), the Neurobehavioral Cognitive Examination (Cognitstat[48]), or the BNI Screen for Higher Cerebral Functions[49] are helpful to determine the level of severity of cognitive impairment and grossly identify areas of deficit. It is important to note that none of these instruments necessarily have adequate sensitivity to the deficits resulting from brain tumors, especially the MMSE.[50,51] Also, focal assessments may be conducted when further clarification is needed to describe a particular area of dysfunction, e.g., further characterization of memory or dysexecutive difficulties. Similarly, screening measures of mood and emotion are also used to have a better description of patients' emotional complaints and the level of severity of psychopathology, including depression and anxiety. Such measures may include the Beck Depression Inventory (BDI-II[52]), Beck Anxiety Inventory (BDI[53]), Patient Health Questionnaire Nine (PHQ-9[54]) the Generalized Anxiety Disorder Seven (GAD-7[55]), and for individuals over 65 years old, the Geriatric Depression Scale (GDS[56,57]).

Patients seen for neuropsychologic evaluation in the outpatient setting will usually undergo a full neuropsychologic workup, which will typically involve evaluation of the different neuropsychologic domains as well as a more complete evaluation of mood and personality functioning than is possible in the inpatient setting. These evaluations will likely involve measures of intellectual and academic functioning, as well as several measures of attention/concentration, language, memory, visuospatial/visuoconstructional skills, fine motor skills, and executive functioning, as well as personality/psychopathology inventories, and other measures as guided by the referral question. Such procedures have been thoroughly described in primary sources on neuropsychologic assessment.[58]

COGNITIVE REMEDIATION THERAPY FOR BRAIN TUMORS

George Prigatano, a pioneer in the field of neuropsychologic rehabilitation, has defined cognitive rehabilitation as "a teaching activity that helps restore higher cerebral functioning by facilitating processes responsible for partial recovery and by avoiding processes responsible for deterioration after brain injury."[59] Cognitive rehabilitation relies heavily on the concept of neuroplasticity and purports to improve the everyday functioning and quality of life of individuals who have sustained acquired brain injury by means of restoring functions impaired by means of drill exercises and the acquisition and mastery of compensatory skills for attention, memory, and executive functions.[60]

The efficacy of cognitive rehabilitation has been demonstrated in the clinical populations from which it was originated, i.e., TBI and stroke. However, there is a scarcity of studies assessing the effectiveness of this intervention modality in patients with brain tumors, and the few studies available have usually dealt with gliomas. No studies involving patients with meningiomas were found during the literature search. In a relatively recent critical review of the current literature, Bergo et al. [61] points out the weaknesses of the few empirical studies available. Some studies lack a control group, none included a placebo group, different types of brain tumors were analyzed, patients were studied at different times during the treatment, and the training programs used were not comparable.

However, some of the few studies available suggest that cognitive remediation may have a positive effect on patients with gliomas, including beneficial effects on self-perceived cognitive functioning in the short term, and after a 6-month follow-up, on objective measures of attention, verbal memory, and mental fatigue in a relatively large sample of adult patients with low-grade and anaplastic gliomas exposed to an intervention program consisting of computer-based attention retraining and compensatory skills training of attention, memory, and executive functions.[62] A preliminary study involving three patients with low-grade glioma who were exposed to a computerized training program for working memory to demonstrate its efficacy exhibited improvement in working memory and attention measures compared with their baseline scores.[63] Additional evidence of the potential beneficial effect of cognitive remediation was observed in the study by Maschio et al.,[64] which sought to evaluate the effect of cognitive rehabilitation in a sample of patients with brain tumor–related epilepsy and cognitive deficits and resulted in improvement in short-term verbal memory, episodic memory, fluency, and long-term visuospatial memory at two different points in time. Overall, these studies suggest that cognitive retraining involving computer-based cognitive retraining tasks with or without additional training in compensatory skills can provide a measureable degree of improvement in cognitive functioning among patients with low- or high-grade gliomas.

MEDICATIONS TO TREAT COGNITIVE IMPAIRMENTS

Given that the current treatment options offered to patients with cancer have the potential to cause cognitive impairments, it is crucial to have an understanding of medications that can be utilized to try to improve and treat these impairments. Although there is no extensive amount of research behind all of these medications, it is important to know their roles and limitations. One proposed mechanism of treatment of these cognitive impairments is the reduction of overall chemotherapy-induced side effects by decreasing the oxidative stress. It has been shown that antioxidant supplementation can reduce chemotherapy-related toxicities.[65] Some medications that are used to help reduce oxidative stress are melatonin, 2-mercaptoethane, and N-acetylcysteine, and Ginkgo biloba are believed to reduce some of this oxidative stress.[66] In particular, one study looked at the medication doxorubicin, which is an anthracycline that is typically used in multi-agent treatments for a vast number of cancers and is known to produce intracellular reactive oxygenated species.[25] By creating this caustic environment inside the cell, it is able to terminate malignant cells. However, it also affects the extracellular environment as well. 2-mercaptoethane, a sulfhydryl-containing antioxidant, is not readily taken up into cells. Therefore, it is able to protect plasma proteins from the increased oxidative stress from medications such as doxorubicin.[25]

Another option that has been studied in reducing oxidative stress is Ginkgo biloba, a tree species originally from China that is believed to be over 200 million years old.[40] With two main components, flavonoids and terpenoids, Ginkgo biloba is believed to have antioxidant stress, increases cerebral blood flow, improves glucose utilization, and stimulates hippocampal choline uptake.[40,67] Studies in the dementia and Alzheimer's population have shown some positive results in treating cognitive impairments in this population, but have not had similar results in the individuals with cancer who experience cognitive impairments.

Moreover, there are medications that have shown to have a beneficial effect in helping cognitive impairments related to the cancer itself and its treatments including fluoxetine, donepezil, modafinil, methylphenidate, dextromethorphan, memantine, and medications stimulating neurogenesis, such as insulin-like growth factor and fluoxetine.[66] Selective serotonin reuptake inhibitors (SSRIs) have been shown to improve memory in individuals with a variety of conditions.[24,68] Fluoxetine, in particular, has been shown to help prevent some of the cognitive impairments that may be a result of certain treatments, such as 5-fluorouracil. This medication is used in a variety of cancer treatments and readily crosses the blood-brain barrier, negatively affecting cell proliferation and hippocampal-dependent working memory. 24 Fluoxetine has been shown to increase hippocampal neurogenesis and improve spatial memory.[24,69,70] In the study conducted, the administration of the SSRI fluoxetine before or during the 5-FU treatment, counteracted the cognitive impairments caused by this chemotherapeutic agent, warranting further studies to be completed.[24]

Additionally, pharmacologic treatments of cognitive impairments in other disorders, such as neurodegenerative diseases, dementia, depression, attention deficit/hyperactivity disorder, have been looked at for individuals with cancer that experience cognitive impairments. This being said, there have been very few psychostimulants that have shown some promise in treating or preventing these cognitive impairments. The effectiveness of these psychostimulants, such as methylphenidate and modafinil, has not yet been fully established, requiring additional research.[66] Another medication, an anticholinesterase, donepezil, also received a lot of attention after initial preclinical findings; however, more recent findings seem to be conflicting.[66] More rigorous studies need to be produced in order to determine the true effectiveness of all of these medications, as counteracting some of the detrimental effects of cancer treatments with these medications has shown some early promise.

COMMUNITY AND EDUCATIONAL RESOURCES FOR FAMILIES AND PATIENTS

The advent of the Internet has allowed the general public to have significant access to relevant information about just about any possible topic, including brain tumors. Browsing over the Internet may offer the interested individuals a wealth of information on resources for individuals suffering from brain tumors. General information about different brain tumors, their etiology, diagnostic methods and techniques, current treatment options, trends in research, resources, and support can all be found on diverse websites from research and academic institutions in the United States and around the world. Information may also be found on free-access online encyclopedias (e.g., Wikipedia) and community and grass roots initiatives dedicated to addressing the informational needs of patients suffering from this condition and their relatives. Such websites remain a relatively constant and an easily accessible source of information which intends to provide information that for different reasons (e.g., care providers' busy schedules, the initial state of shock and lack of readiness when the diagnosis is given to patients and their relatives, lack of institutional support) may not be available to help increase awareness and knowledge about different aspects of the diagnosis and treatment of brain tumors. Consultation of such websites does not go without limitations, as the information may be too technical for the intended audience[71] or the website may be underutilized or not at all due to lack of computer literacy/technologic challenges or patients' cognitive deficits.[72] An exhaustive listing of such resources would be impossible to present in the current chapter; however, some helpful resources will be presented and briefly discussed.

American Brain Tumor Association (www.abta.org; 800-886-2282). Possibly the first advocacy organization committed to funding brain tumor research and education on all tumor types and age groups.

The Brain Tumor Foundation (www.braintumorfoundation.org; 212-265-2401) was founded in 1998 by NYU School of Medicine professor, Patrick Kelly, MD, FACS, with the purpose of treating the whole patient by addressing social, financial, and emotional needs.

Children's Brain Tumor Foundation (www.cbtf.org; 866-228-4673): This organization was founded in 1988 by dedicated parents, physicians, and their friends and is dedicated to improve treatment, quality of life, and long-term outlook of children with brain and spinal cord tumors by means of research, support, education, and advocacy.

End Brain Cancer Initiative/Chris Elliot Fund (www.endbraincancer.org; 800-574-5703) was founded by a terminal brain tumor patient, Chris Elliot, in May 2002 with the purpose of assisting individuals suffering from this condition to gain immediate access to advanced treatments, studies, and clinical trials.

Mission4Maureen (www.mission4maureen.org; 440-840-6497): This grass root organization was also founded by the relatives and friends of another tumor cancer victim, Maureen, soon after her departing in 2005, and aims at assisting qualifying brain cancer patients with everyday expenses.

The National Brain Tumor Society (www.braintumor.org; 800-253-6530) was created in 2008 when two previously existing organizations, the San Francisco–based National Brain Tumor Foundation and the Boston-based Brain Tumor Society, merged bringing together healthcare providers and people affected by brain tumors. Provision of comprehensive resources and support services and raising funds for research of brain tumors are the mission of this organization.

Pediatric Brain Tumor Foundation (www.curethekids.org; 800-253-6530) was created in Atlanta in 1991, following several fund-raisers for childhood brain tumor research organized by Mike and Diane Traynor (Ride for Kids).

Relevant information about brain tumors may also be accessed through the websites of national cancer organizations, in which sections on brain cancer or tumors can be found. Some of these include research and clinical institutions such as the National Cancer Institute (www.cancer.gov; 800-422-6237) and the many medical schools around the country, and other organizations such as Cancer Care (www.cancercare.org; 800-813-4673) and Cancer Net (www.cancer.net).

PATIENT AND FAMILY COMMUNICATION

There are few professional scenarios that may be more challenging than when a healthcare provider has to disclose and discuss with a patient or his or her concerned relatives an adverse or life-threatening diagnosis. For professionals that have not been trained to directly deal with the emotional pain and suffering that a life-threatening condition produces, there is usually little in their professional skills repertoire that prepares them for this task. For the patient and his or her family the situation may not be any easier, especially in advanced, technologic societies where health, youth, and autonomy are highly valued, and any threat to those values is perceived in catastrophic terms. Therefore, how the healthcare professional deals with what the patient knows or does not know becomes crucial to how the patient will cope with his or her diagnosis.

In the acute rehabilitation setting, this situation is particularly challenging given the relatively optimistic tone inherent to the rehabilitation situation, where a general expectation is improvement of function and potential resumption of some sense of normality. Although brain injury rehabilitation professionals, from the physiatrists to the nurses to the different therapists involved, are generally prepared to help the patient and his or her family to gradually come to terms with the fact that rehabilitation will not bring the patient to preinjury normality, there is still the expectation of recovery and increase in functionality, and possibly a life expectancy close to the rest of the population. This is not necessarily different from the situation of many brain tumor patients referred to acute rehabilitation. However, it is important to note that patients with brain tumors need and tolerance to comprehensive therapy is in turn related to their tolerance of their tumor treatment. Actually, there is evidence that brain tumor patients in such a setting recover comparably to acquired brain injury or stroke patients.[73]

Another consideration is about the fact that the professional, the patient, and his or her family are usually aware of the diagnosis, but different factors may contribute to faulty communication about it and its implications. First, it is not the rehabilitation professional's responsibility but that of the oncologist to openly discuss the prognosis and implications of the brain tumor diagnosis, including life expectancy and potential end-of-life decisions. Instead, the conversation in physiatry is about how to improve functions lost or impaired to regain some degree of independence and quality of life. Second, even under the best circumstances the patient and his or her family may still be in a state of shock after the initial diagnosis and the need for tumor resection surgery or biopsy, and not ready to deal with the likely negative prognosis and the fact that other interventions with potential debilitating side effects will follow soon after acute rehabilitation ends. Supportive counseling is usually available in acute rehabilitation contexts and may help the patient and his or her relatives to cope with the cognitive and emotional reactions to the diagnosis and provide a safe environment to discuss their concerns and further the process of awareness and prepare them for a more reality-based coping approach.

Aside from Kübler-Ross's[74] model of the stages of grief, the literature points to the need for professionals to be aware of how to handle communication of such an adverse diagnosis which can be helpful in the rehabilitation setting. Langbecker and Janda[75] found that interventions that include an educational component can improve the provision of information and knowledge for individuals with brain tumors as well as their relatives and caregivers, typically resulting in satisfaction with them. Such an approach can take place in a supportive or educational group embedded within the rehabilitation program. Regarding healthcare provider-patient communications, Sterckx, Coolbrandt, Clement et al.[76] recommend that professionals be "more considerate and supportive of patients with this life-changing diagnosis" and acknowledge their personhood and empower them to enhance their personal strengths. Lobb, Halkett, and Nowak[77] point to the importance of a balance between honesty and hope when such a negative prognosis is disclosed and encourage an individualized delivery of information considering patients' preferences for the amount and type of information, and favor senior staff or advanced trainees with adequate communication skills to discuss the prognosis.

CONCLUSION

Cognitive impairment commonly occurs from malignant and benign intracranial cortical tumors and affects the function and quality of life of not just the patient but also caregivers and family members. Neuropsychologic deficits have been found in multiple cognitive domains. Etiology of these deficits may be due to a consequence of the tumor itself or the effect of radiation or chemotherapy, but also likely multifactorial and each of these factors may contribute to a synergistic effect.

Cognitive effects due to radiation therapy can be delayed at onset for several years. Targeted radiation therapy has a significantly less risk of neurocognitive sequelae compared with whole brain radiation. Chemotherapy is believed to cause cognitive deficits that are dose dependent. In addition to this, side effects of treatment for seizures and edema may exacerbate cognitive deficits.

Neuropsychologic evaluation is essential to obtain an accurate understanding of a patient's cognitive and emotional profile and guide therapeutic treatment measures. There is a limited amount of literature on the effect of cognitive remediation in patients with brain tumors, but does exhibit quantifiable benefit in frontal cognitive impairments. Antioxidant medications may help improve cognition by reducing free radicals. Also, medications targeting the treatment of specific cognitive symptoms that a patient with a brain tumor is exhibiting can be of significant benefit.

In addition to education and support from medical professionals, there are a number of Internet resources that serve the purpose of providing education, advice, and support services for patients and their families. The goal of the rehabilitation team is to maximize patient function. Evidence shows that patients with brain tumors exhibit similar rates of functional gains as patients with stroke or TBI.

REFERENCES

1. Ostrom QT, Gittleman H, Xu J, et al. CBTRUS statistical report: primary brain and other central nervous system tumors diagnosed in the United States in 2009–2013. *Neurooncology*. 2016;18(Suppl. 5):v1–v75.
2. Ricard D, Idbaih A, Ducray F, et al. Primary brain tumors in adults. *Lancet*. 2012;379:1984–1996.
3. Ostrum QT, Bauchet L, Davis FG, et al. The epidemiology of glioma in adults: a "state of the science" review. *Neurooncology*. 2014;16(7):896–913.
4. Rasmussen BK, Hansen S, Laursen RJ, et al. Epidemiology of glioma: clinical characteristics, symptoms, and predictors of glioma patients grade I–IV in the Danish neurooncology registry. *J Neurooncol*. 2017;135(3):571–579.
5. Pignatti F, van den Bent M, Curran D, et al. Prognostic factors for survival in adult patients with cerebral low-grade glioma. *J Clin Oncol*. 2002;20:2076–2084.
6. Weller M, van den Bent M, Hopkins K, et al. EANO guideline for the diagnosis and treatment of anaplastic gliomas and glioblastoma. *Lancet Oncol*. 2014;15:e395–403.
7. Rogers L, Barani I, Chamberlain M, et al. Meningiomas: knowledge base, treatment outcomes, and uncertainties. A RANO review. *J Neurosurg*. 2015;122(1):4–23.
8. Fathi AR, Roelcke U. Meningioma. *Curr Neurol Neurosci Rep*. 2013;13(4):337.

9. Simpson D. The recurrence of intracranial meningiomas after surgical treatment. *J Neurol Neurosurg Psychiatry.* 1957;20(1):22–39.
10. Pollock BE, Stafford SL, Link MJ. Gamma knife radiosurgery for skull base meningiomas. *Neurosurg Clin N Am.* 2000;11(4):659–666.
11. Anderson SW, Ryken TC. Intracranial tumors. In: Morgan JE, Ricker JH, eds. *Textbook of Clinical Neuropsychology.* New York, NY: Taylor & Francis; 2008.
12. Hendrix P, Hans E, Griessenauer CJ, et al. Neurocognitive status in patients with newly diagnosed brain tumors in good neurological condition: the impact of tumor type, volume, and location. *Clin Neurol Neurosurg.* 2017;156: 55–62.
13. van Kessel E, Baumfalk AE, van Zandvoort MJE, et al. Tumor-related neurocognitive dysfunction in patients with diffuse glioma: a systematic review of neurocognitive functioning prior to anti-tumor treatment. *J Neurooncol.* 2017;134:9–18.
14. Cochereau J, Herbet G, Duffau H. Patients with incidental WHO grade II glioma frequently suffer from neuropsychological disturbances. *Acta Neurochir.* 2016;158: 305–312.
15. Froklage FE, Oosterbaan LJ, Sizoo EM, et al. Central neurotoxicity of standard treatment in patients with newly-diagnosed high grade glioma: a prospective longitudinal study. *J Neurooncol.* 2014;116:387–394.
16. Johnson DR, Sawyer AM, Meyers CA, et al. Early measures of cognitive function predict survival in patients with newly diagnosed glioblastoma. *Neurooncology.* 2012; 14(6):808–816.
17. Meskal I, Gehring K, Rutten GM, et al. Cognitive functioning in meningioma patients: a systematic review. *J Neurooncol.* 2016;128:195–205.
18. Zweckberger K, Hallek E, Vogt L, et al. Prospective analysis of neuropsychological deficits following resection of benign skull base meningiomas. *J Neurosurg.* 2017; 127(6):1242–1248 [Epub 2017 Feb 10].
19. Abel TJ, Manzel K, Bruss J, et al. The cognitive and behavioral effects of meningioma lesions involving ventromedial prefrontal cortex. *J Neurosurg.* 2016;124(6): 1568–1577.
20. Gerstenecker A, Nabors LB, Menses K, et al. Cognition in patients with newly diagnosed brain metastasis: profiles and implications. *J Neurooncol.* 2014;120:179–185.
21. Saad S, Wang TJ. Neurocognitive deficits after radiation therapy for brain malignancies. *Am J Clin Oncol.* 2015; 38(6):634–640.
22. Wefel JS, Kayl AE, Meyers CA. Neuropsychological dysfunction associated with cancer and cancer therapies: a conceptual review of an emerging target. *Br J Cancer.* 2004;90(9):1691–1696.
23. Ahles TA, Saykin AJ. Candidate mechanisms for chemotherapy-induced cognitive changes. *Nat Rev Cancer.* 2007;7(3):192–201.
24. ElBeltagy M, Mustafa S, Umka J, et al. Fluoxetine improves the memory deficits caused by the chemotherapy agent 5-fluorouracil. *Behav Brain Res.* 2010;208(1):112–117.
25. Aluise CD, Miriyala S, Noel T, et al. 2-Mercaptoethane sulfonate prevents doxorubicin-induced plasma protein oxidation and TNF-alpha release: implications for the reactive oxygen species-mediated mechanisms of chemobrain. *Free Radical Biol Med.* 2011;50(11):1630–1638.
26. Taphoorn MJ, Klein M. Cognitive deficits in adult patients with brain tumours. *Lancet Neurol.* 2004;3(3):159–168.
27. Meyers CA, Hess KR, Yung WK, Levin VA. Cognitive function as a predictor of survival in patients with recurrent malignant glioma. *J Clin Oncol.* 2000;18(3):646–650.
28. Tucha O, Smely C, Preier M, et al. Preoperative and postoperative cognitive functioning in patients with frontal meningiomas. *J Neurosurg.* 2003;98(1):21–31.
29. Butler JM, Rapp SR, Shaw EG. Managing the cognitive effects of brain tumor radiation therapy. *Curr Treat Opt Oncol.* 2006;7(6):517–523.
30. Crossen JR, Garwood D, Glatstein E, Neuwelt EA. Neurobehavioral sequelae of cranial irradiation in adults: a review of radiation-induced encephalopathy. *J Clin Oncol.* 1994;12(3):627–642.
31. Lee AW, Kwong DL, Leung SF, et al. Factors affecting risk of symptomatic temporal lobe necrosis: significance of fractional dose and treatment time. *Int J Radiat Oncol Biol Phys.* 2002;53(1):75–85.
32. Constine LS, Konski A, Ekholm S, McDonald S, Rubin P. Adverse effects of brain irradiation correlated with MR and CT imaging. *Int J Radiat Oncol Biol Phys.* 1988;15(2): 319–330.
33. Armstrong CL, Hunter JV, Ledakis GE, et al. Late cognitive and radiographic changes related to radiotherapy: initial prospective findings. *Neurology.* 2002;59(1):40–48.
34. Torres IJ, Mundt AJ, Sweeney PJ, et al. A longitudinal neuropsychological study of partial brain radiation in adults with brain tumors. *Neurology.* 2003;60(7):1113–1118.
35. Vigliani MC, Sichez N, Poisson M, et al. A prospective study of cognitive functions following conventional radiotherapy for supratentorial gliomas in young adults: 4-year results. *Int J Radiat Oncol Biol Phys.* 1996;35(3):527–533.
36. Brown PD, Buckner JC, Uhm JH, et al. The neurocognitive effects of radiation in adult low-grade glioma patients. *Neurooncology.* 2003;5(3):161–167.
37. Konat GW, Kraszpulski M, James I, et al. Cognitive dysfunction induced by chronic administration of common cancer chemotherapeutics in rats. *Metab Brain Dis.* 2008;23(3):325–333.
38. Ahles TA, Saykin AJ, Furstenberg CT, et al. Neuropsychologic impact of standard-dose systemic chemotherapy in long-term survivors of breast cancer and lymphoma. *J Clin Oncol.* 2002;20(2):485–493.
39. Wefel JS, Lenzi R, Theriault RL, et al. The cognitive sequelae of standard-dose adjuvant chemotherapy in women with breast carcinoma: results of a prospective, randomized, longitudinal trial. *Cancer.* 2004;100(11):2292–2299.
40. Barton DL, Burger K, Novotny PJ, et al. The use of Ginkgo biloba for the prevention of chemotherapy-related cognitive dysfunction in women receiving adjuvant treatment for breast cancer, N00C9. *Support Care Cancer.* 2013; 21(4):1185–1192.

41. Ginos JZ, Cooper AJ, Dhawan V, et al. [13N] cisplatin PET to access pharmokinetics of intra-arterial versus intravenous chemotherapy for malignant brain tumors. *J Nucl Med*. 1987;28(12):1844–1852.
42. Mitsuki S, Diksic M, Conway T, et al. Pharmacokinetics of 11C-labelled BCNU and SarCNU in gliomas studied by PET. *J Neurooncol*. 1991;10(1):47–55.
43. Gangloff A, Hsueh WA, Kesner AL, et al. Estimation of paclitaxel biodistribution and uptake in human-derived xenografts in vivo with (18)F-fluoropaclitaxel. *J Nucl Med*. 2005;46(11):1866–1871.
44. Damasio H, Tranel D, Anderson SW. Neuropsychological impairments associated with lesions caused by tumor or stroke. *Arch Neurol*. 1990;47(4):397–405.
45. Meyers CA, Geara F, Wong PF, Morrison WH. Neurocognitive effects of therapeutic irradiation for base of skull tumors. *Int J Radiat Oncol Biol Phys*. 2000;46(1):51–55.
46. Folstein MF, Folstein SE, McHugh PR. "Mini-mental state". A practical method for grading the cognitive state of patients for the clinician. *J Psychiatr Res*. 1975;12(3): 189–198.
47. Nasreddine ZS, Phillips NA, Bédirian V, et al. The montreal cognitive assessment, MoCA: a brief screening tool for mild cognitive impairment. *J Am Geriatr Soc*. 2005;53(4): 695–699.
48. Kiernan RJ, Mueller J, Langston JW, Van Dyke C. The neurobehavioral cognitive status examination: a brief but differentiated approach to cognitive assessment. *Ann Intern Med*. 1987;107(4):481–485.
49. Prigatano GP, Amin K, Rosenstein L. *Administration and Scoring Manual for the BNI Screen for Higher Cerebral Functions*. Phoenix, AZ: Barrow Neuropsychological Institute; 1995.
50. Meyers CA, Wefel JS. The use of the mini-mental state examination to assess cognitive functioning in cancer trials: No ifs, ands, buts, or sensitivity. *J Clin Oncol*. 2003; 21(19):3557–3558.
51. Påhlson A, Ek L, Ahlström G, Smits A. Pitfalls in the assessment of disability in individuals with low-grade gliomas. *J Neurooncol*. 2003;65(2):149–158.
52. Beck A, Steer R, Brown G. *Beck Depression Inventory-II*. 1996: 12–15. San Antonio.
53. Beck AT, Steer RA. Manual for the Beck anxiety inventory. *Behav Res Ther*. 1990;37:25–74.
54. Kroenke K, Spitzer RL, Williams JBW. The PHQ-9: validity of a brief depression severity measure. *J Gen Intern Med*. 2001;16(9):606–613.
55. Spitzer RL, Kroenke K, Williams JBW, Löwe B. A brief measure for assessing generalized anxiety disorder: the GAD-7. *Arch Intern Med*. 2006;166(10):1092–1097.
56. Yesavage JA, Brink TL, Rose TL, et al. Development and validation of a geriatric depression screening scale: a preliminary report. *J Psychiatr Res*. 1982;17(1):37–49.
57. Sheikh JI, Yesavage JA. Geriatric depression scale (GDS) recent evidence and development of a shorter version. *Clin Gerontol*. 1986;5(1–2):165–173.
58. Lezak MD, Howieson DB, Bigler ED, Tranel D. *Neuropsychological Assessment*. 5th ed. New York, NY: Oxford; 2012.
59. Prigatano GP. *Principles of Neuropsychological Rehabilitation*. New York, NY: Oxford; 1999.
60. Sohlberg MM, Mateer CA. *Cognitive Rehabilitation: An Integrative Neuropsychological Approach*. New York, NY: Guilford; 2001.
61. Bergo E, Lombardi G, Pambuku A, et al. Cognitive rehabilitation in patients with gliomas and other brain tumors: state of the art. *Biomed Res Int*. 2016:2016.
62. Gehring K, Sitskoorn MM, Gundy CM, et al. Cognitive rehabilitation in patients with gliomas: a randomized, controlled trial. *J Clin Oncol*. 2009;27(22):3712–3722.
63. Sacks-Zimmerman A, Duggal D, Liberta T. Cognitive remediation therapy for brain tumor survivors with cognitive deficits. *Cureus*. 2015;7(10):e350.
64. Maschio M, Dinapoli L, Fabi A, Giannarelli D, Cantelmi T. Cognitive rehabilitation training in patients with brain tumor-related epilepsy and cognitive deficits: a pilot study. *J Neurooncol*. 2015;125(2):419–426.
65. Kennedy DD, Tucker KL, Ladas ED, et al. Low antioxidant vitamin intakes are associated with increases in adverse effects of chemotherapy in children with acute lymphoblastic leukemia. *Am J Clin Nutr*. 2004;79(6):1029–1036.
66. Wefel JS, Kesler SR, Noll KR, Schagen SB. Clinical characteristics, pathophysiology, and management of noncentral nervous system cancer-related cognitive impairment in adults. *Cancer J Clin*. 2015;65(2):123–138.
67. Nada SE, Shah ZA. Preconditioning with Ginkgo biloba (EGb 761(r)) provides neuroprotection through HO1 and CRMP2. *Neurobiol Dis*. 2012;46(1):180–189.
68. Horsfield SA, Rosse RB, Tomasino V, et al. Fluoxetine's effects on cognitive performance in patients with traumatic brain injury. *Int J Psychiatry Med*. 2002;32(4):337–344.
69. Kodama M, Fujioka T, Duman RS. Chronic olanzapine or fluoxetine administration increases cell proliferation in the hippocampus and prefrontal cortex of adult rat. *Biol Psychiatry*. 2004;56(8):570–580.
70. Song L, Che W, Min-Wei W, et al. Impairment of the spatial learning and memory induced by learned helplessness and chronic mild stress. *Pharmacol Biochem Behav*. 2006;83(2):186–193.
71. Druce I, Williams C, Baggoo C, Keely E, Malcolm J. A comparison of patient and health-care professional views when assessing quality of information on pituitary adenoma available on the internet. *Endocr Pract*. 2017 (aop):EP171892.OR.
72. Piil K, Jakobsen J, Juhler M, Jarden M. The feasibility of a brain tumour website. *Eur J Oncol Nurs*. 2015;19(6): 686–693.

73. Vargo M. Brain tumor rehabilitation. *Am J Phys Med Rehabil.* 2011;90(Suppl. 5).
74. Kubler-Ross E. *On Death and Dying*. Vol. 1. 1969.
75. Langbecker D, Janda M. Systematic review of interventions to improve the provision of information for adults with primary brain tumors and their caregivers. *Front Oncol.* 2015;5.
76. Sterckx W, Coolbrandt A, Clement P, et al. Living with a high-grade glioma: a qualitative study of patients' experiences and care needs. *Eur J Oncol Nurs.* 2015;19(4): 383–390.
77. Lobb EA, Halkett GKB, Nowak AK. Patient and caregiver perceptions of communication of prognosis in high grade glioma. *J Neurooncol.* 2011;104(1):315–322.

CHAPTER 7

Communication and Swallowing Impairments in Brain Cancer

MARILYN FROST RUBENSTEIN, MA, CCC-SLP • BRITTANY SCHENKE-REILLY, MA, CCC-SLP, CBIS

DYSPHAGIA IN PERSONS WITH BRAIN CANCER

Swallowing is a complex process which involves cortical and subcortical mediation of motor and sensory fibers. Dysphagia, or swallowing impairment, is a variable but not uncommon symptom in patients with brain tumors.[1–3] The cognitive and sensory-motor impairments that accompany brain tumors, whether pre- or post-treatment, have been shown to have a negative impact on swallowing function.[1] Dysfunction may also occur due to the side effects of radiation, including tissue fibrosis, lymphedema, pain, and xerostomia. Cognitive impairment, a risk factor for dysphagia, may be present as a primary result of the tumor, post-surgical brain edema, or due to the side effects of chemotherapy. Complications of dysphagia include malnutrition, dehydration, and aspiration pneumonia. Dysphagia also has implications for reduced quality of life.

To understand the swallowing deficits that often accompany brain tumor, it is important to have insight into how the normal swallow works. The functional anatomy and physiology involved in swallowing may be represented in four stages which include (1) the anticipatory/pre-oral phase, (2) the oral phase, (3) pharyngeal phase, and (4) esophageal phase. Each phase relies on varying degrees of cognitive, sensory, and motor function. In the anticipatory or pre-oral stage, there must be adequate attention focused on the task of eating or drinking. Cognitive awareness of the food or drink within the environment also excites saliva production. Cranial nerves are activated which will assist in deglutition once food or liquid is introduced into the mouth. During the oral stage, the muscles of the lips, tongue, cheeks, and jaw must effectively accept and remove food from the utensil, as well as be able to move food laterally and medially to facilitate mastication and cohesive bolus formation. The labial and lingual muscles must maintain the food or liquid bolus within the oral cavity both anteriorly and posteriorly until it is ready for transit. Anterior to posterior transit of the bolus is then facilitated in the oral stage by intact lingual and buccal muscles. During the oral phase, the airway remains open and nasal breathing is maintained until the pharyngeal stage begins. Under normal circumstances, the pharyngeal swallow is triggered reflexively when the bolus head passes the line of the mandible (as seen in lateral view radiographically).[4] Once the pharyngeal phase is initiated, velopharyngeal closure must occur to prevent nasal regurgitation and timely closure of the laryngeal vestibule must occur to ensure effective airway protection. Retraction of the base of tongue, hyolaryngeal elevation and anterior movement, epiglottic retroflexion, pharyngeal wall contraction, as well as relaxation and opening of the upper esophageal sphincter (UES) effect pressure on the bolus, propelling it into the cervical esophagus. Adequate timing and duration of the UES opening allows the bolus to clear from the hypopharynx at which time breathing may resume via the mouth or nasal passages.

Assessment of swallowing function may be initiated via a clinical swallowing evaluation (CSE). This typically involves a cranial nerve assessment focused on CN V, VII, IX, X, and XII which play a significant role in oral and pharyngeal swallow function. The CSE will also note how the patient presents in terms of level of arousal and overall mentation, respiratory status, vocal quality, oral awareness of food/utensil, oral management of the bolus, as well as overt signs suggestive of pharyngeal dysfunction. For example, on a bedside examination, multiple swallows may be indicative of pharyngeal residue; throat clearing, cough, and wet vocal and/or breath sounds may be suggestive of laryngeal penetration or aspiration. When the CSE is not conclusive, an objective instrumental assessment may be indicated. The modified barium swallow study (MBS) and the flexible endoscopic evaluation of swallow (FEES) are both considered gold standard tools for the assessment of oropharyngeal dysphagia. The MBS and FEES are helpful in determining presence, absence, and risk for aspiration. If there is increased risk for aspiration, effectiveness of compensatory swallow strategies can be evaluated. Information can be obtained as to whether positional changes or diet modification may improve airway protection. The MBS and FEES are able to reveal specific aspects of dysfunction that are not evident during the clinical bedside examination. Among other findings, silent aspiration, unilateral pharyngeal weakness, pharyngeal residue, incomplete or absent epiglottic retroflexion, UES dysfunction, and pharyngoesophageal backflow of food or liquids may be suspected, however not definitively identified unless visualized fluoroscopically or endoscopically. Additionally, FEES can provide useful information in regard to secretion management, condition of mucosa, and structure and function of the vocal folds. These objective studies are often essential in directing therapy goals and in determining reliable measures of improvement.

Oral, pharyngeal, and pharyngoesophageal dysphagia can be caused by reduced motor control of muscles and structures, reduced sensation, as well as reduced processing of sensation. Bilateral or unilateral labial, lingual, and buccal weakness can result in poor management of food or liquid in the mouth resulting in oral dysphagia. Drooling may also occur. Spillage of material either out of the mouth anteriorly or prematurely to the oro and hypopharynx can occur from reduced strength and sensation of labial and lingual structures. Reduced buccal strength or sensation can result in pocketing of material in the lateral and anterior sulci. Reduced sensation in the pharynx can cause the pharyngeal swallow reflex to be delayed, thus leaving the airway exposed to penetration or aspiration of food and liquid as the material advances before airway closure is initiated. Weak base of tongue movement, reduced pharyngeal wall contractility, and reduced hyolaryngeal movement can result in significant pharyngeal residue which may be susceptible to entering the airway.

Although dysphagia can occur in individuals with cortical and subcortical lesions, those with brainstem lesions often present with significant dysphagia due to the fact that the central pattern generator for swallowing is located in the medulla.[5] The pons acts as a relay station for sensory nerve impulses from oral, pharyngeal, and laryngeal receptors.[5] The pons contains the nuclei of cranial nerves V (trigeminal) and VII (facial), whereas the medulla houses the nuclei of CN IX-XII. Because of impact to the glossopharyngeal (IX), vagus (X), and hypoglossal nerves (XII), lesions localized to the medulla may result in relatively normal oral function in the setting of a profoundly impaired pharyngeal swallow.[5] Studies also indicate high risk for dysphagia along with its sequela of malnutrition, dehydration, and aspiration following surgery, particularly for posterior fossa tumors in both children and adults.[6,7]

Dysphagia may occur due to the side effects of radiation. Tissue fibrosis, lymphedema, pain, and xerostomia can limit normal movement of the oral, pharyngeal, and laryngeal structures and can impact patients' ability to obtain adequate nutrition and hydration. Providing medications via oral route can also be challenging.[8,9]

Cognitive impairment may be present as a primary result of brain tumor, postsurgical brain edema, or due to the side effects of chemotherapy. Impaired cognition is generally correlated with oral stage dysfunction due to cortical involvement and can result in reduced attention to the feeding process, reduced awareness of food/liquid in the mouth, inadequate mastication and/or oral bolus formation, and inadequate oral control of food or liquid with potential for premature spillage over the base of the tongue. Agnosia, reduced attention, reduced insight into deficits, and overall reduced executive functioning can put patients at risk for inadequate nutrition and hydration and may increase risk for aspiration.[8]

Various rating scales, such as the MD Anderson Dysphagia Inventory (MDADI) and the Swallowing Quality of Life questionnaire (SWAL-QOL), allow for a subjective evaluation of the impact of dysphagia on quality of life for cancer patients.[10] Although there is evidence supporting validity of these rating scales, some researchers have found that the degree to which patients reported swallowing difficulties was not necessarily indicative of the actual level of impairment for patients with primary brain tumors, and thus was not predictive of risk for aspiration or risk for inadequate nutritional intake.[11] These findings highlight the importance of thorough clinical assessment through the use of subjective and objective swallowing evaluations.

Incidence of dysphagia and response to rehabilitation in patients with brain tumor has been found to be similar to that of patients with stroke.[1] In a retrospective study, Park et al. found that swallowing dysfunction was comparable in brain tumor and stroke patients and that lesion location was a determining factor in dysphagia. Dysphagia was noted in 72.5% of patients with brain tumor versus 77.5% of stroke patients, and when lesion location was taken into account, findings supported increased risk for dysphagia in patients with infratentorial lesions (90.5%) versus those with supratentorial lesions (52.6%). Vallecular and pyriform residue was a more frequent finding in patients with infratentorial lesions as was lower scores on the ASHA NOMS rating scale. More restrictive diet consistencies and higher supervision levels were also indicated for patients with infratentorial lesions.[1]

Evidence suggests that rehabilitation efforts comparable to those provided for stroke patients will benefit brain tumor patients as well.[12] There is expectation of some initial spontaneous recovery after medical management followed by the benefit of rehabilitative services lasting anywhere from several weeks to several months. Patients with tumors of a progressive nature or frequent recurrence (e.g., glioblastomas) may warrant a greater focus on maximizing independence through the use of compensatory techniques; however, improvement in productivity and quality of life as a result of therapy may occur despite the patient's poor prognosis.[12] Repeat objective studies may be indicated in keeping with disease progression and recommendation for alternative means of nutrition, hydration, and medications may warrant either placement of nasogastric or percutaneous gastrostomy tube. Palliative or hospice considerations may be appropriate and will impact recommendations for diet consistencies as well as oral versus nonoral means.

Dysphagia, especially in the acute stages, can often be remediated through the use of compensatory strategies and/or modifications to diet consistency. Depending on the specific deficit, risk for aspiration can often be reduced with postural changes such as chin tuck positioning or head rotation. Maneuvers can be employed to improve airway protection, reduce pharyngeal residue, or increase extent and duration of UES opening (see Fig. 7.1). Safety and efficiency of swallow can also be improved with the use of thickened liquids or modified food textures such as purees. Although compensatory techniques are often effective in managing immediate concerns, actual rehabilitation of the swallow may be more effectively achieved through active exercise. Traditionally, dysphagia therapy has focused on strength building, which may be appropriate if weakness is the cause of the disordered swallow pattern. If components of apraxia or spasticity exist, then a focus solely on strength building will be a misguided approach. Evidence-based practice suggests that rehabilitation of the swallow may be most effective if it follows the principles of exercise science with intensity and specificity of task designed to reach functional goals.[13,14] In much the same way a physical therapist may work with a patient to improve their mobility, building coordination, speed, and endurance to facilitate functional motor movement in swallowing, which may be as important as building strength.

Leading researchers in the field of speech pathology have questioned whether many commonly used dysphagia exercises currently have an adequate evidence base to support long-term efficacy. In a critique of the literature, Langmore and Pisegna[15] found that one out of five "swallow exercises" and two out of four "nonswallow exercises" had evidence of long-term efficacy for treatment of dysphagia. According to the critique, adequate evidence existed only for the Mendelsohn maneuver, the Shaker head-lift exercise, and expiratory muscle strength training. Swallow and nonswallow exercises may be further defined as maneuvers (which incorporate active swallowing) versus exercises (which do not) (Fig. 7.1). Some techniques have both compensatory and rehabilitative value. The supraglottic and super-supraglottic maneuvers can be used during oral intake to prevent aspiration and can also be used as part of an exercise regimen to produce lasting improvement in airway protection.[16]

The principles of exercise science suggest that the reacquisition of a functional swallow should include three essential components of motor learning: practice in the specific task, progressively increasing difficulty, and the inclusion of feedback.[14,17] Whether visual, verbal, or tactile, and additionally whether it is intrinsic or extrinsic, feedback is necessary to promote attempts at correction on repeated trials. Neuromuscular electrical stimulation (NMES) is often employed to improve oral, pharyngeal, and laryngeal responses during intensive and repetitive swallowing drills. Therapy incorporating this modality typically meets the motor learning requirements of overload and specificity. Recent studies show significant gains in swallowing during therapy with NMES, although evidence supporting efficacy of NMES versus traditional therapy or other techniques alone continues to be mixed.[18]

The McNeill Dysphagia Therapy Program offers skill-based training protocols that incorporate the concepts of task specificity and task challenge.[19,20] There is increasing support for the use of a feedback modality such as surface electromyography (sEMG) in conjunction with targeted skill-based training in order to achieve functional gains in swallowing.[21] It should be noted that newer NMES devices do in fact have

Exercise	Intended Purpose	Swallow (maneuver)	Nonswallow (exercise)
Supraglottic swallow	Prevents aspiration by volitional airway closure at the level of the vocal folds prior to and during the swallow; followed by cough to clear any penetrated material	✓	
Super-supraglottic swallow	Prevents aspiration by promoting anterior movement of the arytenoids and closure of the laryngeal vestibule before and during the swallow	✓	
Mendelsson maneuver	Maximizes laryngeal elevation to increase degree and duration of the UES opening	✓	
Effortful swallow	Improves tongue base retraction to promote bolus clearance	✓	
Shaker exercise	Increases anterior and superior hyolaryngeal excursion for improved UES opening		✓
Masako or Tongue hold	Increases movement and strength of the posterior pharyngeal wall for effective bolus propulsion and clearance		✓

FIG. 7.1 Dysphagia exercises/maneuvers. *UES*, upper esophageal sphincter.

integrated sEMG capabilities. Ongoing research is needed to develop more efficacious therapy techniques. Speech pathologists, in collaboration with multidisciplinary teams, must incorporate current evidence with their clinical expertise in order to develop individualized plans of care that take into consideration patient care needs and values. The specific physiologic impairments of the patient and goals of care should dictate the particular swallowing interventions provided.

MOTOR-SPEECH IMPAIRMENTS IN PERSONS WITH BRAIN CANCER

Speech is comprised of the particular articulatory movements required to produce intelligible phonemes, or individual sounds, as well as the subsystems which allow for each sound to be created. To produce an intelligible sound, the patient must first be able to achieve adequate respiratory support and coordination by inhaling and exhaling with sufficient tidal volume. The patient must then be able to plan and execute the movements of muscles associated with speech articulators (i.e., lips, tongue, jaw, cheeks, velum). Injury secondary to brain tumors, site dependent, as well as the medical treatment of brain tumors may result in two forms of speech disorders: acquired apraxia of speech (AOS) and dysarthria.

AOS is a "neurologic speech disorder that reflects an impaired capacity to plan or program sensorimotor commands necessary for directing movements that result in phonetically and prosodically normal speech."[22] Site of lesion for AOS typically involves the motor cortex and supplementary motor area.[33] It is not caused by weakness, rather the inability to effectively plan and execute motor movement.

Dysarthria is a motor speech disorder wherein a patient's articulatory muscles are too weak or have been surgically removed resulting in the inability to produce normal speech. Conditions causing dysarthria include the atrophy, fibrosis, edema, surgical removal, and reduced sensation of musculature involving the lips, tongue, jaw, cheeks, and velum. Dysarthria could also be caused by medications which act on the "central nervous system, such as narcotics, phenytoin, or carbamazepine."[23] There are seven different types of dysarthria (see Fig. 7.2).

Both AOS and dysarthria impact a patient's ability to communicate effectively, which may negatively influence patient safety and quality of life. Reduced speech intelligibility minimizes the response acuity necessary for relaying important information between patient and caregiver (i.e., pain, personal history). It also impacts the patient's quality of life (i.e., social interaction, attitude toward engaging in therapy). The speech-language pathologist will assess for AOS and dysarthria utilizing both a formal and informal evaluation to create a personalized plan of care and provide education to both the patient and patient's family.[33]

Classification	Site of Lesion	Symptoms
Spastic	UMN	Spasticity
Flaccid	LMN	Weakness
Ataxic	Cerebellum	Incoordination
Hyperkinetic	Basal ganglia	Involuntary movements
Hypokinetic	Basal ganglia	Rigidity and reduced muscle movement
Mixed	Two or more sites	Two or more symptoms
Unilateral UMN	UMN	Weakness, incoordination, spasticity

FIG. 7.2 Types of dysarthria. *UMN*, Upper Motor Neuron; *LMN*, Lower Motor Neuron.

Causation of AOS and dysarthria is the primary indicator of treatment and prognosis. Individual plans of care with be tailored to restorative or supportive outcome measures dependent upon whether the speech disorder was caused by a change in tissue integrity or the removal of tissue. Current practice utilizes oral motor exercises (OMEs) as a restorative means to treat atrophy resulting in slurred or imprecise articulation. Research has provided evidence that OMEs do increase muscular strength when compared with those who did not do the exercises.[24–27] However, there is ongoing criticism of OMEs, specifically detraining effects post discontinuation and that "nonspeech OMEs often do not adhere to accepted principles of muscle training."[28–30] OMEs are comprised of the following movements, either against resistance or in sets of repetitions: buccal, labial retraction/protrusion, labial lateralization, cheek puff, alternating cheek puff, lip press, lingual excursion, lingual lateralization, lingual elevation/depression, lingual-palatal sweep. Ultimately, greater research into strength training of particular orofacial musculature is needed.

Tactile-kinesthetic speech motor treatment [e.g., prompts for reconstructive oral muscular phonetic targets (PROMPT)] is a current practice utilized to treat motor planning disorders resulting in AOS. Research is finding positive outcomes for patients who utilized PROMPT for improving "speech movements in utterances of varying linguistic complexity."[31] However, limited research has been completed with patients specifically diagnosed with brain tumor.

A supportive therapeutic approach will be taken during an inpatient rehabilitation stay if permanent damage is incurred as the result of surgery or nerve impingement from a nonoperative tumor left intact.[33] Supportive approaches include augmentative and alternative communication (AAC) devices (i.e., communication boards, tablets, computers). The inpatient speech-language pathologist's role is to assess the patient's ability to utilize a simple communication board and create an appropriate and functional board tailored to the individual while providing training for functional use. Simple boards are often comprised of basic elements, highlighting basic wants and needs (i.e., pain, site of pain, bathroom, hunger/thirst, etc.). If functional speech cannot be improved, outpatient therapy may address high-tech augmentative devices to facilitate communication.[33] Communication boards can be effective in conveying simple, basic needs; however, they are often limited as to what can be expressed and in the timeliness of expression.

LANGUAGE IMPAIRMENTS IN PERSONS WITH BRAIN CANCER

Language is comprised of both the comprehension and expression of ideas through vocalization, writing, gesture, and if necessary, by utilizing AAC devices.[33] To successfully communicate an idea, a patient must complete a multitude of steps in a fraction of a second. First, the patient must be able to receive the message through auditory, visual, or tactile stimuli. This requires the ability to attend to the stimuli, hear, see, or feel the stimuli, and remember the stimuli. That same patient must encode the meaning of the stimuli, and then decode an appropriate response. To deliver a response, the patient must be physically able to complete one or more of the following tasks: innervate the muscles responsible for breathing, producing voice, moving articulators, holding a writing utensil, and/or moving his or her arms, eyes, and head for gestural purposes. Injury secondary to brain tumors, as well as the medical treatment of brain tumors may result in neoplastic aphasia. Research into neoplastic aphasia has not been widely published as compared with aphasia secondary to stroke and, although there are some similarities, there are important differences to consider.

Aphasia, although it impedes complete understanding or conveyance of a message, does not result in the loss of intelligence. Research has found that approximately "30%–50% of patients with primary brain tumors experience aphasia."[32] There are eight different

Type of Aphasia	Comprehension	Spontaneous Speech	Naming	Repetition
Anomic	Good	Fluent with paraphasia	Poor	Good
Broca's	Good	Nonfluent	Poor	Poor
Transcortical motor	Good	Nonfluent	Poor	Good
Conduction	Good	Fluent with paraphasia	Poor	Poor
Wernicke's	Poor	Fluent with paraphasia	Poor	Good
Transcortical Sensory	Poor	Fluent with paraphasia	Poor	Poor
Global	Poor	Nonfluent	Poor	Good

FIG. 7.3 Types of aphasia.

types of aphasia (see Fig. 7.3). Diagnosis is typically site dependent and not always static, especially when secondary to brain tumors. Subtle changes in pressure due to edema or tumor movement, and the resection or growth of the tumor, can change presenting symptoms.

Typically, a brain tumor affecting the posterior-superior temporal lobe, arcuate fasciculus, and supramarginal gyrus will present with a receptive aphasia.[33] Symptoms include varying degrees of difficulty understanding verbal, written, or visual language.[33] This impacts a patient's quality of life and safety by reducing his or her ability to understand medical recommendations, follow safety precautions, and engage with family or friends. Typically, a brain tumor affecting the posterior-inferior frontal lobe, inferior parietal lobe, and angular gyrus will present with expressive aphasia.[33] Symptoms include varying degrees of anomia, paraphasias, jargon, and neologisms.[33] Expressive aphasia can be fluent or nonfluent and impacts a patient's ability to request help, provide reliable information, articulate pain, and engage with family, friends, or support groups. The most common neoplastic aphasia is anomic aphasia and is typically mild as compared with chronic poststroke aphasia.[32,34] In a recent study of glioma patients, Banerjee et al. [35] utilized voxel-based lesion-symptom mapping to identify correlation between site of lesion and language performance. Banerjee et al.[35] found that "observed associations with left middle and superior temporal gyri including Wernicke's area were consistent with [previous studies associating areas of comprehension with such structural anatomy."[35] Expressive language, however, was "associated with largely independent brain regions, suggesting that expressive language abilities may be quite task dependent and thus much more distributed within the brain."[35] Additionally, the study noted that unlike receptive deficits relating to those areas known to be associated with comprehension (i.e., Wernicke's), expressive language deficits were within the temporal lobe, but "did not include Broca's area [...] suggesting that the etiology of expressive language deficits in glioma patients may be more commonly due to difficulty with category-specific semantic organization and semantic knowledge [...] rather than difficulty with strategic word retrieval."[35]

The speech-language pathologist will assess a patient's ability to communicate through informal and formal evaluation utilizing complete assessment batteries or a compilation of subsections. Evaluation should occur preoperatively, intraoperatively, and postoperatively to establish a baseline, minimize postoperative impairment, and monitor function, respectively.[34] Not only is assessment important for creating personalized plans of care, but preoperative and intraoperative assessment has been shown to have "strong predictive value of postoperative language outcomes."[34] There are numerous assessment batteries available to evaluate a patient's degree and form of aphasia, but the most common include, but are not limited to, the following scales: Boston Diagnostic Aphasia Examination-Third Edition (BDAE-3); Boston Naming Test (BNT); Western Aphasia Battery-Revised (WAB-R). In a recent study by Wilson et al.,[36] the WAB-R was used pre- and postoperatively to assess language function in people with brain tumors. The study found that, although the WAB is a "comprehensive and validated aphasia battery that yields" a quantitative score, the naming subsection of the WAB was insensitive to deficits in patients with brain tumors.[36] Instead, they supplemented the naming section from the BNT for evaluation purposes.[36] The WAB-R is also only appropriate for monolingual English-speaking patients.[33] Similarly, the BDAE-3, although comprehensive for examining auditory/reading comprehension and oral/written expression, is limited by number of items used in each subsection for evaluation.[33]

Treatment of neoplastic aphasia should consider both restorative and supportive means depending on a neuro-oncologist's prognosis. The speech-language pathologist will work closely with a multidisciplinary group to provide appropriate services based on functional goals. Counseling should begin at the time of diagnosis to provide compensatory strategies preoperatively and to review the possibilities of persisting symptoms postoperatively. Unlike stroke-related aphasia, neoplastic aphasia typically remediates within 3 months of surgery.[37] However, if a tumor is inoperable or recurrent, symptoms may persist or worsen.[34] In some cases, neuroplasticity begins as the body's response to slow-growing tumor development. Plasticity, in this way, has been observed to shift language sites, such that when tissue and tumor are removed surgically, the patient may not experience expected language impairments at all.[38]

Restorative therapy aims to improve functional communication. Current therapeutic techniques include, but are not limited to, repetition priming treatment; melodic intonation therapy (MIT); semantic feature analysis (SFA); script therapy; and verb network strengthening treatment (VNeST). These modalities are initiated during acute rehabilitation, but are continued in both homecare and outpatient therapy settings.

During repetition priming treatment, the patient is prompted to name semantically related, phonologically related or unrelated pictures to improve word retrieval and comprehension. MIT utilizes neuroplasticity through music and singing to promote language. Patients with nonfluent aphasia and good auditory comprehension may benefit from this technique. Patients will practice functional phrases while changing intonation, voicing, and producing rhythmic tapping. SFA focuses on improving word retrieval in patients with anomia. Patients are trained how to describe features of a particular word they are having difficulty retrieving to self-cue or cue their listener for the word. Similar to SFA, VNeST focuses therapy around a word, in this case verbs. This therapeutic approach asks the patient to correlate people, places, or actions to a verb, which in turn improves the mental network associated with the verb. This approach has been found to generalize across words that may not have been practiced to improve overall word retrieval. However, the literature shows that this modality is only appropriate for patients who can understand the directives and have a baseline expressive language at the single word level through speaking or writing.[39] Current research has shown each of these therapeutic techniques to be beneficial for short-term improvement; however, there is need for research to support long-term improvement.[40–43] Additionally, there is little to no research differentiating the effectiveness of each technique for brain tumor patients versus stroke patients.[40–43]

Functional communication for activities of daily living (ADLs) can also be trained through script therapy. Script training is comprised of repetitive rehearsal of words, phrases, and sentences presented to the patient in the format of a dialog. Recently, Fridriksson et al.[44] found that the benefits of script training only exist when the clinician presents stimuli both auditorily and visually, whereas visual stimuli alone yield little to no improvement. It is important for the clinician to keep this in mind since both visual and auditory deficits may present as either premorbid or comorbid diagnoses.

Conversely, supportive therapy provides patients with compensatory means to overcome symptoms that cannot be remediated. Supportive means may need to be considered depending on type of lesion and prognosis. It is the role of the speech-language pathologist and the therapeutic team to include the patient and the patient's family in discussing realistic expectations and obtainable goals in therapy. Supportive means may include training in writing, gesture, sign language, using communication boards, or computer programs.

There are two types of AAC systems: aided and unaided. Aided systems require the use of a tool, such as a pen, whereas unaided systems work solely on the patient's own body. The speech-language pathologist will evaluate the patient and recommend the least restrictive supportive means. This may change over the course of a patient's therapy and with disease progression. Longitudinal evaluation is essential in continuing to provide for each individual with the most appropriate plan of care.

COGNITIVE-LINGUISTIC IMPAIRMENTS IN PERSONS WITH BRAIN CANCER

In the rehabilitative setting, cognitive status is evaluated along with language function and may have a significant impact on a patient's ability to communicate effectively. Cognitive impairment is widely reported as a common symptom in patients with brain tumor.[45,46] Decline in functioning of cognitive domains may result from the presence of disease, the impact of tumor resection, or from the side effects of radiation and chemotherapy. Impairment in executive functioning and memory impairment appear to be hallmarks of advanced disease in patients with brain tumor, whereas more subtle changes in behavior have been associated with early-stage disease.[47] Comorbidities such as a history of dementia, stroke, or general learning disabilities will be taken into consideration during evaluation and in the process of choosing appropriate therapeutic goals. Speech language pathologists and neuropsychologists are uniquely qualified to address deficits in cognition. The diagnosis and treatment of cognitive aspects of communication (e.g., memory, problem-solving, reasoning and organization, judgment, and insight) along with related aspects of language (e.g., comprehension and expression) is within the scope of practice of speech-language pathologists. While there are areas of overlap between speech pathology and neuropsychology, referrals to neuropsychology often stem from concerns over a patient's emotional and psychologic behavior.[48]

Depending on a patient's previous level of functioning, age, and level of education, a speech language pathologist will employ screening tools along with formal testing to identify areas of cognitive decline that may be amenable to retraining, facilitation, or compensation. The Mini Mental State Examination (MMSE) and the Montreal Cognitive Assessment (MoCA) are often used in whole or in part. Although the MMSE is widely employed, there is research to suggest that the test has relatively low sensitivity for detection of mild cognitive impairment, which is typical in patients with brain tumor, especially in the early stages.[49] While Roalf et al.[50] and Robinson[49] agree that the MoCA has increased sensitivity in detecting cognitive impairment related to Alzheimer's- and Parkinson's-related dementia, Robinson et al.[49] notes that the MoCA has poor detection of cognitive impairments in patients with a wide variety of brain tumor types and stages. Both Robinson[49] and Roalf[50] note that screening tools may be most effective if used in conjunction with other domain specific portions (e.g., verbal fluency, short story recall) of formal tests such as the Boston Diagnostic Aphasia Examination (BDAE) and the Ross Information Processing Assessment (RIPA). As in other areas of rehabilitation, the primary goal of cognitive intervention is to improve skills that allow a patient to participate in ADLs (e.g., bathing, dressing, toileting) and life skills management (IADLs) (e.g., managing finances). The importance of initial and ongoing assessment that is sensitive to cognitive decline in patients with brain tumor may be seen in the findings of Meyers and Hess.[51] In a study of 56 patients with recurrent brain tumor, cognitive function began to decline prior to tumor progression being detected on MRI.[51] Measures of quality of life and ADLs did not show correlation with a decline in cognitive function or tumor progression.[51] These findings suggest that appropriate screening and assessment of cognitive function can provide an early indication of possible tumor growth or recurrence. Results of studies are often confounded by the lack of baseline assessments prior to tumor removal, radiation treatment, or chemotherapy.[47]

Adequate arousal and attention provide a basis for communication and life participation. Memory, problem-solving, reasoning, judgment, and insight are essential components of functional discourse and of effective completion of self-care tasks. Cognitive impairment can often have a negative impact on rehabilitation potential across all therapeutic disciplines, as patients may not be able to attend well to tasks during therapy. Reduced participation, reduced recall of compensatory strategies, and reduced adherence to a prescribed home exercise program may confound prognosis. Additionally, studies have begun to investigate impaired theory of mind in patients with brain tumor.[47] Theory of mind, or the ability to understand the mental and emotional state of others, can have a direct impact on social relationships and quality of life.[47] Ongoing research into the sensitivity of screening and evaluation tools for cognitive decline is needed. Additional focus on areas such as social cognition may have clinical significance due to its impact on quality of life. Improved accuracy in identifying impairments and early detection of changes that may indicate tumor growth will help to direct the multidisciplinary team to more specific and efficacious rehabilitation treatments in the future.

EDUCATION AND COUNSELING FOR PERSONS WITH BRAIN CANCER

The loss of basic functions due to disease process can be devastating to patients and family members as they attempt to adjust to new and difficult realities. Roles and responsibilities of patients and their caregivers invariably change as they attempt to manage functional decline directly relating to the disease process and complicating factors such as anxiety, depression, and pain.[52] In providing education and counseling, understanding the emotional and psychologic impact of impairment on patients and their family members along with their medical and therapeutic needs is paramount for members of the interdisciplinary care team.[52]

Studies involving the needs of patients with brain tumor and their caregivers have indicated that what patients and family members want most from their healthcare team, aside from effective medical treatment, is information.[52,53] Caregivers reported that information from healthcare providers "helped them to make sense of the illness" and aided in developing coping strategies.[52] In educating patients and family members, the concept of *patient-centered care* as defined by the IOM (Institute of Medicine) can be a useful guide: "Providing care that is respectful of and responsive to individual patient preferences, needs, and values, and ensuring that patient values guide all clinical decisions.[54]" The constraints of time as well as language and sociocultural differences can confound the process of delivering information. Effective communication is best achieved with open-ended questions, reiteration of information, and ongoing confirmation that accurate understanding was achieved by all parties.[55]

In regard to swallowing impairments, patients and family members will need to be fully educated about the relative risks and benefits of modified diets and oral versus nonoral means of nutrition and hydration; to be fully aware of the caregiver burden if patient is to accept or reject specific recommendations for feeding; and to understand the potential impact of decisions on quality of life. Well-informed decision-making by patients and family members, even in some instances when it goes against clinical recommendations, should be respectfully honored by the healthcare team.

Impairments in communication and cognition place an extra burden on family members and healthcare providers to ensure that patient concerns and wishes are being met. Within the interdisciplinary team, speech pathologists are uniquely qualified to support effective communication between patients, caregivers, and interdisciplinary team members. With an in-depth knowledge of how to facilitate communication in persons who have language and speech impairment, speech pathologists can be instrumental in maximizing communication not only in support of a patient's daily living activities but also in support of their involvement in the medical decision-making process, including end-of-life considerations.[56]

CONCLUSION

Ongoing research is fundamental to maximizing therapy outcomes and improving quality of life in the care of persons with brain tumors. Research correlating many of the traditional therapeutic approaches to successful outcomes for persons with brain tumors is lacking compared with that available for survivors of strokes. Future research should focus on the efficacy of known treatment as it relates to the brain tumor population. What has been concluded through current research is the necessity of a multidisciplinary approach during treatment. Persons with brain tumors benefit from both supportive and restorative therapy, in conjunction with continuing education and counseling for themselves and their families.

REFERENCES

1. Park DH, Chun MH, Lee SJ, Song YB. Comparison of swallowing functions between brain tumor and stroke patients. *Ann Rehabil Med.* 2013;37(5):633–641.
2. Jennings KS, Siroky MS, Jackson CG. Swallowing problems after excision of tumors of the skull base: diagnosis and management in 12 patients. *Dysphagia.* 1992;7:40–44.
3. Weisling MW, Brady S, Nickell M, Statkus D, Escobar N. Dysphagia outcomes in patients with brain tumors undergoing inpatient rehabilitation. *Dysphagia.* 2003;18:203–210.
4. Logemann JA. *Evaluation and Treatment of Swallowing Disorders.* 1998:31–32.
5. Daniels SK, Pathak S, Mukhi SV, Stach CB, Morgan RO, Anderson JA. The relationship between lesion localization and dysphagia in acute stroke. *Dysphagia.* 2017;32:777–784.
6. Wadhwa R, Toms J, Chittiboina P, et al. Dysphagia following posterior fossa surgery in adults. *World Neurosurg.* 2014;82(5):822–827.
7. Lee WH, Oh BM, Seo HG, et al. One year outcome of postoperative swallowing impairment in pediatric patients with posterior fossa brain tumor. *J Neurooncol.* 2016;127(1):73–81.
8. Raber-Durlacher JE, Brennan MT, Verdonck-de Leeuw IM, et al. *Support Care Cancer.* 2012;20:433–443.
9. (a) Burger PC, Mahley MS, Dudka L, Vogel FS. The morphologic effects of radiation administered therapeutically for intracranial gliomas: a postmortem study of 25 cases. *Cancer.* 1979;44;

   (b) Rinkel RN, Verdonck-de Leeuw IM, Langendijk JA, et al. The psychometric and clinical validity of the SWAL-QOL questionnaire in evaluating swallow problems experienced by patients with oral and oropharyngeal cancer. *Oral Oncol.* 2009;45:e67–e71.

10. Rinkel R, Verdonck-de Leeuw I, Langendijk J. The psychometric and clinical validity of the SWAL-QOL questionnaire in evaluating swallow problems experienced by patients with oral and oropharyngeal cancer. *Oral Oncol.* 2009;45:e67–e71.
11. Newton HB, Newton C, Pearl D, Davidson T. Swallowing assessment in primary brain tumor patients with dysphagia. *Neurology.* 1994;44:1927–1932.
12. Vargo M. Brain tumor rehabilitation. *Am J Phys Med Rehabil.* 2011;90(suppl):S50–S62.
13. Burkhead Morgan L. *Exercise-based dysphagia rehabilitation: past, present, and future.* In: *Perspectives of the ASHA Special Interest Groups. SIG 13.* Vol. 2 (Part 1). 2017:36–43.
14. Huckabee M, Macrae P. *Rethinking rehab: skill-based training for swallowing impairment.* In: *Perspectives.* Vol. 23 (SIG 13). 2014:46–53.
15. (a) Langmore SE, Pisegna JM. Efficacy of exercises to rehabilitate dysphagia: a critique of the literature. *Int J Speech-Lang Pathol.* 2015;17(3):222–229;
(b) Steele CM, Bennett JW, Chapman-Jay S, Cliffe Polacco R, Molfenter S, Oshalla M. Electromyography as a biofeedback tool for rehabilitating swallowing muscle function in dysphagia. In: Steele C, ed. *Applications of EMG in Clinical and Sports Medicine.* 2012:311–328 [Chapter 19] InTech Publishing.
16. American Speech Language Hearing Association. *Adult Dysphagia;* 2018. http://www.asha.org/public/speech/swallowing/Swallowing-Disorders-in-Adults/.
17. Steele C, Bennett J, Chapman-Jay S, Polacco R, Molfenter S, Oshalla M. Electromyography as a biogeedback tool for rehabilitating swallow muscle function. In: *Applications of EMB in Clinical and Sports Medicine;* 2012. https://www.intechopen.com/books/applications-of-emg-in-clinical-and-sports-medicine/electromyography-as-a-biofeedback-tool-for-rehabilitating-swallowing-muscle-function.
18. Humbert IA. *Point/counterpoint: electrical stimulation for dysphagia: the argument against electrical stimulation for dysphagia.* In: *SIG 13 Perspectives on Swallowing and Swallowing Disorders (Dysphagia).* Vol. 20. 2011:102–108.
19. Crary MA, Carnaby GD, LaGorio LA, Carvajal PJ. Functional and physiological outcomes from an exercise-based dysphagia therapy: a pilot investigation of the McNeill dysphagia therapy program. *Arch Phys Med Rehabil.* 2012;93(7):1173–1178.
20. Sapienza C, Troche M, Pitts T, Davenport P. Respiratory strength training: concept and intervention outcomes. *Semin Speech Lang.* 2011;32(1):21–30.
21. Wheeler-Hegland KM, Rosenbek JC, Sapienza CM. Submental sEMG and hyoid movement during Mendelsohn maneuver, effortful swallow, and expiratory muscle strength training. *J Speech Lang Hear Res.* 2008;51(5):1072–1087.
22. Duffy J. *Motor Speech Disorders: Substrates, Differential Diagnosis, and Management.* St. Louis, MO: Elsevier; 2013.
23. Shelat A. *Dysarthria.* Medline Plus; 2016. https://medlineplus.gov/ency/article/007470.htm.
24. Lof G, Watson M. A nationwide survey of non-speech oral motor exercise use: implications for evidence-based practice. *Lang Speech Hear Serv Sch.* 2008;39:392–407.
25. Lazarus C, Logemann J, Huang C, Rademaker A. Effects of two types of tongue strengthening exercises in young normals. *Folia Phoniatr Logop.* 2003;55:199–205.
26. Logemann J, Pauloski B, Rademaker A, Colangelo L. Speech and swallowing rehabilitation for head and neck cancer patients. *Oncology.* 1997;5:651–656, 659; discussion 659, 663-664.
27. Robbins J, Gangnon R, Theis S, Kays S, Hewitt A, Hind J. The effects of lingual exercise on swallowing in older adults. *J Am Geriatr Soc.* 2005;9:1483–1489.
28. Burkhead L, Sapienza C, Rosenbek J. Strength-training exercise in dysphagia rehabilitation: principles, procedures, and directions for future research. *Dysphagia.* 2007;22(3):251–265.
29. Cerny F, Sapienza C, Lof G, Robbins J. Muscle training principles and resulting changes to speech and swallowing. In: *Paper Presented at: Annual Convention of the American Speech-language-hearing Association Boston, MA.* 2007.
30. Clark H. Clinical decision making and oral motor treatments. *ASHA Lead.* 2005:8–35.
31. Bose A, Square PA, Schlosser R, van Lieshout P. Effects of PROMPT therapy on speech motor function in a person with aphasia and apraxia of speech. *Aphasiology.* 2001;15(8):767–785.
32. Davie G, Hutcheson K, Barringer D, Weinbers J, Lewin J. Aphasia in patients after brain tumour resection. *Aphasiology.* 2009;9:1196–1206.
33. Papathanasiou I, Coppens P, Potagas C. *Aphasia and Related Neurogenic Communication Disorders.* Jones & Bartlett Learning, LLC, An Ascend Learning Company; 2013.
34. Shafi N, Carozza L. Treating cancer-related aphasia. *ASHA Lead.* 2012.
35. Banerjee P, Leu K, Harris R, et al. Association between lesion location and language function in adult glioma using voxel-based lesion-symptom mapping. *NeuroImage Clin.* 2015;9:617–624.
36. Wilson S, Lam D, Babiak M, et al. Transient aphasias after left hemisphere respective surgery. *J Neurosurg.* 2015;123(3):581–593.
37. Wu A, Witgert M, Lang F, et al. Neurocognitive function before and after surgery for insular gliomas. *J Neurosurg.* 2011.
38. Plaza M, Gatignol P, Leroy M, Duffau H. Speaking without Broca's area after tumor resection. *Neurocase.* 2009;4:294–310.
39. Edmonds L. A review of verb network strengthening treatment: theory, methods, results, and clinical implications. *Top Lang Disord.* 2016;2:123–135.
40. Martin N, Fink R, Renvall K, Laine M. Effectiveness of contextual repetition priming treatments for anomia depends on intact access to semantics. *J Int Neuropsychol Soc.* 2006;12(6):853–866.

41. Conklyn D, Novak E, Boissy A, Bethoux F, Chemali K. The effects of modified melodic intonation therapy on nonfluent aphasia: a pilot study. *J Speech Lang Hear Res*. 2012;55: 1463–1471.
42. Boyle M. Semantic feature analysis treatment for anomia in two fluent aphasia syndromes. *Am J Speech Lang Pathol.* 2004;13:236–249.
43. Edmonds L, Nadeau S, Kiran S. Effect of verb network strengthening treatment (VNeST) on lexical retrieval of content words in sentences in persons with aphasia. *Aphasiology*. 2009;23(3):402–424.
44. Fridriksson J, Hubbard H, Hudspeth S, et al. Speech entrainment enables patients with broca's aphasia to produce fluent speech. *Brain*. 2012;12:3815–3829.
45. Gehring K, Aaronson NK, Taphoorn MJ, Sitskoorn MM. Interventions for cognitive deficits in patients with a brain tumor: an update. *Expert Rev Anticancer Ther*. 2010; 10(11):1779–1795. https://doi.org/10.1586/era.10.163.
46. Mukand JA, Blackinton DD, Crincoli M, Lee JJ, Santos B. *Am J Phys Med Rehabil*. 2001;80(5):346–350.
47. Giovagnoli AR. Investigation of cognitive impairments in people with brain tumors. *J Neurooncol*. 2012;108(2): 277–283.
48. Paul-Brown D, Ricker J, American Speech Language Hearing Association. *Evaluating and Treating Communication and Cognitive Disorders: Approaches to Referral and Collaboration for Speech-language Pathology and Clinical Neuropsychology [Technical Report]*; 2003. Available from: www.asha.org/policy.
49. Robinson G, Biggs V, Walker D. Cognitive screening in brain tumors: short but sensitive enough? *Front Oncol.* 2015;5(60). https://doi.org/10.3389/fonc.2015.00060.
50. Roalf D, Moberg P, Xie S, Wolk D, Moelter S, Arnold S. Comparative accuracies of two common screening instruments for classification of alzheimer's disease, mild cognitive impairment, and healthy aging. *Alzheimer's Dementia.* 2012:1–9.
51. Meyers C, Hess K. Multifaceted and points in brain tumor clinical trials: cognitive deterioration precedes MRI progression. *Neurooncology*. 2003;5(2):89–95.
52. Schubart J, Kinzig M, Farce E. Caring for the brain tumor patient: family caregiver burden and unmet needs. *Neurooncology*. 2008:61–72.
53. Hazen RJ, Lazar A, Gennari JH. Assessing patient and caregiver needs and challenges in information and symptom management: a study of primary brain tumors. *AMIA Annu Symp Proc*. 2016:1804–1813.
54. Institute of Medicine. Crossing the Quality Chasm. Wash., D.C: The National Academies Press.
55. Epstein RM, Street RL. The values and value of patient-centered care. *Ann Fam Med*. 2011:100–103.
56. American Speech-Language-Hearing Association. *Scope of Practice in Speech-language Pathology [Scope of Practice]*; 2016. Available from: www.asha.org/policy/.

CHAPTER 8

Spinal Tumors

LISA MARIE RUPPERT, MD

INTRODUCTION

Spinal tumors or their treatments may directly or indirectly cause neurologic impairments that affect the physical, social, vocational, and emotional capabilities of an individual and their caregivers. The available treatment options for these tumors continue to improve and bring with them improved patient survival. This has made it more important than ever for clinicians to be aware of the potential long-term neurologic impact of these potentially devastating disorders.[1]

EPIDEMIOLOGY AND PATHOPHYSIOLOGY

Spinal tumors are classically grouped into three categories, extradural tumors, intradural extramedullary tumors, and intradural intramedullary tumors. These tumors may be primary or secondary to metastatic disease. Primary tumors account for a relatively small percentage of all spinal tumors and generally occupy the intradural spaces, whereas metastatic disease tends to be extradural in nature.[2]

Extradural Tumors

Extradural (epidural) tumors refer to lesions outside of the dura mater, in the vertebral bodies and neural arches (Fig. 8.1). These tumors are more commonly malignant than benign. Primary tumors may arise from osteoblasts, chondrocytes, fibroblasts, and hematopoietic cells. Benign tumors include vertebral hemangiomas, giant cell tumors, osteochondromas, osteoid osteomas, and osteoblastomas. Primary malignant tumors include lymphoma, osteosarcoma, Ewing sarcoma, chondrosarcoma, chordoma, sacrococcygeal teratoma, malignant fibrous histiocytoma, solitary plasmacytoma, and fibrosarcoma.[3]

Metastatic disease is far more common in the extradural space, with up to a 70% prevalence in patients with cancer. Solid tumors such as lung, breast, and prostate cancers are the most common sources of metastases. Renal cell carcinoma, thyroid cancer, and colon cancer are also relatively common. Among hematologic tumors, non-Hodgkin lymphoma is the most common.[3,4] The majority of metastases reaches the spine through hematogenous spread.[4] Direct extension of primary tumors may also occur. For instance, prostate, bladder, and colorectal cancers may become locally aggressive and invade the lumbar or sacral regions of the spine.[5]

Primary and metastatic extradural tumors may be osteolytic, osteoblastic, or mixed in nature. Osteolytic lesions result in bone destruction greater than bone formation, whereas osteoblastic lesions result in bone deposition without breakdown of old bone first. Osteolytic lesions are more common in adults and seen with

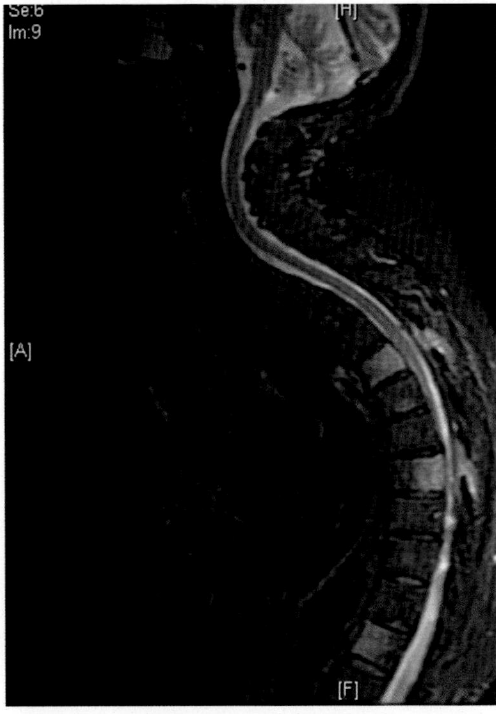

FIG. 8.1 Lung cancer with extradural metastases.

breast, lung, and thyroid cancers. Prostate and bladder cancers and carcinoid tumors are typically osteoblastic in nature. Mixed lytic/blastic lesions can be seen with lung, breast, cervical, and ovarian cancers.[3]

Both osteolytic and osteoblastic lesions alter normal bone architecture, potentially resulting in deformity or collapse of the affected vertebral body. This deformity or collapse may lead to spinal instability by increasing strain on the support elements of the spine, including muscles, tendons, ligaments, and joint capsules.[5] Spinal instability can result in spinal cord compression from retropulsion of bone fragments into the epidural space.

Extradural lesions may grow into the epidural space, resulting in mechanical injury to the axons and myelin of the spinal cord. Growth into the epidural space may also cause vascular compromise of the spinal arteries and epidural venous plexus, resulting in cord ischemia and/or infarction.[4]

Depending on the underlying malignancy, 2%–5% of patients will develop clinical signs and symptoms of epidural spinal cord compression (ESCC) during the course of their disease. Adults with myeloma and prostate cancer have the highest risk of developing ESCC (7.9% and 7.2%, respectively). In the pediatric population, sarcoma and neuroblastoma are the most common malignancies resulting in ESCC.[4] Symptomatic lesions are most often diagnosed in the thoracic region, presenting as incomplete paraplegia; although cadaveric studies have shown the most common site of tumor burden is in the lumbar spine.[5]

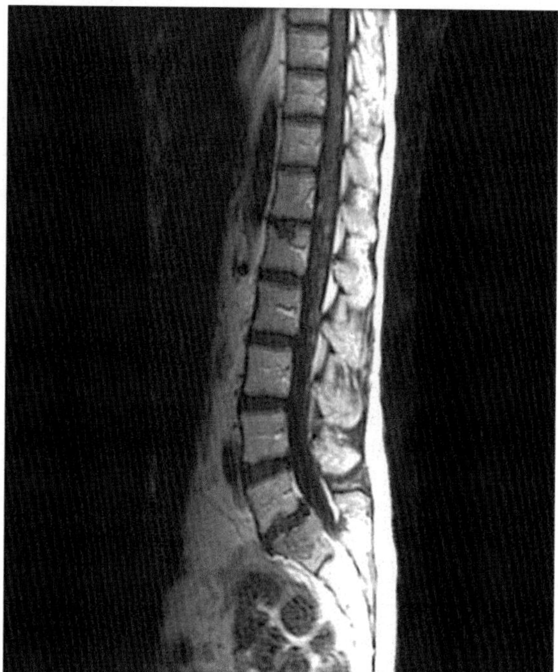

FIG. 8.2 Breast cancer with intradural extramedullary metastases.

Intradural Extramedullary Tumors

Intradural extramedullary tumors (Fig. 8.2) are located within the dura mater but outside the spinal cord parenchyma. These tumors are most commonly benign and can be seen in all regions of the spine. Primary intradural extramedullary tumors arise from peripheral nerves, nerve sheaths, and sympathetic ganglion. Benign tumors include meningioma, schwannoma, neurofibroma, paraganglioma, and ganglioneuroma. Malignant primary tumors include malignant nerve sheath tumors and hemangiopericytoma.[3]

Extramedullary metastases, or leptomeningeal disease (LMD), are a relatively common complication of cancer, occurring in 3%–8% of all patients.[3] Metastatic disease is thought to reach the leptomeninges through hematogenous spread, cerebrospinal fluid (CSF) seeding, or direct extension. CSF seeding can occur spontaneously or as a by-product of surgical intervention. Direct extension can occur along the epineurium or perineurium of spinal nerves, particularly from paravertebral metastases. It can also occur along veins exiting vertebral body bone marrow.[3,6] Glioblastoma, central nervous system (CNS) lymphoma, leukemia, lymphoma, breast cancer, lung cancer, and melanoma are common sources of LMD.[3] The most common site of leptomeningeal involvement is the dorsal aspect of the spinal cord, particularly at the cauda equina.[6]

Similar to extradural lesions, LMD can result in spinal cord compression and vascular compromise. Vascular compromise in this setting can result in ischemia and spinal subarachnoid hemorrhage. The risk of subarachnoid hemorrhage is greatest in patients undergoing treatment with anticoagulants.[3]

Intradural Intramedullary Tumors

Primary intradural intramedullary tumors account for 4%–5% of all primary CNS tumors. They are located within the spinal cord parenchyma and arise from glial cells, neuronal cells, and other connective tissue cells.[3,5] Intramedullary tumors are classified as low, intermediate, or high grade based on cytology.[3] Ependymomas are the most common primary intramedullary tumors in adults and are most often located in the filum terminale and conus medullaris. Astrocytomas are the most common in children and can be located in any region of the spinal cord. Other primary intramedullary tumors include hemangioblastoma, cavernous angioma,

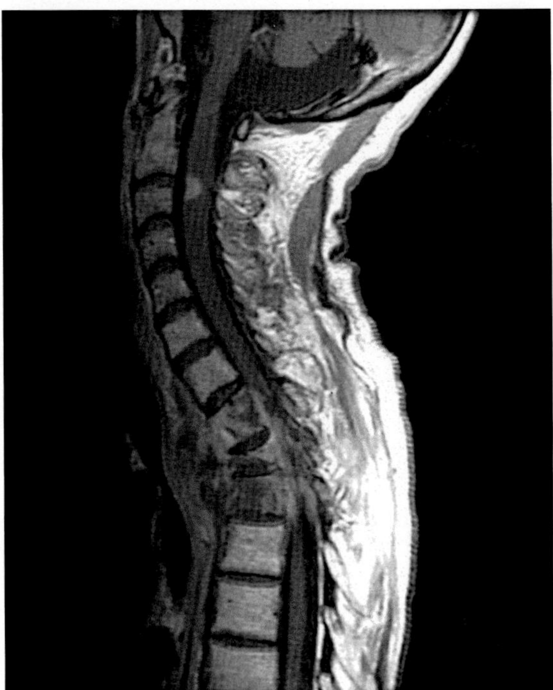

FIG. 8.3 Leiomyosarcoma with intradural intramedullary metastasis.

ganglioglioma, neurocytic tumors, oligodendroglioma, and embryonal neoplasms.[3]

Intramedullary spinal cord metastases usually occur in the setting of extensive metastatic disease and are diagnosed in less than 1% of patients with cancer (Fig. 8.3). Metastatic disease occurs either by hematogenous spread or via the leptomeninges, along nerve roots or through the Virchow-Robin spaces.[4] These lesions can be seen throughout the spinal cord, usually as a solitary lesion. The most common segment involved is the vascular-rich cervical spinal cord.[3]

Lung and breast cancers, melanoma, lymphoma, and renal cell carcinoma can result in intramedullary metastases. Half of all instances are the result of small-cell lung cancer. A majority of patients with intramedullary lesions have concomitant brain metastases and up to 1/4 have known LMD.(HAMMACK) Intramedullary metastases may result in neurologic injury, through direct compression to the surrounding spinal cord and vascular structures.[3]

CLINICAL MANIFESTATIONS

Extradural Tumors

Pain is the most common initial presenting symptom in patients with ESCC (80%–90% of cases) and may precede the development of neurologic symptoms by weeks to months. Individuals with extradural involvement classically describe three types of pain, local, mechanical, and/or radicular pain.[2,5] An individual with epidural involvement may experience one or more of these pain syndromes.

Localized pain, described as a deep "gnawing" or "aching" pain, is thought to be the result of periosteal stretching and inflammation caused by tumor growth. It is often nocturnal in timing and improves with activity and antiinflammatory medications. Percussion or palpation over involved spinous processes may elicit tenderness in individuals with this type of pain.[2,5]

Unlike localized pain, mechanical pain varies with position or activity and is often refractory to antiinflammatory and pain medications. Mechanical pain characteristically occurs with transitional movements or axial loading of the spine. Alternatively, it may be elicited by lying prone or supine, particularly with thoracic spine involvement. This pain is concerning as it is often indicative of impending or established spinal instability. Mechanical pain responds well to stabilization of the spine with bracing or surgical fixation.[2,4,5]

Radicular pain occurs in the setting of nerve root compression either from tumor extension into the neuroforamen or with pathologic fractures that obliterate this space. It is often described as sharp, shooting, or stabbing in nature. With cervical or lumbar lesions, radicular pain is usually unilateral, radiating to the upper or lower extremity, respectively. In the thoracic region, radicular symptoms can be bilateral and are described as a bandlike sensation around the chest or abdomen.[5,7]

Motor weakness is the next most common presenting symptom of epidural cord compression (35%–85% of cases). Similar to traumatic injuries, patterns and distribution of weakness is dependent on the region of cord involvement. Patients with cervical involvement may have a lower motor neuron pattern of weakness in the upper extremities and upper motor neuron pattern in the lower extremities. Thoracic lesions may result in upper motor neuron findings in the lower extremities, with flexor musculature weaker than extensor. Lumbosacral involvement affects the lower extremities in a lower motor neuron pattern.[2,5]

Sensory impairments are rarely the initially reported symptom of epidural cord compression but are usually present at the time of diagnosis. Similar to motor weakness, the distribution of sensory impairments is dependent on the location of nerve root or spinal cord involvement.[2]

Nerve root compression may result in a dermatomal distribution of paresthesias. Compression of the dorsal columns may result in loss of conscious proprioception, vibration and light touch from the ipsilateral body, and information about visceral distension. Individuals may report an ascending pattern of tingling and numbness or a sensation of tightness about the trunk or limb. They may experience ataxia and balance impairments as a result of proprioception loss. Lhermitte's phenomenon, an electric shock sensation that extends into the back and sometimes limbs with changes in neck or head position, can be seen with cervical and upper thoracic dorsal column involvement.[2,4]

Involvement of the lateral spinothalamic tracts results in a loss of pain and temperature perception one or two dermatomes below the level of injury, on the contralateral side of the body. Spinothalamic involvement rarely causes paresthesias.[2]

Autonomic symptoms are unusual as an initial symptom but can be present with epidural cord compression. These symptoms usually correlate with the degree of motor involvement and may include bowel, bladder, and sexual dysfunction, loss of sweating below the level of compression, and orthostatic hypotension.[2,4,5]

Gait and truncal ataxia may occur with compression of the spinocerebellar tracts. Spinocerebellar involvement can be differentiated from cerebellar involvement by the absence of upper extremity ataxia, dysarthria, and nystagmus.[4]

Other clinical findings of epidural cord compression may include the eruption of herpetic zoster at the level of cord involvement, Horner's syndrome (C7-T1 involvement), and neuropathic facial pain (high cervical lesions with involvement of the descending fibers of the trigeminal-thalamic tract).[4]

Intradural Extramedullary Tumors

Patterns of spinal cord injury from extramedullary tumors are similar to those from epidural lesions. Approximately 70%–90% of individuals present with pain as the initial symptoms of cord involvement. This pain is often axial and/or radicular in nature and is worsened in recumbent positions. There is however a higher rate of neurologic impairment with extramedullary involvement. In addition, neurologic impairments may occur in the absence of pain. More than 60% of individuals referred for surgical resection of LMD have some degree of weakness.[3]

Almost all patients with extramedullary cord involvement have some degree of sensory impairments. Bowel, bladder, and sexual dysfunction are also common (30%–80% of cases) and tend to be an early finding. The constellation of symptoms with extramedullary cord compression may resemble those of Brown-Séquard, conus medullaris, or cauda equina injuries.[2]

Intramedullary Tumors

Intramedullary tumors may also present with surprisingly similar symptoms to their epidural counterparts. Pain, the most common initial symptom (30%–85% of cases), is often described as a dull/aching posterior midline pain, paravertebral stiffness/tightness, or radiculopathy. (KIM) Neurologic impairments are also common and typically involve cord segments below the level of tumor involvement. More than 92% of patients with intramedullary tumors have some degree of weakness, 62%–87% sensory deficits and approximately 70% have bowel and/or bladder dysfunction on examination.[2,3]

Similar to extramedullary cord compression, intramedullary lesions may resemble Brown-Séquard, conus medullaris, and cauda equina syndromes. In addition, they may present with central cordlike findings and Horner's syndrome.[2,3]

Spinal Instability

Spinal instability is defined as a loss of spinal integrity as a result of a neoplastic process. Instability is associated with movement-related (mechanical) pain, symptomatic and progressive spinal column deformity, and/or neurologic compromise under a normal physiologic load. Factors considered by treating teams when evaluating the structural stability of the spinal column include presence of mechanical pain, location of the tumor, alignment of involved spinal segments, extent of vertebral body involvement, presence of posterior element involvement, bone lesion quality, and overall bone mineral density.[8]

The presence of multiple contiguous or noncontiguous lesions, loss of intervertebral disc integrity, facet joint arthropathy, prior surgical interventions, and treatments such as radiation therapy and hormonal therapies may also influence the risk for spinal instability. There are various scoring scales available to assess spinal stability in the cancer population. Any concern about potential instability warrants a surgical referral.[2,8]

DIAGNOSIS

Patients with suspected spine or spinal cord tumors should undergo a thorough diagnostic workup. History taking should include inquires about current pain and/

or neurologic symptoms and functional status. It should also include inquires about smoking history, known neurologic injuries, medical comorbidities, environmental or occupational carcinogen exposures, travel history, recent screening examinations, and family history of cancers.[2,5]

Physical examination should include an assessment of strength, sensation, reflexes, autonomic function, and sphincter function. The International Standards for Neurological Classification of Spinal Cord Injury and Autonomic Standards Assessment Form can be used as guides for completing these examinations but not to determine prognosis.[2]

Laboratory testing including a complete blood count, chemistry, and cancer-specific studies such as prostate-specific antigen, breast cancer genes 1 and 2 (BRCA 1 and BRCA2), carcinoembryonic antigen, and serum and urine protein electrophoresis should be completed based on clinical suspicions. Lumbar puncture for CSF analysis can be performed upon completion of neuro-axis imaging for patients with intradural involvement.[2,5]

Diagnostic imaging should be performed. Plain films have long been the mainstay in the initial evaluation of patients with new spine complaints. They are a useful screening test to identify lytic or sclerotic lesions, pathologic fractures, spinal deformities, and large masses. Plain films do however have limitations. Spinal ligament and spinal cord abnormalities cannot be visualized. Also these films may not reveal bony changes until 30%–50% of the vertebral body is involved.[5]

Computerized Tomography (CT) scans provide highly detailed imaging of the osseous anatomy of the spine, degree of tumor involvement, and spinal alignment. The addition of myelography allows for assessment of spaces occupied by neural elements and identification of compressed structures. In addition to CT of the spine, patients with suspected metastatic disease should have CT imaging of the chest, abdomen, and pelvis to establish extent of disease or identify the primary tumor. Angiography can also be incorporated into CT imaging when information about the vascular supply of a tumor is needed, such as prior to surgical interventions.[5]

Magnetic resonance imaging (MRI) is considered the gold standard for assessing spinal involvement. The resolution provided by MR imaging allows for assessment of the soft tissue structures of the spine, including the intervertebral discs, spinal cord, spinal nerve roots, meninges, musculature, and ligaments. MR imaging should include T1- and T2-weighted studies obtained in three planes (axial, sagittal, and coronal) with and without gadolinium contrast. The entire neuro-axis should be imaged when intradural lesions are suspected or diagnosed as concomitant brain lesions are common.[5]

[F]-2-fluoro-2-deoxy-D-glucose positron emission tomography (PET with FDG) is commonly used for whole body detection of metastatic disease and cancer staging. In the spine, PET allows for earlier detection and differentiation of tumor from other processes. Given the limited resolution of PET imaging for anatomic assessment, correlation with CT or MRI imaging is required.[5]

Nuclear scintigraphy (bone scan) is a sensitive method for identifying areas of increased metabolic activity throughout the skeletal system. Bone scans have 62%–89% sensitivity for detection of metastatic disease. However, because nuclear scans detect increased metabolic activity, they are not specific for metastatic lesions, as increased activity may be related to inflammation or infection. Scintigraphy is also limited by poor image resolution requiring correlation with CT or MRI to exclude benign lesions.[5]

Conventional digital subtraction angiography is an important modality as it provides valuable information for decision-making. In patients with highly vascular lesions, such as renal cell, thyroid, angiosarcoma, leiomyosarcoma, hepatocellular, and neuroendocrine tumors, knowledge of the tumor's vascular supply may prove invaluable if surgical intervention is considered. In addition, angiography may permit preoperative embolization to reduce intraoperative blood loss, potentially preventing development of postoperative hematomas and shortening surgical times. Of note, tumor embolization may be considered as an alternative treatment option for patients who are not candidates for surgical intervention.[5]

Biopsy of spinal lesions should be considered in patients without a prior history of cancer, unknown primary tumor, or history of limited stage or "cured" malignancy. If an easily accessible alternative target is identified during workup (i.e., lymphadenopathy, breast lump, lung mass, prostatic nodular), it should be biopsied before treatment decisions are made.[4]

ONCOLOGIC MANAGEMENT

Management of spinal tumors varies according to the stability of the spine, neurologic and functional status, and presence of pain. Treatment options include surgical intervention, radiation therapy, and systemic treatments such as chemotherapy, hormonal manipulation, corticosteroids, and bisphosphonates.

Radiation Therapy

Radiation therapy is a mainstay in treatment for spinal tumors and plays an important role in pain relief, stabilization of neurologic function, and prevention of pathologic fractures.[5] The most common dosing schedule in the United States is 30 Gy in 10 fractions. The goal of dosing is to optimally treat the tumor while minimizing risk for radiation toxicity to the cord. Radiosensitive tumors include myeloma, lymphoma, seminoma, and prostate and breast cancers. Relatively radioresistant tumors include sarcoma and renal cell carcinoma.[2,5]

Spinal stereotactic radiosurgery (SRS) is also being employed as a treatment modality for spinal tumors. SRS is a form of radiation therapy that delivers high-dose precisely targeted radiation therapy to a tumor. It provides treatments in fewer fractions than more traditional forms of radiation therapy. Studies of SRS have suggested favorable outcomes, including halted tumor progression, improved pain, and few adverse effects. Long-term studies on outcomes and adverse effects are ongoing.[4,5]

Unfortunately radiation is not without adverse effects, including gastrointestinal toxicity, mucositis, bone marrow suppression, and radiation-induced myelopathies. Radiation myelopathies albeit rare have been reported with radiation treatment of primary spine/spinal cord tumors, prophylactic radiation for prevention of metastatic disease, and when the spinal cord is included in the field of radiation such as with colorectal cancers.[4,5]

Radiation myelopathies are divided into four subtypes, acute complete radiation myelopathy, lower motor neuron disease, acute transient radiation myelopathy (ATRM), and chronic progressive radiation myelopathy (CPRM). Acute complete radiation myelopathy is rare and presumed to be related to radiation-induced vascular damage resulting in spinal cord ischemia/infarction. Lower motor neuron disease is also rare and presumed to result from anterior horn cell damage.[4,9]

ATRM is the most common. ATRM typically occurs 1–29 months after completion of radiation therapy and is thought to be the result of demyelination of the posterior columns. ATRM is generally associated with radiation to the cervical spine but has been reported in other cord segments. Clinical manifestations include Lhermitte's sign without neurologic changes on examination. Treatment is reassurance as symptoms resolve over weeks to months.[4,9]

CPRM is the most feared radiation myelopathy and occurs in 1%–5% of patients who survive 1 year post treatment. Symptoms can appear 9–15 months post radiation therapy, following a latent period in which the patient is asymptomatic. Clinical onset is usually painless and insidious. Clinical manifestations include ascending weakness, clumsiness, and diminished sensation. Brown Séquard pattern of symptoms has been described. The literature suggests CPRM results in a steady progression of neurologic deficits over the course of weeks to months.[4,9,10]

Diagnosis of CPRM is made via the Pallis criteria, which state that the spinal cord must have been included in the field of radiation therapy, the main neurologic deficit must be consistent with the segment of the cord exposed to radiation, and that metastases or other primary cord lesions have been ruled out.[9]

There is no effective treatment to reverse CPRM. Corticosteroids have been tried with varying results. Anticoagulation and hyperbaric oxygen have occasionally been shown to improve or stabilize symptoms. Bevacizumab has shown anecdotal evidence of benefit. As a result, treatment goals are aimed at alleviating symptoms and maintaining functional status.[4]

Systemic Treatments

Chemotherapy can be considered with lymphomas, neuroblastomas, and germ cell tumors. It can also be used as an adjuvant therapy for metastatic disease from breast and prostate cancers and melanoma. Unfortunately, for most patients, chemotherapy plays a limited role largely because of slow and unpredictable tumor responses and the urgent need to decompress the spinal cord. Spinal metastases may be sensitive to hormonal manipulation, particularly in the setting of breast and prostate cancers.[5,7]

Chemotherapy-induced myelopathy is an exceedingly rare complication most likely to be seen with chemotherapeutic agents administered directly into the CSF, such as methotrexate, cytarabine, and thiotepa. The exact pathogenesis is unknown, but ascending paresthesias, weakness, and sphincter dysfunction may be observed. Lhermitte's phenomenon has been reported after IV administration of cisplatin and is felt to be the result of injury to the dorsal root ganglion. Lhermitte's phenomenon is usually transient, although patients may be left with sensory ataxias after multiple cycles. There is no definitive treatment for chemotherapy-induced myelopathy. Similar to myelopathies from radiation therapy, treatment goals focus on symptom management and function maintenance.[4]

Corticosteroids play a role in the initial treatment for spinal tumors. They provide analgesia for pain, have cytotoxic effects on lymphoma and melanoma, and improve or stabilize neurologic function by reducing tumor and spinal cord edema.[4] Significant variability exists with regard to initial recommended dose and tapering schedule. Reported side effects from corticosteroids include hyperglycemia, increased risk of infection, gastrointestinal irritation, mood disturbances, fluid retention, impaired wound healing, and steroid myopathy.[4,7]

Bisphosphonates, which inhibit osteoclast activity and suppress bone reabsorption associated with spinal metastases, have been proven effective in reducing the risk of pathologic fractures, relieving pain, and reducing malignancy-associated hypercalcemia.[5]

CONCLUSION

As survival rates improve for patients with spinal column and spinal cord involvement, it is important for clinicians to be aware of the potential long-term neurologic impact of these tumors and their treatments.

REFERENCES

1. Kirshblum S, O'Dell MW, Ho C, Barr K. Rehabilitation of persons with central nervous system tumors. *Cancer.* 2001;92(suppl 4):1029–1038.
2. Ruppert LM. Malignant spinal cord compression: adapting conventional rehabilitation approaches. *Phys Med Rehabil Clin N Am.* 2017;28(1):101–114.
3. Kim D, Chang U, Kim S, Bilsky M. *Tumors of the Spine.* 1st ed. Philadephia, PA: Elsevier Health Sciences; 2008.
4. Hammack JE. Spinal cord disease in patients with cancer. *Continuum (Minneap Minn).* 2012;18(2):312–327.
5. Sciubba DM, Petteys RJ, Dekutoski MB, et al. Diagnosis and management of metastatic spine disease. A review. *J Neurosurg Spine.* 2010;13(1):94–108.
6. Clarke JL. Leptomeningeal metastasis from systemic cancer. *Continuum (Minneap Minn).* 2012;18(2):328–342.
7. Raj VS, Lofton L. Rehabilitation and treatment of spinal cord tumors. *J Spinal Cord Med.* 2013;36(1):4–11.
8. Fisher CG, DiPaola CP, Ryken TC, et al. A novel classification system for spinal instability in neoplastic disease: an evidence-based approach and expert consensus from the Spine Oncology Study Group. *Spine.* 2010;35(22):E1221–E1229.
9. Goldwein JW. Radiation myelopathy: a review. *Med Pediatr Oncol.* 1987;15(2):89–95.
10. Schiff D. Spinal cord compression. *Neurol Clin.* 2003;21(1):67–86, viii.

CHAPTER 9

Neurosurgical Management of Spinal Tumors

BLAKE WALKER, MD • DANIEL T. GINAT, MD, MS • R. SHANE TUBBS, MS, PA-C, PHD • MARC D. MOISI, MD, MS

BACKGROUND

Tumors of the spine represent a broad and diverse pathologic process which can present physicians with difficult situations regarding diagnosis and treatment. For the purposes of this chapter, emphasis will be placed on the bony spine and the contents contained within, including meninges, spinal cord, and nerve roots. It is important for physicians to understand the various locations where spinal tumors may arise and the pathologic processes from which they arise. Missed or delayed diagnosis can have a significant impact on quality of life as spinal cord compression is a common cause of pain, loss of mobility, and neurologic deficit.[1]

Tumors are either primary or metastatic. Primary spine tumors arise from the spine or its adjacent tissues (spinal cord or meninges), whereas metastatic tumors arise from distant tissues.[2] Primary tumors of the axial skeleton are rare with an estimated incidence of approximately 2.8–8.5 per 100,000 people per year.[3] Metastatic spinal lesions are a relatively more common entity with approximately 18,000 metastatic lesions alone diagnosed each year; this is not surprising given that 70% of cancer patients have metastatic spinal disease.[4]

It is especially important to recognize symptoms of spinal cord compression because up to 12% of patients with spinal disease will develop symptomatic spinal cord compression; 49% of these patients will have multifocal extradural lesions.[5] With the advent of new surgical approaches and nonsurgical means for managing patients with spinal tumors, it will become increasingly important to be able to identify the early signs and symptoms of spinal lesions and to be able to order the appropriate imaging to aid in expedited diagnosis and treatment. Early signs of disease process should be identified upon patient presentation to clinics or the emergency department, followed by evaluation by orthopedic surgery or neurosurgery. After surgical referral, radiation oncology and medical oncology can make further recommendations at a multidisciplinary tumor board. Rehabilitation services are essential for maximizing postoperative outcomes.

DIAGNOSTICS

There are many diagnostic studies available to assist today's physician with diagnosing a spinal tumor. The physical examination discussed earlier should provide the physician with some guidance as to the first location to image. Care must be taken to not order excessive or unnecessary studies, as patients may not be able to tolerate many examinations.

Plain radiographs are a common imaging study and are frequently ordered in patients with back pain. Unfortunately, the site of pain and structure level of compression do not necessarily correlate.[6] This can present a diagnostic issue if the location of the site of compression is not imaged. In one series, the most frequent plain film requested was the lumbar spine, whereas the most common site of compression was the thoracic spine.[6] Nonetheless, if plain films are to be pursued, the "winking owl sign" (radiolucent area obscuring a pedicle, i.e., absent pedicle sign) is the earliest radiographic sign of an osteolytic metastatic lesion (Fig. 9.1). Other signs of spinal metastasis include vertebral body collapse.[2,6] Plain films have the potential for false-negative results as a tumor must be 1 cm in diameter and there must also be 50% bone mineral loss to be detected; up to 40% of lesions will be undiagnosed.[7]

Computed tomography (CT) scans are another valuable diagnostic tool for the evaluation of patients with suspected spinal pathology. CT scans provide excellent

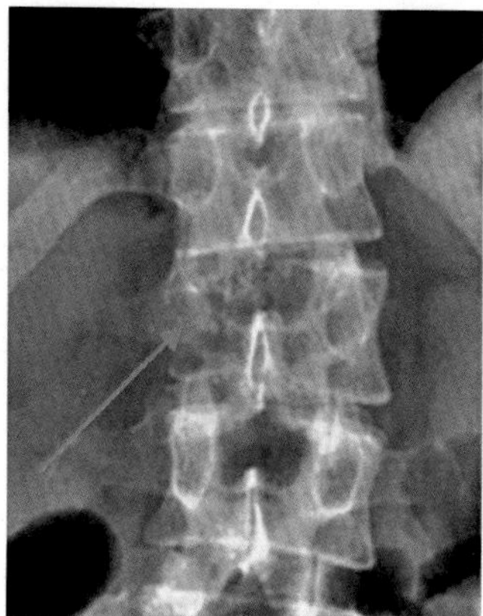

FIG. 9.1 Winking owl sign demonstrating radiolucent area of tumor involvement, obscuring the pedicle.

osseous delineation and can identify bony metastatic lesions 6 months earlier than plain films.[7] Sensitivity and specificity of CT scans for identifying histologically confirmed primary spinal malignancies is 66.2% and 99.3%, respectively, with overall diagnostic accuracy of 88.8%.[8] When ordering CT scans, it is important to remember the risks associated with radiation and contrast exposure to the patient.

Magnetic resonance imaging (MRI) is a powerful tool for assessing the spine. The sensitivity and specificity of MRI for identifying histologically confirmed primary spinal malignancies is 98.5% and 98.9%, respectively, with overall diagnostic accuracy of 98.7%.[8] The ability to directly image the spinal cord without presence of bone artifact (found in CT scans) makes MRI the ideal diagnostic for examining the spinal cord.[9] One thing to consider when ordering an MRI is that the acquisition time is significantly longer than a CT scan; patients with pain or claustrophobia may be very uncomfortable and could possibly require sedation. Contrast is also important to help delineate tissues; contrast allergies must be considered prior to obtaining imaging.

CT myelograms are CT scans obtained after intrathecal administration of contrast (Fig. 9.2). This study is useful in patients who cannot undergo MRI (pacemakers or other non-MRI compatible implants) as it allows the physician to assess osseous integrity and contents within the thecal sac.[7] Intrathecal contrast is administered prior to a traditional CT scan via lumbar puncture and at this time, cerebrospinal fluid may be sent for flow cytometry to assist in diagnosis.

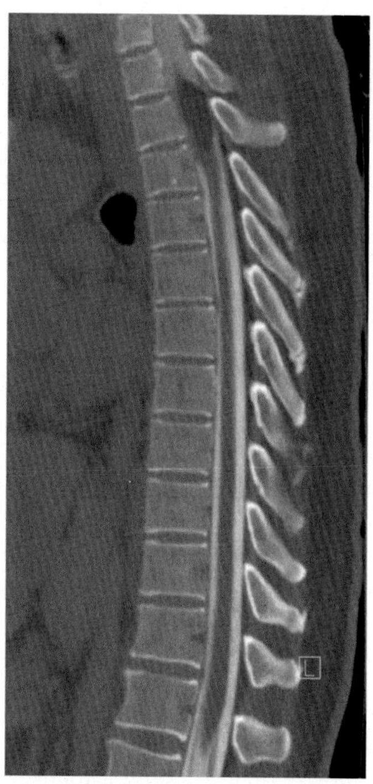

FIG. 9.2 Lipoma: Sagittal CT myelogram image shows a fat attenuation mass in the upper thoracic spinal canal.

SURGICAL MANAGEMENT

The widespread availability of MRI has invariably led to earlier diagnosis of spinal tumors. Radiation can be considered in select patients; however, it is generally not first-line therapy. The potential drawbacks of radiation include limited effectiveness of controlling tumor growth, doses of ionizing radiation to the spinal cord/nerve roots, and impaired wound healing, which can present an issue for surgical candidates.

The mainstay of treatment is surgery; however, the extent of surgery and addition of other components such as fusion hardware is a decision that must be made prior to surgery. It is generally accepted that if a patient's life span is less than 3 months, surgery should not be considered. Surgery is the first option for patients with neurologic deficit and life expectancy greater than 3 months. In general, surgical options are aimed at decompression, i.e., reducing pressure on the spinal cord or nerve roots by removing bone (indirect decompression) or by removing tumor (direct decompression). A laminectomy (removal of the posterior elements (Fig. 9.3) can assist in decompression and

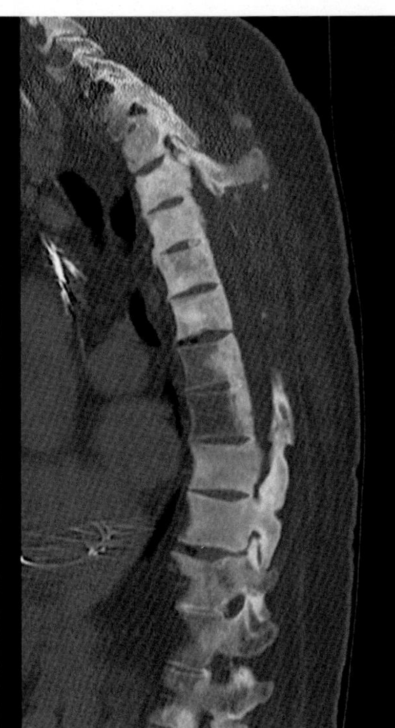

FIG. 9.3 Prostate cancer metastasis: Sagittal CT image shows extensive blastic lesions throughout the spine and prior multilevel thoracic surgical decompression.

TABLE 9.1
Patchell Criteria

INCLUSION
• Tissue-proven cancer, not of CNS or spinal column origin
• Radiographic spinal cord displacement
• >or = 1 neurologic sign, symptom, or pain
• Single area (one level or multiple contiguous spinal levels)
• Estimated survival > or =3 months
EXCLUSION
• Radiosensitive tumors: lymphoma, leukemia, multiple myeloma, germ cell tumor
• Paraplegic >48 h
• Only cauda equina or root compression
• Prior radiation (if 10 × 3 Gy contraindicated)

Adapted from Patchell RA. Direct decompressive surgical resection in the treatment of spinal cord compression caused by metastatic cancer: a randomised trial. *The Lancet*. August 2005;366:643.

tumor debulking when there is posterior involvement. A laminectomy is generally a midline posterior approach which removes the lamina and/or spinous processes; it can be unilateral (hemilaminectomy) or bilateral (laminectomy). Patients are positioned prone on the operating room table when a laminectomy is performed.

A corpectomy/vertebrectomy (removal of the vertebral body) can assist in decompression and tumor debulking when there is anterior tumor involvement. Removal of the anterior vertebral column is more complicated, as a traditional midline posterior approach does not provide enough lateral exposure to access the entire vertebral body. In this instance, modified posterior approaches that provide more posterolateral access may be employed such as a transpedicular approach or lateral extracavitary approach. Once again, prone is the position of choice for posterior approaches. Depending on the level in the thoracic spine, a lateral approach can also be considered when attempting to remove the anterior vertebral column.

Ventral lumbar tumors may also be approached anteriorly. A general surgeon (or anterior access trained orthopedic/neurosurgeon) can gain access to the vertebral body via an anterior retroperitoneal approach, allowing the spine surgeon to decompress, debulk, and instrument the spine via an abdominal incision, where the patient is positioned supine. Similarly, surgically amenable tumors of the spine can be approached via a lateral retroperitoneal transpsoas approach, where a patient is positioned in a lateral decubitus position. It is important to note that when patients have extensive spinal disease with a neurologic deficit that has been present for greater than 48 h, surgery may not be the best option.[10]

In 2005, Patchell et al. compared outcomes of patients with metastatic spinal cord compression who received surgery and radiation versus the previous standard, radiation alone. It was found that 84% of patients who received surgery and radiation were able to walk after treatment versus 54% of patients who received surgery alone. Furthermore, the patients who received surgery and radiation retained the ability to walk for a median of 122 days versus 13 days for those who received radiation alone.[10] From this information, the Patchell criteria was established (Table 9.1).

When assessing a patient with spinal metastatic disease, it is important to determine if the disease causes spinal instability; this allows the surgeon to decide if it is necessary to add instrumentation to provide the patient with additional internal support following a decompressive surgery. There are many forms of instrumentation provided by many manufacturers; the most

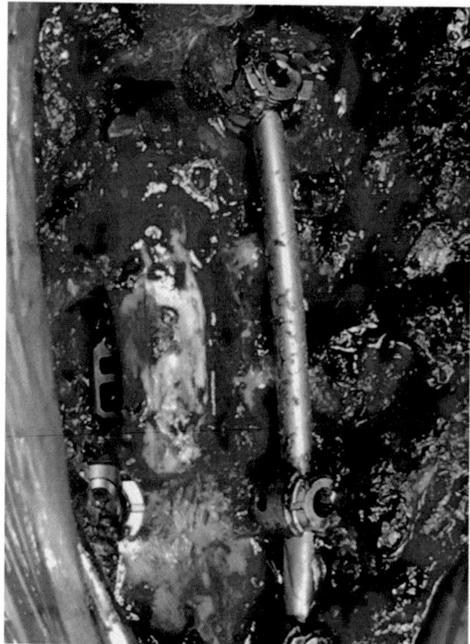

FIG. 9.4 Intraoperative photograph depicting pedicles, rods, and vertebral cage.

commonly encountered form of instrumentation is the pedicle screw, rod, and cage (Fig. 9.4).

The pedicle is the channel between the anterior and posterior elements of each thoracolumbar spinal segment. Metal screws which have recesses for metal rods can be navigated through the pedicle either anatomically or radiographically (using fluoroscopy or neuronavigation). After a pedicle screw is placed, the screw should span the posterior, middle, and anterior elements of the spine. Similarly, metal screws can be placed into the lateral masses of the cervical spine. Following placement of pedicle screws, metal rods are affixed to the screw heads and secured into place using either a locking cap or individual proprietary manufacturer mechanisms depending on the manufacturer. When combined, pedicle screws and rods provide segmental, bilateral instrumentation of the spine. The second component of spinal fusion is bone graft, which is generally laid lateral to the instrumentation to provide more mechanical strength in the form of bony fusion. Bone graft can be either autologous (harvested from the patient) or allogenic (processed and manufactured from cadaver bone). Other forms of instrumentation include biomechanical cages, which replace excised portions of the vertebral body (Fig. 9.5).

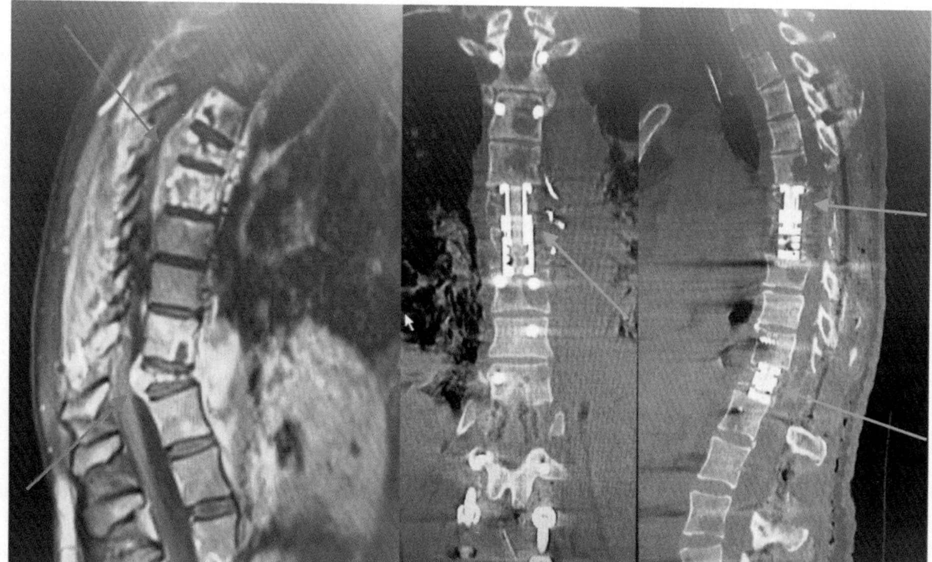

FIG. 9.5 Sagittal MRI T1 postcontrast (Preoperative) demonstrating multiple contrast-enhancing metastatic thoracic lesions (*orange arrows*). Coronal CT and sagittal CT (Postoperative) demonstrating laminectomy, placement of biomechanical cages (*blue arrows*).

TABLE 9.2
Spinal Instability Neoplastic Score

Component	Score
LOCATION	
Junctional (Occiput-C2; C7-T2; T11-L1; L5-S1)	3
Mobile spine (C3–C6; L2–L4)	2
Semirigid spine (T3–T10)	1
Rigid Spine (S2–S5)	0
MECHANICAL PAIN	
Yes	3
No	1
Pain-free lesion	0
BONE LESION	
Lytic	2
Mixed (lytic/blastic)	1
Blastic	0
RADIOGRAPHIC SPINAL ALIGNMENT	
Subluxation	4
Deformity (kyphosis/scoliosis)	2
Normal	0
VERTEBRAL BODY COLLAPSE	
>50% collapse	3
<50% collapse	2
No collapse with >50% vertebral body involved	1
None of the above	0
POSTEROLATERAL INVOLVEMENT	
Bilateral	3
Unilateral	1
None of the above	0

Adapted from Fisher CG, et al. A novel classification system for spinal instability in neoplastic disease: an evidence-based approach and expert consensus from the Spine Oncology Study Group. *Spine*. October 2010;35:E1221.

In 2010, the Spine Oncology Study Group published a tool to assist physicians with the management of spinal metastasis, called the Spinal Instability Neoplastic Score (SINS).[11] SINS (Table 9.2) is a 0–18 numerical scale based on location of neoplasm, mechanical pain, quality of bony lesion, spinal alignment, vertebral body collapse, and posterolateral involvement of spinal elements.[11] SINS scores can be interpreted as follows:

- 0 through 6: likely stable
- 7 through 12: intermediate, warranting surgical consult
- 13 through 18: unstable, warranting surgical consult

The SINS scale is one of many tools employed by physicians in the decision-making process of spinal metastatic management. Higher numerical score likely necessitates instrumented fusion. One benefit of SINS is the high interobserver reliability; a 2017 study found the intraclass correlation coefficient (a value that measures reliability) between independent observers to be 0.990 (a perfectly reliable value is 1.0), indicating that SINS is extremely reliable.[12]

Surgical management of intramedullary spinal cord tumors can be more complicated and carries more significant risks. In addition to the laminectomy required for other spinal lesions, the dura must be opened to expose the spinal cord. The spinal cord must then be incised to remove the tumor, potentially disrupting the many ascending and descending spinal tracts; potential neurologic deficits from surgery include hypesthesia, paresthesias, paresis or paraplegia, loss of urinary sphincter control, loss of proprioception, temperature sensation, etc. As fiber pathways are contiguous across the entire spine, deficits can occur at levels at or below the level of surgery, creating the potential for devastating neurologic injuries. Nonetheless, the presence of intramedullary spinal cord tumors can also cause any of the aforementioned deficits and must be addressed.

POSTOPERATIVE CARE

After completing surgery and returning the patient from the prone position (generally) on the operating room table to the hospital bed, anesthesia will assess the patient's face for edema. Extensive surgical resections may take many hours and patients are prone to developing facial edema, which can indicate airway edema. If the patient is found to have excessive facial edema, the decision may be made to leave the patient intubated until it is safe to extubate.

Surgical times, estimated blood loss, and overall clinical picture must be used to guide postoperative decision-making; however, patients generally go to the intensive care unit (ICU) for their early postoperative care. While in the ICU, fluid balance, Jackson-Pratt Drain (a surgical drain consisting of a channeled tube that is tunneled from the surgical site, out of the skin, and connected to a small compressible bulb suction device) output, postoperative laboratories including electrolytes and complete blood count and neurologic examination are monitored serially. Emphasis is placed on the neurologic examination, and nursing staff is expected to complete a thorough neurologic examination every hour, documenting the examination and reporting any changes to the covering physician.

Physical therapy, occupational therapy, and physical medicine and rehabilitation services are consulted early in the postoperative course to encourage mobility. Postoperative imaging in the form of CT scan is usually obtained to confirm placement of hardware. MRI may be degraded by metal artifact and postsurgical changes, making its utility somewhat limited. The Foley catheter is removed as soon as possible to reduce infection risk and encourage normal bladder use; if bladder training is required, straight catheterization may be employed following a trial of void if the patient fails. When the patient is hemodynamically stable and ready for transfer to the regular unit, invasive blood pressure monitoring is discontinued and neurologic check frequency is relaxed to every 4 h (frequency of neurologic checks allowed on non-ICUs will vary from institution to institution).

While on a regular unit, patients are encouraged to continue working with physical therapy and occupational therapy; many will require inpatient rehabilitation and are counseled on this prior to surgery. Oncology and Radiation Oncology services are consulted early in the postoperative course and determine future medical therapeutics. Chemotherapy and radiation are generally held for the first 2 weeks to allow for wound healing. The Jackson-Pratt Drain is removed when the output is sufficiently low, usually below 50 cc output in a 24-h period. Staples are generally the skin closing agent of choice and are kept in place for 2 weeks following surgery; they are removed prior to initiation of radiation. Individual inpatient stay lengths vary highly between patients because of diversity of pathology and associated medical comorbidities; however, the goal is to minimize hospital stay and discharge as soon as the patient is medically stable. Patients are scheduled for a 2-week follow-up on discharge and continue to be followed closely.

SURGICAL OUTCOMES

The most common presenting symptom for spinal metastatic disease is pain.[13] In one multicenter observational study of 223 patients with spinal metastatic disease managed with surgery, 71% of patients had better pain control, 64% of patients improved by at least one Frankel grade or maintained their preoperative Frankel grade of E, and 53% of patients who were immobile regained their mobility. The presence of an intact neurologic examination on presentation was a positive survival predictor; patients with Frankel grade E on admission had a median survival of 567 days compared with a median survival of 332 days for patients with Frankel grade A through D. Of note, patients who underwent surgery with en bloc or aggressive resection of tumor had better pain control, postoperative mobility, and sphincter control compared with palliative surgery (laminectomy with minimal tumor debulking).[1]

Surgical intervention is not without risk; the same 223 patient series had the following complications: perioperative mortality (5.8%), implant failure (2.2%), wound dehiscence (4%), combined urinary tract infection, pneumonia, deep vein thrombosis (7.6%), and thoracic duct injury/dysphagia (7.2%); the overall complication rate was 21%. It is not surprising that more aggressive surgeries were associated with more complications. The debulking alone group had the fewest overall complications followed by palliative resection groups and en bloc resection groups. Of note, palliative patients tended to have more direct surgical complications because of overall poor health status due to disease burden, resulting in a higher American Society of Anesthesiologists physical status classification (a measure of patients disease burden, with higher numbers indicating higher risk patients).[1]

Intramedullary tumors are more difficult to manage as they are found within the spinal cord and there is a greater risk of neurological deficit associated with assessing the lesion. In one series of 69 patients with surgically managed intramedullary tumors, 68% remained at their baseline neurologic status, 23% had neurologic improvement, and 9% showed neurologic decline from baseline functional status. Patients who could ambulate with or without assistance (ASIA D/E) had favorable outcomes in 90% of cases, whereas patients who could not ambulate (ASIA A/B/C) had favorable outcomes in only 30% of cases.[1] Once again, preoperative functional status is a good indicator of postoperative functional status. United States National Inpatient Sample data showed that the most common postoperative complications following the resection of intramedullary lesions were urinary/renal (3.7%), postoperative hematoma (2.5%), pulmonary (2.4%), and neurologic (1.7%).[14]

Taking the aforementioned studies into consideration, early intervention provides patients with the best chance of maintaining normal functional status if there is no neurologic deficit; if neurologic deficit is already present, outcomes are more favorable with higher functioning patients. Delay in evaluation, diagnosis, and intervention can all contribute to increased morbidity and mortality among patients with spinal tumors. Although most treatment is palliative in nature (as most tumors of the spine are metastatic), pain relief from surgical intervention, preservation of mobility, and preservation of sphincter control can drastically improve quality of life in cancer patients.

CONCLUSIONS

Management of patients with tumors of the spine and spinal cord must start with recognition. Expedited workup, imaging, surgical consultation, and intervention are essential to optimize patient outcomes. A multidisciplinary approach involving primary care physicians, medical oncologists, radiation oncologists, orthopedic/neurosurgeons, physiatrists, physical therapists is necessary to provide patients with spinal disease complete medical and surgical therapy. Each of the respective physicians must understand disease pathophysiology and disease management to appreciate the other managing physician's role in management; each team should have a common goal, which is to preserve neurologic function for as long as possible. Early surgical decompression <48 h after neurologic deficit and preoperative neurologic function are important factors in patient outcomes.[1,10] Unfortunately, most spinal disease is metastatic, and optimum patient selection is difficult as many patients who require emergent surgery are quite ill.

REFERENCES

1. Ibrahim A. Does spinal surgery improve the quality of life for those with extradural (spinal) osseous metastases? An international multicenter prospective observational study of 223 patients. Invited submission from the Joint Section Meeting on Disorders of the Spine and Peripheral Nerves, March 2007. *J Neurosurg Spine*. 2008;8:271.
2. Ciftdemir M, Kaya M, Selcuk E, Yalniz E. Tumors of the spine. *World J Orthop*. 2016;7(2):109–116. https://doi.org/10.5312/wjo.v7.i2.109.
3. Fuchs B, Boos N. Primary tumors of the spine. In: *Spinal Disorders*. Berlin, Heidelberg: Springer; 2008:951–976. https://doi.org/10.1007/978-3-540-69091-7_33.
4. Jacobs WB. Evaluation and treatment of spinal metastases: an overview. *Neurosurg Focus*. 2001;11.
5. Heldmann U. Frequency of unexpected multifocal metastasis in patients with acute spinal cord compression. Evaluation by low-field MR imaging in cancer patients. *Acta Radiol*. 1997;38:372.
6. Levack P. Don't wait for a sensory level—listen to the symptoms: a prospective audit of the delays in diagnosis of malignant cord compression. *Clin Oncology*. 2002;14:472.
7. Shah LM, Salzman KL. Imaging of spinal metastatic disease. *Int J Surg Oncol*. 2011;2011:769753. https://doi.org/10.1155/2011/769753.
8. Buhmann S, Becker C, Duerr HR, Reiser M, Baur-Melnyk A. Detection of osseous metastases of the spine: comparison of high resolution multi-detector-CT with MRI. *Eur J Radiol*. 2009;69(3):567–573. https://doi.org/10.1016/j.ejrad.2007.11.039. ISSN 0720-048X.
9. Norman D, Mills CM, Brant-Zawadzki M, Yeates A, Crooks LE, Kaufman L. Magnetic resonance imaging of the spinal cord and canal: potentials and limitations. *Am J Roentgenol*. 1983;141(6):1147–1152.
10. Patchell RA. Direct decompressive surgical resection in the treatment of spinal cord compression caused by metastatic cancer: a randomised trial. *The Lancet (British Edition)*. 2005;366:643.
11. Fisher CG, et al. A novel classification system for spinal instability in neoplastic disease: an evidence-based approach and expert consensus from the Spine Oncology Study Group. *Spine*. 2010;35:E1221.
12. Fox S. Spinal instability neoplastic score (SINS): reliability among spine fellows and resident physicians in orthopedic surgery and neurosurgery. *Glob Spine Journal*. 2017;7(8):744.
13. Camins M, Oppenheim J, Perrin R. Tumors of the vertebral axis benign, primary, malignant and metastatic tumors. In: Winn HR, ed. *Youmans Neurological Surgery*. 5th ed. Philadelphia, Pennsylvania: Saunders; 2004:4835–4868.
14. Patil CG. Complications and outcomes after spinal cord tumor resection in the United States from 1993 to 2002. *Spinal Cord*. 2008;46:375.

CHAPTER 10

Inpatient Rehabilitation of Persons With Spinal Cord Injury due to Cancer

MIGUEL XAVIER ESCALÓN, MD, MPH • THOMAS N. BRYCE, MD

INTRODUCTION

A spinal cord injury (SCI) is a life-changing event. Regardless of the cause or the time course of presentation, the patient will be affected dramatically as will his or her support system.

Perhaps the most important aspect of rehabilitative care of a person with SCI due to cancer is to understand the goals of inpatient rehabilitation (IPR) in this population. These goals can be affected by diagnosis, with, for example, the needs of a person with complete C4 tetraplegia are much different than that of a person with incomplete T11 paraplegia, but also by prognosis. A patient with an excellent prognosis could maximize his/her time in IPR in order to try and achieve a goal of going home with independence or modified independence. However, for a patient with a prognosis of less than 6 months, IPR of SCI would be better focused on family training, patient education, and discharge home as soon as possible with focus of optimizing the remaining quality of life. These goals and lengths of stay vary from situation to situation, but it is generally accepted that with appropriate family involvement and training for care of a person with SCI due to cancer, length of stay can be as short as 10 days or less.

All patients discharged from IPR require a plan for ongoing care called a discharge plan. The goal of which is to anticipate not only the current medical and physical needs of the patient but also those medical and physical needs that will exist or develop in the coming months and design a plan to meet those needs. The rehabilitation team determines, in collaboration with the oncology team, who can give insight into the specific prognosis for cancer progression, a projection of functional recovery or decline which in turn dictates durable medical equipment (DME) and ongoing therapy needs post discharge. Successful implementation of the discharge plan is affected by a host of factors. For example, patient resources can play a role in discharge planning and continuity of rehabilitative care after discharge. In some cases, a patient may require a hospital bed, commode, or transfer assistance device such as a hydraulic patient lift for safe discharge home, but this DME may not fit inside the home or may be unaffordable, making a safe discharge plan less than optimal. Another example is that a lack of access to an automobile or public transportation can affect a plan for continued rehabilitation in an outpatient setting after discharge.

The successful rehabilitation of a person with SCI due to cancer relies upon teamwork and constant communication between the rehabilitation team, the patient, and the family. Ultimately, IPR is only the first step in an arduous road to medical, physical, and psychologic recovery or decline and a manageable death.

SPINAL CORD INJURY AND CANCER DIAGNOSIS

Tumors of the spine often lead to SCI; tumors of the spinal cord by definition cause SCI. Any part of the spinal cord can be affected and to varying degrees. As such patients can present with complete or incomplete paraplegia or tetraplegia. SCI related to tumors and cancer of the spine is most often due to direct compression, although vascular insults are possible as well.

Persons with SCI due to cancer often present with a variety of symptoms including those common to any cancer patient such as pain, fatigue, malaise, and weight loss in addition to neurologic dysfunction including focal weakness of one or more extremities, difficulty walking or standing, sensory losses, dysesthesias, and bowel and bladder incontinence or retention. These neurologic signs and symptoms may present insidiously or appear suddenly. Pain related to SCI and cancer can be localized to the spine at the level of the tumor or metastasis or may appear in a dermatomal or radicular distribution. Back pain related to cancer is often characterized as dull or achy, which is not an uncommon presentation for noncancer-related back pain; however, if a patient complains of back pain that is worse at night or with lying down, clinicians should have a high suspicion for cancer as a cause.

A patient's history is also important in diagnosing SCI due to cancer. For example, a patient with a prior history of cancer merits workup of possible metastases to the spine when presenting with the aforementioned symptoms. First and foremost a thorough physical examination is important in diagnosing spinal metastases or tumors. A full neurologic examination should be completed and should include strength examination and sensory examinaton and should include a digital rectal examination to test for sensation, tone, and volitional contraction. The International Standards for Neurological Classification of Spinal Cord Injury (ISNCSCI) is an examination used to quantitatively score the motor and sensory impairment, determine a neurologic level of injury, and determine the severity of SCI by assigning an American Spinal Injury Association Impairment Scale (AIS) ranging from "A" to "E" (Fig. 10.1). Persons without any sensation or motor function in the lowest sacral dermatomes (S4-5) would be classified under the 2011 ISNCSCI revision as having a complete injury and designated AIS "A." Those who have sensory function in the lowest sacral dermatomes (S4-5) but no motor function more than three levels below the neurologic level of injury would be classified as having an incomplete sensory injury and designated as AIS "B." Persons with sensory function in the lowest sacral dermatomes (S4-5) and motor function more than three myotomal levels below the motor level would be classified as having an incomplete motor injury and designated as AIS "C," or "D." If at least

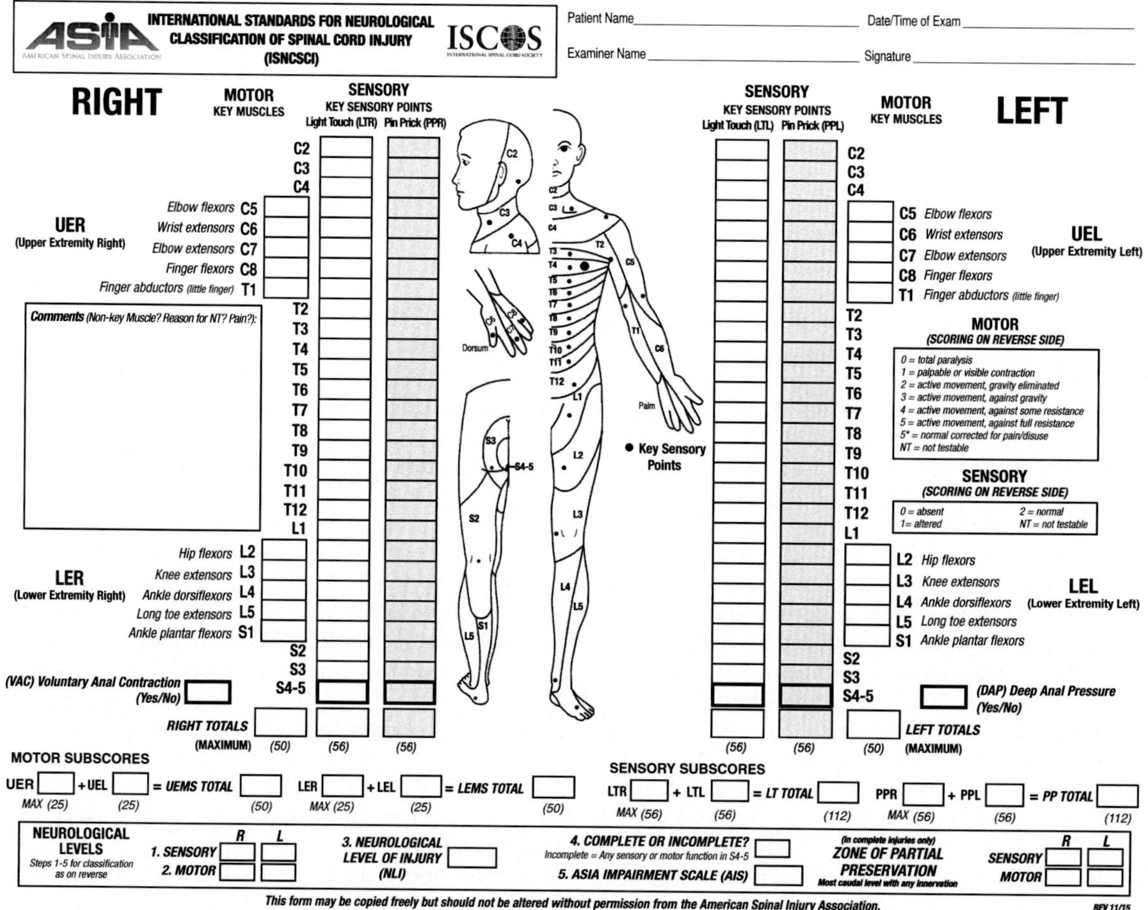
ASIA AMERICAN SPINAL INJURY ASSOCIATION
INTERNATIONAL STANDARDS FOR NEUROLOGICAL CLASSIFICATION OF SPINAL CORD INJURY (ISNCSCI)
ISCoS INTERNATIONAL SPINAL CORD SOCIETY

Patient Name ____________ Date/Time of Exam ____________
Examiner Name ____________ Signature ____________

RIGHT

MOTOR KEY MUSCLES | SENSORY KEY SENSORY POINTS: Light Touch (LTR) Pin Prick (PPR)

C2, C3, C4

UER (Upper Extremity Right): Elbow flexors C5; Wrist extensors C6; Elbow extensors C7; Finger flexors C8; Finger abductors (little finger) T1

Comments (Non-key Muscle? Reason for NT? Pain?):

T2, T3, T4, T5, T6, T7, T8, T9, T10, T11, T12, L1

LER (Lower Extremity Right): Hip flexors L2; Knee extensors L3; Ankle dorsiflexors L4; Long toe extensors L5; Ankle plantar flexors S1

S2, S3, S4-5

(VAC) Voluntary Anal Contraction (Yes/No)

RIGHT TOTALS (MAXIMUM) (50) (56) (56)

LEFT

SENSORY KEY SENSORY POINTS: Light Touch (LTL) Pin Prick (PPL) | MOTOR KEY MUSCLES

C2, C3, C4

UEL (Upper Extremity Left): C5 Elbow flexors; C6 Wrist extensors; C7 Elbow extensors; C8 Finger flexors; T1 Finger abductors (little finger)

T2, T3, T4, T5, T6, T7, T8, T9, T10, T11, T12, L1

MOTOR (SCORING ON REVERSE SIDE)
0 = total paralysis
1 = palpable or visible contraction
2 = active movement, gravity eliminated
3 = active movement, against gravity
4 = active movement, against some resistance
5 = active movement, against full resistance
5* = normal corrected for pain/disuse
NT = not testable

SENSORY (SCORING ON REVERSE SIDE)
0 = absent; 2 = normal
1 = altered; NT = not testable

LEL (Lower Extremity Left): L2 Hip flexors; L3 Knee extensors; L4 Ankle dorsiflexors; L5 Long toe extensors; S1 Ankle plantar flexors

S2, S3, S4-5

(DAP) Deep Anal Pressure (Yes/No)

LEFT TOTALS (MAXIMUM) (56) (56) (50)

MOTOR SUBSCORES
UER ☐ + UEL ☐ = UEMS TOTAL ☐ MAX (25) (25) (50)
LER ☐ + LEL ☐ = LEMS TOTAL ☐ MAX (25) (25) (50)

SENSORY SUBSCORES
LTR ☐ + LTL ☐ = LT TOTAL ☐ MAX (56) (56) (112)
PPR ☐ + PPL ☐ = PP TOTAL ☐ MAX (56) (56) (112)

NEUROLOGICAL LEVELS (Steps 1-5 for classification as on reverse): R L; 1. SENSORY; 2. MOTOR
3. NEUROLOGICAL LEVEL OF INJURY (NLI)
4. COMPLETE OR INCOMPLETE? Incomplete = Any sensory or motor function in S4-5
5. ASIA IMPAIRMENT SCALE (AIS)
(In complete injuries only) ZONE OF PARTIAL PRESERVATION Most caudal level with any innervation: R L; SENSORY; MOTOR

This form may be copied freely but should not be altered without permission from the American Spinal Injury Association.

REV 11/15

FIG. 10.1 International Standards for Neurological Classification of Spinal Cord Injury examination.

half of the key muscles, where a single key muscle is defined for each of five upper extremity myotomes from C5-T1 and five lower extremity myotomes from L2-S1 on both sides of the body, below the neurologic level of injury have a muscle grade strength of at least 3 out of 5, the AIS would be designated "D," if not the SCI would be designated as AIS "C." The AIS "E" designation is reserved for those with SCI who make full recovery of motor strength and sensation within all dermatomes and key muscle myotomes. The ISNCSCI examination is utilized to track neurologic function and should be performed at minimum yearly on patients with SCI to ensure no neurologic deterioration requiring neurologic workup. Special consideration and more frequent ISNCSCI examinations should be performed on those patients with SCI due to cancer as these patients are prone to progressive or worsening SCI by the very nature of their disease state. Should neurologic deterioration be discovered in a patient with SCI due to cancer, immediate workup including imaging should be performed.

After obtaining a thorough history and physical, if a clinician has suspicion that his or her patient has cancer or a tumor that is causing or has the potential to lead to compromise of the spinal cord, the next diagnostic step should be urgent imaging. Imaging should include magnetic resonance imaging (MRI) and computed tomography (CT) of the area of the spine (cervical, thoracic, or lumbosacral) thought to be affected. MRI is the best modality for evaluation for neural compromise, whereas CT is the best modality for evaluating bony destruction and spinal stability. MRIs should be ordered with contrast since almost all intrinsic spinal cord tumors and metastases enhance with gadolinium. Should the MRI elucidate tumor or metastatic lesion, MRIs of the remaining segments of the spine should be considered to rule out other tumor or metastasis along the spine as well. Positron emission tomography (PET) scans are mostly used for surveillance and are not used to diagnose cancer of the spine but can be used to assess for any new metastatic disease.

SPINAL CORD INJURY AND CANCER PROGNOSIS

With improved medical and oncologic care, persons with cancer are living longer with less cancer-related morbidity. However, this also means that some persons are living with deficits and issues that previously would have been untreatable. This is apparent in the reported 18,000 new cases of spinal tumor per year in North America of which 85% are metastatic. Cancer is thought to metastasize to the spine either via the lymphatic or vascular system. Some studies suggest that up to 70% of those with cancer will have metastases to the spine. In fact, spinal tumors account for 26% of nontraumatic SCI admissions to IPR units. Cancer of the spine can be primary (cancer or tumor arising in the spine) or secondary (metastatic). The most common forms of cancer that metastasize to the spine are lung, breast, kidney, prostate, and thyroid. Spine lesions are most commonly diagnosed in the thoracic spine, despite cadaveric studies showing they are more common in the lumbar spine. This may be due to the narrowed spinal canal and vascular anatomy making mass lesions in this area more likely to lead to symptoms of complete or incomplete paraplegia.

Spinal tumors can be classified into three man subtypes by location: intramedullary, intradural-extramedullary, and extradural. Different subtypes of tumor have different prognoses and different types of tumor or cancer (See Chapter 8 for more information on tumors of the spine). It is important to note that given that intramedullary tumors arise from within the spinal cord itself, even a small intramedullary tumor can have dramatic neurologic effects.

Spinal tumors, by nature of their classifications, cause SCI and neurologic dysfunction in different ways. The most common cause of dysfunction due to primary tumors (intramedullary or intradural-extramedullary) involves direct destruction of the nervous system by tumor invasion. The most common cause of dysfunction due to secondary tumors (metastatic disease) is compression of neural tissue within the spinal canal. Metastatic lesions of the cervical and thoracic spine are most often the result of lung and breast disease, whereas lumbosacral involvement is most often due to prostate, colon, or pelvic involvement. Survival rates for common metastatic cancers to the spine include the following:

- Lung metastases to the spine with 50% survival rate at 1 month and at best 16% after 24 months.
- Breast cancer with metastases to the spine with 44% survival rate after 24 months.
- Prostate cancer with metastases to the spine with 25% survival rate at 24 months.
- Patients with primary spine tumors who completed IPR programs had a median survival of 9.5 months with 1-year survival of 47.4% and 5-year survival of 10.5%.
- Patients with secondary spine tumors had a median survival of 2.8 months with 1-year survival of 21.4% and 5-year survival of 3.6%.

Cancer may also cause SCI indirectly. According to the American Cancer Society, the incidence of cancer from 2008 to 2012 was 454.8 per 100,000 persons. With cancer being so prevalent, these indirect causes of SCI become more common as well.

Paraneoplastic syndromes are a group of syndromes that are an autoimmune response to a primary cancer or tumor. Via this pathway these syndromes lead to medical issues at sites of the body distant from the cancer's actual location. Paraneoplastic syndromes have been known to cause cerebellar degeneration, myasthenia gravis, as well as transverse myelitis (TM), which is an inflammatory disorder of the spinal cord that results in SCI. In over 50% of cases of TM, a specific cause of the inflammatory condition is not found; however, paraneoplastic syndrome should be considered within the differential diagnosis of a patient presenting with TM of unknown etiology, especially if this patient has a history of cancer.

Treatment of cancer can also cause SCI. Radiation-induced SCI is a possibility when radiation is used in the treatment of cancer adjacent to the spinal cord. Irradiation of lung cancers and cancers of the head and neck leave the spinal cord particularly susceptible to radiation-induced SCI. Depending on the anatomic area irradiated, different levels of the spine (cervical, thoracic, or lumbosacral) could be affected. As such, radiation-induced SCI could lead to paraplegia or tetraplegia. Radiation-induced SCI can present in multiple fashions. It could present as a transient myelitis, a limited SCI that most often presents 2–4 months after irradiation and most commonly presents with electric shock–like neuropathic pain and can also be accompanied by varying degrees of weakness. Transient myelitis induced by radiation is self-limiting and does not require treatment to resolve. Despite the self-correcting nature of transient myelitis, recovery can take up to 40 weeks, and depending on level of impairment, these patients could benefit from intense rehabilitation. Patients who have had irradiation to treat cancer can also develop chronic progressive radiation myelopathy (CPRM) that most often first appears 9–15 months following irradiation, but has been reported to present as long as 3 years following irradiation. CPRM is hallmarked by demyelination of the spinal cord leading to white matter necrosis and atrophy of the spinal cord itself. Radiation can also lead to vascular injury in the spine leading to SCI. The likelihood of developing CPRM is thought to be related to the volume of the spinal cord exposed to radiation and the total dose of radiation received. The accepted dosing of radiation to the spinal cord is not to exceed 45 Gy, although if it is necessary for successful treatment of the cancer, a small volume of cord is allowed to receive a higher dose. Studies have shown that patients that received 50–55 Gy to the spinal cord had a 1% chance of developing CPRM after 2 years, whereas those that received 55–60 Gy to the spinal cord had a 5% chance of developing CPRM after 2 years, and those that received 68–73 Gy to the spinal cord had a 50% chance of developing CPRM. It is generally accepted that the risks of radiation to the spinal cord outweigh the benefits above 60 Gy. There is no treatment known to reverse CPRM, and neurologic dysfunction is usually permanent.

SECONDARY CONDITIONS OF SPINAL CORD INJURY AND CANCER

In order to provide the most effective IPR of a patient with SCI due to cancer, it is important to be aware of the secondary conditions unique to SCI and how to best manage these. These medical considerations can vary based on the type of cancer diagnosis and location; however, there are some more commonly experienced medical conditions that will be discussed in the following section.

Neurogenic Bladder

Before discussing neurogenic bladder, and neurogenic bowel, further, it is important to understand that patients with SCI can present with either upper motor neuron (UMN) or lower motor neuron (LMN) injuries. It is important to differentiate the two types of SCI in order to provide the proper medical management. Lower motoneurons are cells whose axons leave the central nervous system (CNS) and connect to skeletal muscle fibers. LMN dysfunction arises from damage to the anterior horn cells within the spinal cord, specifically to the cell bodies of the LMNs or to the motoneuron axons within the cauda equina. With injury to LMNs, affected muscles are typically flaccid and there is loss of reflex activity. UMN dysfunction arises from damage to neurons proximal to the LMNs which reside entirely within the CNS. Reflex activity typically is preserved below the level of injury for UMN injuries. Most SCIs with the exception of injuries to the conus medullaris, such as may occur with a chordoma, or cauda equina compression, or cord infarction in which segments of the cord are damaged due to ischemia can be expected to present as UMN injuries. In order to assess for a UMN SCI, the practitioner should complete an anal examination that includes assessing for bulbocavernosus and anocutaneous reflexes. If these reflexes are intact and there is normal resting or increased anal sphincter tone on physical examination, then a patient has a UMN SCI. If these reflexes cannot be elicited and the anal sphincter is flaccid on examination, then a patient has an LMN SCI. With few exceptions, those persons with tetraplegia or mid- to high-level paraplegia have UMN injuries and those with low-level paraplegia have UMN, LMN, or a combination of injuries.

Neurogenic bladder is common after SCI, and lack of proper management can lead to significant morbidity with life-threatening infections and even renal failure. A neurogenic bladder can be either a UMN or LMN type, and the management approach for each type is different; however, if there is any doubt about the appropriate bladder management for a patient with SCI, it is always acceptable to insert a Foley catheter transurethrally and consult urology for further recommendations. Consultation to and follow-up with a urologist with experience in neurogenic bladder is standard of care for any SCI patient.

Upper motor neuron bladder management

Those patients with UMN lesions and neurogenic bladder typically have a spastic detrusor muscle (the muscle within the bladder wall responsible for contracting and expelling urine) and spastic urinary sphincter (the muscle responsible for maintaining continence at rest and allowing expulsion of urine by relaxing during normal voiding). This invariably results in variable degrees of detrusor sphincter dyssynergia, a condition in which a spastic detrusor muscle contracts but the sphincter does not relax at the same time. When a spastic detrusor muscle is triggered to contract against a closed sphincter the pressures generated within the bladder may exceed the capacity of the sphincter to maintain closure allowing urine to be expelled and incontinence especially if bladder sensation is also impaired. If the pressures are not excessive (<50 cm H_2O) and most of the urine is expelled leaving a post void bladder residual volume less than 200–250 mL, then this involuntary reflex emptying of the bladder can be considered "safe" or "balanced." If the pressures are sustained and exceed 50 cm H_2O, the risk for upper urinary tract deterioration with the potential for the development of hydronephrosis and renal insufficiency increases and reflex emptying alone would not be considered a "safe" bladder management technique. In this latter case or in the situation where urine is largely or completely retained within the bladder, emptying of the bladder with a urinary catheter is essential.

There are four basic ways for patients with UMN neurogenic bladder to empty: normal voiding, reflex voiding, intermittent catheterization, and continuous indwelling catheter drainage with a Foley catheter. Reflex voiding is a reasonable goal for a male patient without normal control whose bladder empties involuntarily or with incomplete control at safe pressures as noted earlier. In this situation, the individual would continuously wear a condom catheter over his penis. In order to ensure this management remains "safe," periodic bladder residual urine checks (several time daily in the beginning) should be performed, the serum creatinine monitored (weekly in the beginning), bladder pressures assessed with urodynamic study (if there is any suspicion that voiding is not "safe"), upper urinary tracts imaged (at baseline and yearly) with a renal sonogram to screen for hydronephrosis, and the patient queried for the presence of autonomic dysregulation (discussed in autonomic dysregulation section) as well as the frequency of urinary tract infections. Should a patient managing his bladder with reflex voiding have low 24-h output in the drainage bag attached to the catheter (indicating perhaps the patient is retaining urine) or elevated bladder volumes on scanning for residual urine within the bladder, then the patient should be intermittently catheterized. Many patients with SCI will develop worsening spasticity over the first few months after SCI that will make it more likely for them to be able to reflex void. Also α-1 blockers, such as tolterodine, can be used to "relax" the urinary sphincter presumably decreasing sphincter outlet resistance and improve the chances of successful reflex voiding.

Intermittent catheterization is the preferred method of management for persons, both men and women, who retain urine and are able to perform the technique safely themselves. It is typically performed every 4–6 hours depending on the volume consumed and the bladder capacity before reflex voiding is triggered. It is important to note that new onset leaking in between catheterizations can be caused by urinary tract infection, overingestion of liquids, and evolution (changing spasticity) of bladder after SCI. If a patient is leaking in between catheterizations and the bladder capacity before reflex voiding is triggered is low (<400 mL), a bladder-specific anticholinergic, such as oxybutynin, or a β 3 adrenergic agonist, such as mirabegron, can be added and titrated to promote continence.

Indwelling catheters are indicated for those individuals who retain urine and are unable to perform intermittent catheterization or for those who reflex void without control and are unable to maintain an external urine collection appliance and are at risk for skin breakdown.

Lower motor neuron bladder management

LMN bladders are flaccid by nature and treated almost exclusively by intermittent catheterization every 4–6 hours.

Special considerations

A patient with a lesion causing progressive mass effect or a patient that could develop new metastatic lesions has the potential to have changing bladder management needs over time, and as such should be followed closely by a urologist and physiatrist. A patient with SCI due to cancer prognosis is also a consideration. If a patient has a poor prognosis (on the order of a few months), an indwelling catheter is often chosen for quality-of-life reasons.

Neurogenic Bowel

Neurogenic bowel is also common after SCI and like neurogenic bladder, it also has different treatment considerations based on whether a patient has UMN or LMN SCI. Having control over when a patient might have a bowel movement not only allows therapy sessions to go uninterrupted but also allows the patient to learn to have more control over his or her life and avoid embarrassing situations. A patient with UMN bowel can be considered to have regular, albeit slow, functioning of his or her intestines through the transverse colon. This is due to the fact that the gastroenterologic (GI) tract from esophagus to splenic flexure is innervated by the vagus nerve, whereas the pelvic and pudendal nerves innervate the GI tract for the remainder of the colon and rectum. Connections to these lower nerves are often interrupted in SCI. The goal for these patients is to have soft, but formed stool. These patients require stool softeners, laxatives (osmotic or irritant), and suppositories or mini-enemas in combination with digital stimulation in order to evacuate their bowels completely. An example of a medication regimen for these patients would be

- Docusate sodium 100 mg by mouth twice daily
- Senna 17.2 mg by mouth at bedtime
- Bisacodyl suppository with digital stimulation daily

When scheduling these medications, it is important to note that one should expect the laxative (in the above example senna) to take approximately 8 h to work. As such, the suppository should be scheduled accordingly. The combination of the suppository and digital stimulation of the anus takes advantage of the recto-colic reflex that is still intact in a person with UMN SCI. Other reflexes can also be leveraged, such as the gastrocolic reflex with bowel routines being scheduled after breakfast or dinner. Patients with sufficient manual dexterity and with the use of specialized commodes can learn to perform their own suppository insertion and digital stimulation. Many patients with UMN bowel will not have the manual dexterity to perform their own bowel routines. In these scenarios, a family member or caregiver should be trained to perform the bowel routine. Patients with LMN injuries have a flaccid bowel. As such they do not respond to irritant laxatives, suppositories, or digital stimulation. In addition, these patients have a flaccid sphincter and are prone to accidents or anal leakage. With this in mind, the goal for these patients is to have hard stool formed in the shape of small pebbles. These patients normally do not take medications, but could take stool softeners or stool-bulking agents, such as psyllium, as needed to obtain the appropriate stool texture. Persons with LMN SCI require manual disimpactions for bowel management. These patients are prone to accidents after meals, and for that reason they may need to perform several bowel routines per day. Most patients with LMN bowel are able to perform their own bowel routines; however, should they not be able to for any reason, a caregiver or family member should be trained on how to do so for that patient. There are special considerations for those patients with SCI secondary to cancer. A patient with a lesion causing progressive mass effect or a patient that could develop new metastatic lesions has the potential to form changing bowel management needs over time and as such should be followed closely by a physiatrist. Patients on chemotherapy may develop nausea or diarrhea. They may also be on opioid medications for pain control that can slow bowel transit time for these patients even further. Laxatives, stool softeners, and stool-bulking agents should be adjusted as needed.

Spasticity

Patients with UMN SCI typically will develop spasticity. Spasticity is a form of hyperreflexia manifesting in muscle tightness, especially with rapid passive or active movement and stretch. These spasms can become powerful enough to hinder physical and occupational therapies, make it difficult to dress or clean a patient, and make transfers dangerous. Spasticity often increases in the early weeks to months following an SCI and either will remain or dissipate over time. Initial management of spasticity is via therapy and stretching; however, often this alone is not enough. Oral baclofen is the pharmacologic agent of choice for spasticity. It is usually started at a dose of 5–10 mg three to four times per day and gradually increased as tolerated. Side effects that can affect tolerability include sedation and confusion. It is not uncommon for persons with SCI to take doses of up to 40 mg at a time. Should oral baclofen not be sufficient to control the spasms, then secondary oral agents such as tizanidine can be tried [caution with orthostatic hypotension(OH)] or intrathecal baclofen via an intrathecal pump should be considered. Cancer patients with spasticity may not be medically able to undergo pump implantation, and in this case benzodiazepines or dantrolene could also be considered to treat spasm. Of note, dantrolene can lead to hepatotoxicity, and as such liver function tests should be followed closely and it should be avoided in those with liver disease.

Autonomic Dysfunction

Autonomic dysreflexia

Patients with SCI at thoracic level 6 or higher are at increased risk of autonomic dysfunction. This can present in several ways, the most serious of which is autonomic dysreflexia (AD). AD is defined as a sudden rise in systolic blood pressure (20–40 mm Hg above baseline) that is frequently associated with bradycardia. Of note, the normal range of systolic blood pressure for a person with SCI at T6 or above may be as low as 90–110 mm Hg. AD is a response to a noxious stimulus below the level of SCI, most commonly related to distal bowel (e.g., constipation) or bladder (e.g., elevated bladder pressure) irritation. It results in a reflex sympathetic response above the neurologic level of injury leading to hypertension and tachycardia. Baroreceptors are then able to regulate heart rate often leading to bradycardia in an attempt to mitigate the rapid rise in blood pressure. The body makes an attempt to trigger a parasympathetic response to counter the hypertension, but because these patients have SCI lesions at T6 or above, there is impaired parasympathetic control of the splanchnic vasculature and hypertension remains until the noxious stimulus is removed. Often the only sign of AD are a patient's subjective complaints that often include headache, flushing, or sweating above the lesion, itchiness, or stuffy nose. AD is a potentially life-threatening condition and can result in hemorrhagic stroke. Treatment of AD primarily involves removal of the noxious stimulus. If a practitioner suspects AD, the following steps should be taken (Fig. 10.2):

Once the source of AD has been identified and blood pressure normalized, it is important to take note of the inciting factors so that the patient's treatment plan could be adjusted accordingly. In patients with SCI due to metastatic disease and persistent AD, it is important to consider that the metastases themselves may be irritating by compressing upon muscle, bone, or otherwise. The body could interpret this invasion as noxious. In this case, scheduled pain medications may provide relief from AD.

Orthostatic hypotension

AD is not the only cardiovascular consideration in persons with SCI due to metastatic disease. Again patients with SCI lesions at T6 or above are particularly susceptible to OH, again for lack of appropriate vascular control. OH cause subjective light-headedness and dizziness limiting therapy but can also be severe enough to cause syncope. Patients that may be susceptible to, or develop, OH should be fitted with thigh high compression stockings and an abdominal binder before sitting up. Should a patient fail conservative management of OH, medications could be used as well. Sodium chloride tablets, midodrine, and fludrocortisone are all acceptable in treating OH secondary to SCI. Given the steroidal properties of fludrocortisone, it should be used with caution in certain types of cancer or in patients already on steroid medication.

Venous Thromboembolic Disease

Venous thromboembolism (VTE) is a leading cause of morbidity and mortality in SCI. Following SCI, patients are transiently hypercoagulable and are particularly susceptible to Virchow's triad. Rates of VTE have been reported to be as high as 100% in patients with SCI not being treated with thromboprophylactic medications. Moreover, those with greater levels of impairment are more susceptible to developing VTE. For traumatic SCI, guidelines suggest initiating sequential compression devices and low molecular weight heparin as soon after injury as possible. Warfarin and direct-acting anticoagulants are also acceptable in the rehabilitation setting. Typically these thromboprophylactic methods would be used for 8 weeks following acute SCI. Given that patients with cancer are considered to be in a hypercoagulable state, it is generally thought best, assuming acceptable risk of bleeding, to prophylax based on the more aggressive treatment plan. That is to say, should the SCI guidelines offer more and longer coverage for thromboprophylaxis, then those would be followed or should the standard of care for a particular cancer have stronger guidelines for thromboprophylaxis, then those should be followed.

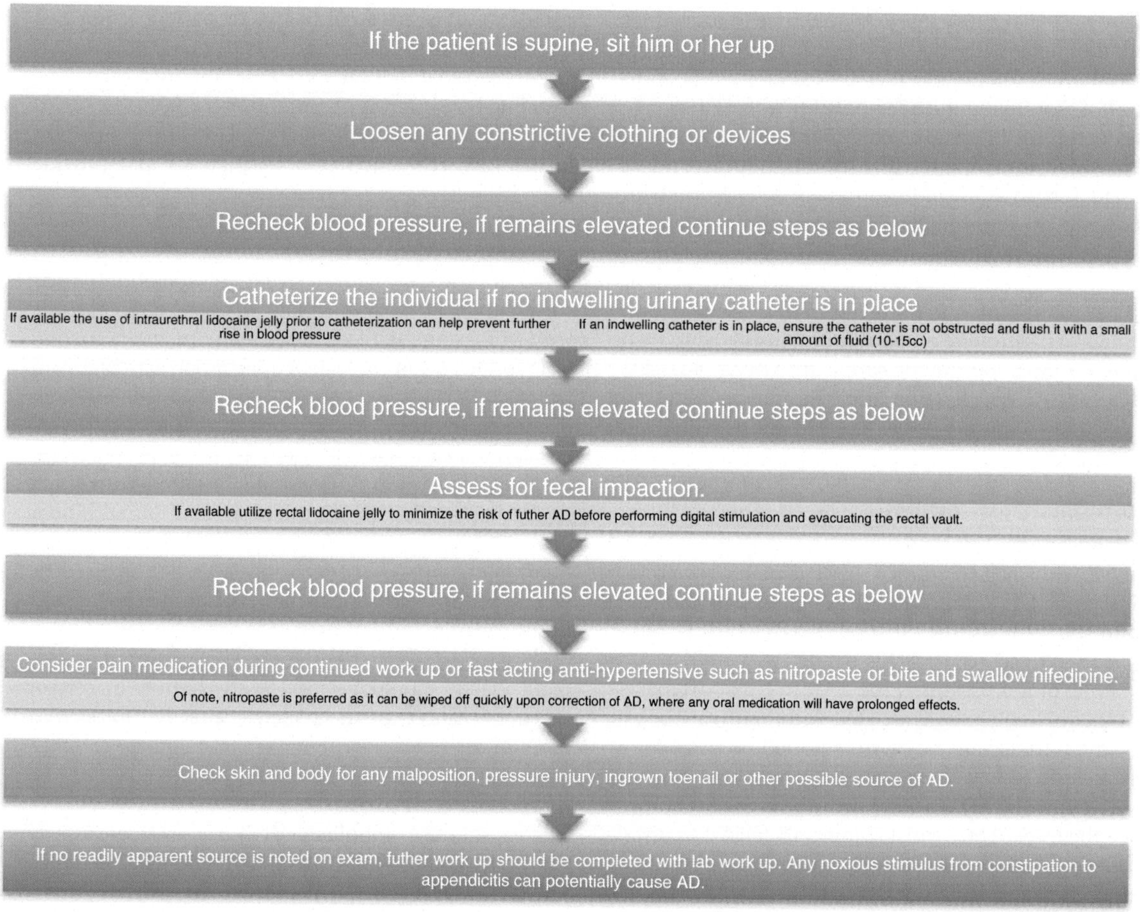

If the patient is supine, sit him or her up

↓

Loosen any constrictive clothing or devices

↓

Recheck blood pressure, if remains elevated continue steps as below

↓

Catheterize the individual if no indwelling urinary catheter is in place

If available the use of intraurethral lidocaine jelly prior to catheterization can help prevent further rise in blood pressure

If an indwelling catheter is in place, ensure the catheter is not obstructed and flush it with a small amount of fluid (10-15cc)

↓

Recheck blood pressure, if remains elevated continue steps as below

↓

Assess for fecal impaction.

If available utilize rectal lidocaine jelly to minimize the risk of futher AD before performing digital stimulation and evacuating the rectal vault.

↓

Recheck blood pressure, if remains elevated continue steps as below

↓

Consider pain medication during continued work up or fast acting anti-hypertensive such as nitropaste or bite and swallow nifedipine.

Of note, nitropaste is preferred as it can be wiped off quickly upon correction of AD, where any oral medication will have prolonged effects.

↓

Check skin and body for any malposition, pressure injury, ingrown toenail or other possible source of AD.

↓

If no readily apparent source is noted on exam, futher work up should be completed with lab work up. Any noxious stimulus from constipation to appendicitis can potentially cause AD.

FIG. 10.2 Flowchart for management of autonomic dysreflexia.

Osteoporosis and Pathologic Fractures

Patients with SCI alone are at greater risk of osteoporosis and heterotopic ossification (HO). Many patients with metastatic disease are also at risk for fracture (pathologic) and osteoporosis (chronic medication use or in the case of prostate cancer, androgen depravation). Studies in both patients with SCI and those with metastatic disease have shown little benefit to bisphosphonates in preventing osteoporosis. Vitamin D supplementation in both populations has shown benefit in overall bony health but not in preventing osteoporosis. In patients with SCI, those that are able to bear weight on their legs to stand or on their arms to transfer can reverse osteoporotic changes in those bones that are weight bearing, but those who do not regain functional use enough to weight bear will develop osteoporosis over time. The most common site of fragility fracture after SCI is in the femur. Patients with chronic SCI have been known to fracture this bone performing low-impact tasks such as crossing their legs or transferring. Owing to decreased sensation, patients may not notice these fractures until redness and swelling develop in the area. These are also signs of infection, VTE, and HO. Should a patient develop redness and swelling with no obvious abscess or fracture, a workup should be undertaken to determine the cause of the redness and swelling. The gold standard for diagnosis of HO is a triple phase bone scan. HO is treated aggressively since if left unchecked it can limit movement and even ankylose a joint. The preferred treatment for HO is etidronate, and it is most often dosed at 20 mg/kg daily for 2 weeks followed by 10 mg/kg daily for 10 weeks. Phosphorus levels should be monitored while on etidronate, and the dose of this medication may need to be decreased or even weaned entirely for persistent hyperphosphatemia.

Pulmonary Dysfunction

Patients with tetraplegia are at high risk for developing pneumonia and other pulmonary issues. Respiratory complications are the number one cause of death in persons with SCI. IPR for persons with tetraplegia and higher level paraplegia should include focused strengthening of accessory muscles of breathing such as pectoralis major and sternocleidomastoid. In addition, muscles of inspiration and expiration can be trained with inspiratory and expiratory resistive devices as well as aerobic exercise. Patients with complete tetraplegia at level C4 or above often need ventilator support for neurogenic respiratory failure. Some of these patients can be weaned from a ventilator but others may not. A diaphragm pacemaker can be used but is not always practical in those with metastatic disease. Generally those patients with high-level tetraplegia due to invasive tumor or cancer have very poor prognoses. Predictors of prognosis of weaning from the ventilator for those patients that require ventilator support include forced vital capacity (FVC) and negative inspiratory force (NIF). Those patients with FVC less than 800 cc or with NIF less than 40 cm H_2O are less likely of being able to wean from the ventilator. These prognostic indicators can be useful in decisions regarding appropriateness for admission to IPR and, if admitted, goal setting for these patients. In addition to potential need for ventilator support, patients with tetraplegia and mid-to-high level paraplegia suffer from difficulty clearing secretions. This is due to weakness of expiratory muscles, such as abdominals. These patients require abdominal binders when sitting up in bed to optimize the position of the diaphragm and may require regular chest percussion, nebulizers, postural drainage, and assistive cough in order to clear these secretions appropriately in order to avoid atelectasis and infection. Assistive cough can be performed manually by a nurse, caregiver, or family member or can be performed by using a cough assist machine. Even with proper care, patients with SCI will always be at increased risk of respiratory issues, including infection. This risk increases in the setting of primary lung cancer, metastases to the lungs, or metastases to any other part of the body that effect expansion of the lungs or function of the diaphragm. In addition, many patients with cancer are immunosuppressed and at higher risk of infection, a fact that makes proper respiratory care even more essential in this population.

Pressure Injuries

Pressure injuries are of particular concern in patients with SCI secondary to cancer. Any person with impaired sensation or mobility is at risk of pressure injuries. Pressure injuries can become infected. The presence of pressure injuries increases calorie and protein needs substantially. This can be an issue in the population of patients with SCI due to cancer given that increased caloric intake is required for strength gaining and muscle rebuilding in the first 2–3 months after SCI, but these patients often suffer from decreased appetite due to the cancer itself or even a paraneoplastic syndrome too. In addition, the tumor and host will battle for nutrients. A pressure injury acts as another competitor for these nutrients, a complication that could worsen the prognosis for such a patient. Patients with SCI with impaired mobility or sensation should be turned every 2 hours while in bed and should perform pressure reliefs every 20 minutes while sitting in order to prevent pressure injuries It is also important for these patients to avoid contact with hard surfaces for prolonged periods (e.g., feet abutting foot of hospital bed). Should a pressure injury develop, a physiatrist specialized in SCI or a wound care physician should be consulted.

Immunosuppression and Risk of Infection

Those patients with cancer often have cytopenia or are at higher risk of infection from chemotherapy, concurrent steroid use, and hypogammaglobulinemia secondary to hematologic disorders. While there is no literature to suggest that persons with SCI have depressed immune systems, they are more prone to infections given physiologic changes in respiration and bladder function and propensity to pressure injuries. Patients involved in IPR often perform exercises in a shared gymnasium with other patients. If a patient is at particularly high risk of infection, then proper precautions should be taken with that patient.

Pain of Spinal Cord Injury and Cancer

Perhaps the most common complication with either SCI or cancer is pain. Patients with SCI are prone to neuropathic and nociceptive pain as are patients with cancer affecting the nervous system. Patients with metastases may also experience visceral pain. For patients with SCI secondary to metastases or tumor and poor prognosis that have pain, opioid medications should be strongly considered in order to maximize quality of life. While opioid medication may be necessary in the acute phases of SCI, if a patient has a good prognosis and pain not related to metastases, these medications are best weaned before discharge from IPR. The most common pain in SCI due to cancer is nociceptive axial spine pain. It is often described as dull, achy, or throbbing. It is often made worse by sneezing, coughing, or any increase in intra-abdominal or intrathoracic pressure. It is also commonly made worse by lying down, facing up, or in a recumbent position. This type of pain is most often related to tumor burden itself. Neuropathic pain is a common occurrence following SCI for any reason. Neuropathic pain related to SCI is classified either as *at-level SCI pain* if it is localized at or within three dermatomes below the neurologic of injury or *below-level SCI* pain if it is localized to an area more than three dermatomes below the neurologic level, although it can also be present in the levels at or immediately below the neurologic level as well. Common descriptors of *at-level* and *below-level SCI pain* include "electric shock like," "numb," "tingling," "burning," or "tight pressure." First-line pharmacologic treatments for these types of pain include the gabapentinoids, pregabalin and gabapentin, and tricyclic antidepressants. A second-line treatment is the combination of weak opioid and serotonin-norepinephrine reuptake inhibitor (SNRI) tramadol. Other treatments that can be considered include other SNRIs such as duloxetine, although the evidence is weak for its effectiveness for the treatment of pain after SCI. Pain management is particularly important for participation in physical and occupational therapy. Pain control should be sufficient to allow patients to participate fully in therapies, but still allow the patient to be alert enough to follow commands and have carryover of techniques learned during therapies.

Blood and Electrolyte Disorders

Blood disorders are common in patients with different types of malignancies. Most notably for considerations in IPR is pancytopenia. Patients may present with low levels (white blood cells, hemoglobin, and platelets) or any combination of these. Patients with anemia will be more prone to OH and will appear more fatigued and less able to participate in IPR. Symptomatic anemia is most often treated with blood transfusion, but levels of hemoglobin below which a particular patient should be transfused should always be discussed with a patient's hematologist/oncologist. Patients with thrombocytopenia may be at risk of bleeding with certain types of rehabilitation. Safe levels of platelets to avoid bleeding should be established with a patient's hematologist/oncologist. Vital signs should be followed closely in these patients, and signs of hypovolemia (either from anemia or bleeding) such as tachycardia and hypotension should be taken seriously and assessed. Laboratory work should be followed weekly at minimum and more often in patients known to have or be at risk of pancytopenia or any other blood disorder.

Hypercalcemia often occurs in patients with cancer, especially those with breast cancer, lung cancer, and multiple myeloma. Severe hypercalcemia can be life-threatening, and a high index of suspicion is required to diagnose this condition. The most common subjective complaints of hypercalcemia are muscle cramps and associated pain. Laboratory workup is required for diagnosis, and treatment most often involves hydration, calcitonin, denosumab, and/or bisphosphonates. Patients with known kidney disease may require hemodialysis for hypercalcemia. A patient's oncologist should be called for any patient with symptomatic hypercalcemia or hypercalcemia greater than 12 g/dL.

Nutritional Considerations

Diet and nutritional considerations play a role in the IPR of persons with SCI due to cancer. The acute phase of SCI and paralysis results in a negative nitrogen balance (NB) and a state of hypercalcemia due to metabolic breakdown and processes. A negative NB is particularly important since nitrogen is essential in building muscle. Studies have shown that in patients with acute SCI even increasing protein intake to 2.4 g of protein per kilogram of ideal body weight per day could not prevent negative NB. Other nutritional deficiencies in acute SCI include albumin, carotene, transferrin, ascorbate, folate, and copper.

Accordingly, increased calorie and protein intake is essential for persons with SCI to maintain ideal body weight, replenish metabolites, and build muscle while healing from neurologic insult. This is even truer in persons with SCI due to cancer given competing nutritional needs: basal caloric needs, caloric needs for healing from SCI, and caloric needs of the cancer or tumor. This increased caloric need can become particularly difficult to address adequately in patients with cancer that often have decreased appetite as well as side effects from chemotherapy and radiation that make it difficult for them to eat. Without appropriate nutrition, these patients with both SCI and cancer can become malnourished more quickly than they would with either diagnosis alone.

Of note, after the acute phase of SCI, these persons require a decreased caloric intake relative to their amount of paralysis. Studies have shown that persons with tetraplegia require approximately 23 kcal/kg/day and those with paraplegia require 28 kcal/kg/day to maintain ideal body weight. This caloric intake often needs to be increased in those patients with cancer.

Mood Disorders

Patients with SCI due to cancer are at risk of depression, anxiety, and other mood disorders. The potential of permanent physical disability or death can be overwhelming and lead to a variety of mood disorders. It is essential to incorporate psychology in the IPR plan for these persons to discuss and help mediate these issues. It can be difficult to balance the need to motivate persons with SCI due to cancer to participate fully in IPR while addressing these psychologic needs, especially given the short lengths of stay allowed by insurances for the IPR of persons with SCI. Communication with the family and patient to establish goals for IPR is important from the outset of admission.

Initiation of antidepressant or anxiolytic medications should be strongly considered in these patients, especially in those patients with pain issues. Consult to psychiatry is beneficial in more difficult cases. Social work can also provide some degree of psychotherapy as well as be a welcome resource for the patient and family to coordinate continued care after discharge from IPR.

End-of-Life Considerations

Most patients admitted to IPR have experienced a traumatic event, but can look forward to improved medical status, functionality, and psychosocial state. This is not always the case for those patients admitted to IPR for SCI secondary to cancer as many of them will have poor long-term prognosis. This often necessitates difficult conversations that physiatrists are not accustomed to having.

For example, patients with SCI due to cancer should be educated on different considerations for resuscitation. Many of these patients may choose to become do not resuscitate (DNR) or do not intubate (DNI) status, but in order for them to make such a decision, not only is a thorough understanding of the meaning of DNR or DNI required but these patients should also have a full appreciation of their diagnosis and prognosis.

There are times that patients with SCI due to cancer are transferred to IPR without a complete diagnosis, perhaps from pending pathology, or without a full understanding of their prognosis. It is advised that on initial history and physical examination, the physiatrist take inventory of a patient's understanding of his or her medical status, especially regarding his or her prognosis in relation to both the SCI and the cancer diagnosis.

In the event that a diagnosis is pending upon transfer to IPR, it is best to discuss the diagnosis and prognosis with the patient's hematologist/oncologist when it is available. In a scenario in which the patient has no or incomplete knowledge of his or her diagnosis or prognosis related to cancer, it is advised to coordinate a meeting with the patient, any family members or friends the patient would like to attend, the patient's hematologist/oncologist, psychology, and hospice palliative care (if poor prognosis). This meeting should revolve around ensuring the patient understands his or her prognosis, the treatment options and plan, and the importance and goals of IPR (see the following section for further information on IPR goal setting). Occasionally, there are situations where other specialties are not available in person or over the phone to help discuss prognoses. In these cases the physiatrist is tasked with having these discussions. One should be honest without overstepping expertise. It is acceptable to give a diagnosis of cancer, but explain that a prognosis would be best given by a hematologist/oncologist and offer to coordinate this type of consult or conversation as soon as possible. Regardless of how this news is delivered, it will be emotional, and it is important to allow the patient time to process any information given and to ask any follow-up questions. It is also recommended that one ask the patient and his or her chosen family and friends whether they understand the information that was portrayed and even to ask them to speak back their interpretation of the news delivered. The meeting should close by reassuring the patient and any family or friends present that you are available for continued conversations and questions.

INPATIENT REHABILITATION

Goal Setting

The goals of IPR of persons with SCI secondary to cancer are largely driven by SCI level and by prognosis of the cancer or tumor. In order to qualify for IPR, a patient must have both medical and rehabilitative needs. Medical needs require daily physician oversight and may include but are not limited to management of pain, neurogenic bowel and bladder, and anticoagulation or blood glucose, for example. Rehabilitative needs require physical therapy (PT) plus either occupational or speech therapy. Specific needs that fall within the purview of PT include functional mobility tasks such as getting in and out of bed, transferring, and walking. Specific needs that fall within the purview of occupational therapy (OT) include the performance of activities of daily living (ADL) such as getting dressed and brushing one's teeth or bathing. It can also encompass cognitive tasks and evaluations, some of which are termed instrumental ADL, which may include the ability to make correct change or balance a checkbook. Speech therapy focuses on speech quality, swallow, and cognition.

IPR also optimally includes other members to make up a patient's care team. On SCI specialized units this would normally include recreational therapy, neuropsychology, and social work. Recreational therapy's focus lies in leveraging community integration as a form of rehabilitation for a patient with SCI. For example, a recreational therapist may take a patient with SCI to a movie theater during IPR. In the process of going to the movies the patient will need to either transfer into a vehicle or take public transportation, maneuver through a crowded movie theater, and carry a soda or snacks while pushing a wheelchair (WC). These are all important learning experiences for navigating everyday events and form a critical part of reintegration into society. A psychologist with experience in SCI is an essential team member. A patient with SCI secondary to cancer will have many psychologic hurdles related to his or her cancer prognosis and to his or her deficits related to SCI. The psychologic toll can be difficult to overcome and at times can be a hindrance to participation in therapies. Motivation, insight, and care given to the patient by the neuropsychology team can help patients optimize their time in IPR and help patients and their family members with the ultimate transition home.

Different levels of SCI can expect different outcomes. When first assessing a patient with SCI due to cancer for IPR, it is important to consider short- and long-term goals for that patient. Short-term goals normally begin with the plan for a safe discharge and education of the patient on how to care for himself or herself and how to guide others in best helping him or her. These short-term goals can be modified in persons with a poor prognosis from cancer to educate the family on some or all of the proper care for the patient. In these cases, the primary goal of IPR becomes family training and equipment assessments. This does not mean that the patient does not work toward goals of maximal independence during his or her IPR stay, but it does mean that the focus of the team should be to discharge the patient home to maximize his or her time in the home with his or her family. Table 10.1 shows expected maximal, long-term goals for patients with complete

TABLE 10.1
Goals for Persons With Complete Spinal Cord Injury due to Cancer

	C4 or Above	C5	C6	C7	C8 or Below
Feeding and grooming	Dependent	Modified independent to minimal assistance	Modified independent	Modified independent to independent	Independent
Dressing	Dependent	Assistance with upper body, dependent lower body	Some assistance with lower body	Modified independent to independent	Independent
Bathing	Dependent	Moderate to maximal assistance	Minimal assistance	Modified independent to contact guard assistance	Modified independent to independent
Bed mobility	Dependent	Moderate to maximal assistance	Close supervision or contact guard assistance	Modified independent	Independent
Transfers	Dependent	Moderate to maximal assistance	Contact guard assistance to minimal assistance	Modified independent	Independent
Wheelchair (WC)	Can drive power WC	Independent with power WC, may be able to use manual WC with adaptations	Use of manual WC with adaptations	Modified independent	Independent
Toileting	Dependent	Dependent	Modified independent	Modified independent	Independent

SCI based on injury level. For patients with good prognosis and complete SCI these goals should be attainable either during IPR or within the first 6 months of injury with proper outpatient follow-up and therapies. Patients with SCI secondary to tumor or cancer and incomplete injuries could achieve goals above and beyond those listed in the table. More than 70% of persons with traumatic SCI and an AIS of "D" and about 40% of those with traumatic SCI and AIS of "C" that receive IPR and proper outpatient follow-up after discharge will achieve ambulation with or without an assistive device. There are no studies to prognostic ambulation in patients with SCI secondary to cancer, but the aforementioned statistics could be used to set inpatient and long-term rehabilitation goals. Rehabilitation has been shown to have positive outcomes in persons with benign or malignant tumors of the spine leading to SCI. One study suggests that over 84% of those patients with SCI due to neoplasm were able to discharge home and at least maintained their functional level for 3 months after discharge. There have also been studies to suggest that how far a patient progresses functionally during IPR can influence prognostic survival. Poorer survival has been linked to those that gain less than 13 on the functional independence measure (FIM) and have an overall FIM score of less than 65.

Patients with SCI secondary to cancer may not be able to achieve all expected functional goals for a variety of reasons. Cancer-related fatigue is a significant issue during IPR. It is often best to front-load therapies earlier in the day when a patient is less likely to be experiencing symptoms of fatigue. Side effects of radiation or chemotherapy itself may also limit ability to participate in IPR. Common side effects such as nausea, diarrhea, and mood changes should be treated symptomatically and aggressively to ensure maximal quality of life and tolerance of therapies. Chemotherapy-induced peripheral neuropathy is also a serious problem. Peripheral neuropathies can lead to decreased sensation and proprioception making walking difficult for any person, especially those with SCI. These symptoms can arise many months following completion of chemotherapy and should be treated pharmacologically if painful. They should also be discussed with the patient's oncologist, especially if the patient is still undergoing chemotherapy as this could lead to a change in the patient's chemotherapy regimen.

The coordination of chemotherapy and radiation while on IPR can often be difficult for a variety of reasons. Foremost an IPR facility is typically reimbursed based upon a negotiated rate that typically does not include the costs of chemotherapy and radiation that can be significant and potentially cost prohibitive in this setting. This prevents many patients from being able to receive the care they need; either preventing them from receiving IPR or keeping them on a different hospital unit to receive chemotherapy. Radiation and chemotherapy can often cause fatigue and as such are best coordinated to be done later in the day after inpatient therapies have been completed. In the case of chemotherapy that is given once weekly or less, then the medication could be given on the evening prior to a day with little to no therapy staff present. Often this would be a Saturday evening leading into a Sunday.

A patient's cancer prognosis should guide the team's approach to the patient. Those patients with poor prognosis should have shorter lengths of stay focused on quality of life and family training. Palliative care, oncology, and neuropsychology should be heavily involved. Patients with the possibility of progressive disease should be followed closely after discharge from IPR as their functional needs could decline over time. For example, a patient could be discharged with a manual WC, but many months or years later may decline functionally and require a power WC. In the event of expected rapid decline, equipment should be ordered which can accommodate an anticipated lower functional level.

DISCHARGE PLANNING

Discharge planning should start on the day of a patient's admission to IPR. As noted, IPR length of stay and goal expectations will vary based on patients' injury level and prognosis of the tumor or cancer that led to his or her SCI. A family meeting (Table 10.2) is an essential part of discharge planning and of guiding family expectations of the immediate and long-term future. Family meetings are gatherings held with the patient, the patient's family or loved ones, and all members of the rehabilitation team. They are led by the physiatrist and should touch upon the patient's current status, the plan for IPR, and the plan for continued therapies upon discharging home.

Maximizing home and outpatient therapies is essential to achieving maximal functional recovery in patients with SCI secondary to cancer. Commonly, patients are discharged home with home PT and OT services. This aids in the transition home and also allows for therapists to assess a patient in his or her permanent environment and work on any problems that may arise in the home, for example, difficulty transferring in a bathroom that is more cramped than those in the hospital.

TABLE 10.2
Outline of Family Meeting

FAMILY MEETING		
Discuss Current Medical State/ Condition	**Discuss Goals for Inpatient Rehabilitation (IPR)**	**Discuss Long-Term Goals**
Ask the patient and family what his/her/their understanding is about the patient's status Fill in gaps of medical state condition as relates to the spinal cord injury • Prognosis, bowel, bladder, pain, etc. It is important to hear the patient and family and acknowledge any fears or apprehensions they have at several points during the meeting	Ask the patient and family what his/her/their expectations are • Include patient-specific desires (e.g., cooking if the patient was a chef) Physician to discuss overall goals of IPR discharge home as independent as possible, family training as needed, etc. Physical therapy, occupational therapy, and any other therapists to give their insights for goals during IPR and the next several months after discharge • Including equipment needs such as wheelchair and hospital bed	Ask the patient and family what his/her/their long-term goals are • Include patient-specific desires Physician to discuss achievable goals based on examination and current progress If appropriate, reassure the patient that goals are an educated estimation and they may be surpassed with hard work. If poorer prognosis, palliative care may be included in the meeting Neuropsychology to discuss their experience with the patient Social work to discuss equipment and home care options offered by the patient's insurance

After a brief period of transition, usually a month or less, the patient should transition to outpatient therapies in order to work on higher level goals and tasks.

Patients should also follow up regularly with a physiatrist specialized in SCI that can not only continue to coordinate outpatient therapies but also continue to communicate with patients and families regarding resources, expectations, equipment, pain, patient decline, and any other new or changing issues that arise after discharge from IPR. The management and rehabilitation of patients with SCI secondary to tumor or cancer is difficult and unpredictable. No two patients are the same, and a watchful eye is necessary to achieve the best quality-of-life outcome.

CONCLUSION

IPR for persons with SCI due to cancer is unique and requires an understanding of the medical issues specific to this population and an interdisciplinary approach not only enveloping the classical IPR model but also including necessary medical teams, such as hospice and palliative care or oncology, which can vary patient to patient. A patient's and said patient's family's goals are always important to consider, but it is the physician's responsibility to help navigate attainable quality-of-life goals within any prognostic and/or time restrictions given the nature of the patient's disease state. The impact of IPR for persons with SCI due to cancer is invaluable and can give people the opportunity to maximize their life moving forward after a life-changing diagnosis.

FURTHER READING

1. Carr J, Finlay P, Pearson D, Thompson K, White H. Neurological tumours and associated conditions. In: Rankin J, Robb K, Murtagh N, Cooper J, Lewis S, eds. *Rehabilitation in Cancer Care*. Oxford: Blackwell Publishing Ltd; 2008: 99–108.
2. Kirshblum S, O'Dell MW, Ho C, Barr K. Rehabilitation of persons with central nervous system tumors. *Cancer*. 2001;92(4 suppl):1029–1038.
3. Abrahm JL, Banffy MB, Harris MB. Spinal cord compression in patients with advanced metastatic disease: 'all I care about is walking and living my life. *JAMA*. 2008; 299(8):937–946.
4. Guo Y, Young B, Palmer JL, Mun Y, Bruera E. Prognostic factors for survival in metastatic spinal cord compression: a retrospective study in a rehabilitation setting. *Am J Phys Med Rehabil*. 2003;82(9):665–668.
5. Fitzsimmons A, Wen P. *Tumors of the Spinal Cord* [Chapter 99]; 2015. https://clinicalgate.com/tumors-of-the-spinal-cord/.

6. McKinley WO, Seel RT, Hardman JT. Nontraumatic spinal cord injury: incidence, epidemiology, and functional outcome. *Arch Phys Med Rehabil.* 1999;80(6):619–623.
7. McKinley W. Rehabilitation of patients with spinal cord dysfunction. In: Stubblefield MD, O'Dell MW, eds. *Cancer Rehabilitation: Principles and Practice.* New York: Demos Medical Publishing, LLC; 2009:533–550.
8. Heary RF, Bono CM. Metastatic spinal tumors. *Neurosurg Focus.* 2001;11(6):E1.
9. Bowers DC, Weprin BE. Intramedullary spinal cord tumors. *Curr Treat Options Neurol.* 2003;5(3):207–212.
10. Tan M, New P. Survival after rehabilitation for spinal cord injury due to tumor: a 12-year retrospective study. *J Neurooncol.* 2011;104(1):233–238.
11. Drudge-Coates L, Rajbabu K. Diagnosis and management of malignant spinal cord compression: Part 1. *Int J Palliat Nurs.* 2008;14(3):110–116.
12. Cowap J, Hardy JR, A'Hern R. Outcome of malignant spinal cord compression at a cancer center: implications for palliative care services. *J Pain Symptom Manage.* 2000; 19(4):257–264.
13. Sundaresan N, Sachdev VP, Holland JF, et al. Surgical treatment of spinal cord compression from epidural metastasis. *J Clin Oncol.* 1995;13(9):2330–2335.
14. Rades D, Karstens JH. A comparison of two different radiation schedules for metastatic spinal cord compression considering a new prognostic factor. *Strahlenther Onkol.* 2002;178(10):556–561.
15. Woodley R, Martin D. Chronic nontraumatic myelopathies. In: Lin V, ed. *Spinal Cord Medicine: Principles and Practice.* New York: Demos Medical Publishing, LLC; 2002:419–427.
16. Rampling R, Symonds P. Radiation myelopathy. *Curr Opin Neurol.* 1998;11(6):627–632.
17. Drudge-Coates L, Rajbabu K. Diagnosis and management of malignant spinal cord compression: part 2. *Int J Palliat Nurs.* 2008;14(4):175–180.
18. Nagata M, Ueda T, Komiya A, et al. Treatment and prognosis of patients with paraplegia or quadriplegia because of metastatic spinal cord compression in prostate cancer. *Prostate Cancer Prostatic Dis.* 2003;6(2):169–173.
19. Rades D, Rudat V, Veninga T, et al. A score predicting posttreatment ambulatory status in patients irradiated for metastatic spinal cord compression. *Int J Radiat Oncol Biol Phys.* 2008;72(3):905–908.
20. Le H, Balabhadra R, Park J, Kim D. Surgical treatment of tumors involving the cervicothoracic junction. *Neurosurg Focus.* 2003;15(5):E3.
21. Raco A, Esposito V, Lenzi J, Piccirilli M, Delfini R, Cantore G. Long-term follow-up of intramedullary spinal cord tumors: a series of 202 cases. *Neurosurgery.* 2005; 56(5):972–981.
22. Washington CM, Leaver DT. *Principles and Practices of Radiation Therapy.* 2nd ed. St Louis, MO: Mosby; 2004.
23. Baumann M, Budach V, Appold S. Radiation tolerance of the human spinal cord. *Strahlenther Onkol.* 1994;170(3): 131–139.
24. Nieder C, Andratschke NH, Grosu AL. Effects of radiotherapy and chemotherapy on sensory deficits from spinal cord damage. *Acta Oncol.* 2005;44(4):412–414.
25. McKinley WO, Conti-Wyneken AR, Vokac CW, Cifu DX. Rehabilitative functional outcome of patients with neoplastic spinal cord compression. *Arch Phys Med Rehabil.* 1996;77(9):892–895.
26. Foley KM. The treatment of pain in the patient with cancer. *CA Cancer J Clin.* 1986;36(4):194–215.
27. Bach F, Larsen BH, Rohde K, et al. Metastatic spinal cord compression, occurrence, symptoms, clinical presentations and prognosis in 398 patients with spinal cord compression. *Acta Neurochir (Wien).* 1990;107(1–2): 37–43.
28. Helweg-Larsen S, Sorensen PS. Symptoms and signs in metastatic spinal cord compression: a study of progression from first symptom until diagnosis in 153 patients. *Eur J Cancer.* 1994;30A(3):396–398.
29. Donnelly C, Eng JJ. Pain following spinal cord injury: the impact on community reintegration. *Spinal Cord.* 2005; 43(5):278–282.
30. Jadad AR, Browman GP. The WHO analgesic ladder for cancer pain management. Stepping up the quality of its evaluation. *JAMA.* 1995;274(23):1870–1873.
31. Mirrakhimov A. Hypercalcemia of malignancy: an update on pathogenesis and management. *North Am J Med Sci.* 2015;7(11):483–493.
32. Laven G, Chi-Tsou H, DeVivo M, Stover S, Kuhlemeir K, Fine P. Nutritional status during the acute stage of spinal cord injury. *Arch Phys Med Rehabil.* 1989;70(4):277–282.
33. Cox SA, Weiss SM, Posuniak EA, Worthington P, Prioleau M, Heffley G. Energy expenditure after spinal cord injury: an evaluation of stable rehabilitating patients. *J Trauma.* 1985;25(5):419–423.
34. Rodriguez D, Clevenger F, Osler T. Obligatory negative nitrogen balance following spinal cord injury. *J Parenter Enter Nutr.* 1991;15(3):319–322.
35. Stiens SA, Bergman SB, Goetz LL. Neurogenic bowel dysfunction after spinal cord injury: clinical evaluation and rehabilitative management. *Arch Phys Med Rehabil.* 1997;78(3 suppl):S86–S102.
36. Schiff D. Spinal cord compression. *Neurol Clin.* 2003; 21(1):67–86.
37. Miaskowski C, Cleary J, Burney R. *Guideline for the Management of Cancer Pain in Adults and Children. APS Clinical Practice Guideline Series, No 3.* Glenview, IL: American Pain Society; 2005.
38. Henry RF, Rilart R. Tumors of the spine and spinal cord. In: Kirshblum SK, Campagnolo DI, DeLisa JA, eds. *Spinal Cord Medicine.* Philadelphia: Lippincott Williams & Wilkins; 2002:480–497.
39. Davis A, Nagelhout MJ, Hoban M, Barnard B. Bowel management: a quality assurance approach to upgrading programs. *J Gerontol Nurs.* 1986;12(5):13–17.
40. Zejdlik CP. Reestablishing bowel control. In: Zejdlik CP, ed. *Management of Spinal Cord Injury.* 2nd ed. Boston: Jones and Bartlett; 1992:397–416.

41. Spinal Cord Medicine Consortium. Neurogenic bowel management in adults with spinal cord injury: a clinical practice guideline for healthcare providers. *J Spinal Cord Med.* 1998;21(3):248–293.
42. Reitz A, Haferkamp A, Wagener N, Gerner HJ, Hohenfellner M. Neurogenic bladder dysfunction in patients with neoplastic spinal cord compression: adaptation of the bladder management strategy to the underlying disease. *NeuroRehabilitation.* 2006;21(1):65–69.
43. Consortium for Spinal Cord Medicine. Bladder management for adults with spinal cord injury: a clinical practice guideline for health-care providers. *J Spinal Cord Med.* 2006;29(5):527–573.
44. Krassioukov A, Fulran J, Fehlings M. Autonomic dysreflexia in acute spinal cord injury: an under-recognized clinical entity. *J Neurotrauma.* 2004;20(8):707–716.
45. Consortium for Spinal Cord Medicine. *Acute Management of Autonomic Dysreflexia.* 2nd ed. 2001.
46. Krassioukov A, Eng J, Warburton D, Teassell R. A systematic review of the management of orthostatic hypotension following spinal cord injury. *Arch Phys Med Rehabil.* 2009;90(5):876–885.
47. Klastersky J. From best supportive care to early palliative care. *Curr Opin Oncol.* 2011;23(4):311–312.
48. Vargo MM, Gerber LH. Rehabilitation for patients with cancer diagnoses. In: DeLisa JA, ed. *Physical Medicine & Rehabilitation: Principles and Practice.* Philadelphia: Lippincott Williams & Wilkins; 2005:1771–1794.
49. Consortium for Spinal Cord Medicine Clinical Practice Guidelines. *Pressure Ulcer Prevention and Treatment Following Spinal Cord Injury: A Clinical Practice Guideline for Health-care Professionals.* 2nd ed. 2014.
50. Freifeld AG, Kaul DR. Infection in the patient with cancer. In: Abeloff MD, ed. *Abeloff's Clinical Oncology.* 4th ed. Philadelphia: Churchill Livingstone Elsevier; 2008:717–718.
51. Dworkin RH, O'Connor AB, Backonja M, et al. Pharmacologic management of neuropathic pain: evidence-based recommendations. *Pain.* 2007;132(3):237–251.
52. Levendoglu F, Ogun CO, Ozerbil O, Ogun TC, Ugurlu H. Gabapentin is a first line drug for the treatment of neuropathic pain in spinal cord injury. *Spine.* 2004;29(7): 743–751.
53. Cardenas DD, Warms CA, Turner JA, Marshall H, Brooke MM, Loeser JD. Efficacy of amitriptyline for relief of pain in spinal cord injury: results of a randomized controlled trial. *Pain.* 2002;96(3):365–373.
54. Siddall PJ, Cousins MJ, Otte A, Griesing T, Chambers R, Murphy TK. Pregabalin in central neuropathic pain associated with spinal cord injury: a placebo controlled trial. *Neurology.* 2006;67(10):1792–1800.
55. Levack P, Graham J, Kidd J. Listen to the patient: quality of life of patients with recently diagnosed malignant cord compression in relation to their disability. *Palliat Med.* 2004;18(7):594–601.
56. Murray PK. Functional outcome and survival in spinal cord injury secondary to neoplasia. *Cancer.* 1985;55(1): 197–201.
57. Eriks IE, Angenot EL, Lankhorst GJ. Epidural metastatic spinal cord compression: functional outcome and survival after inpatient rehabilitation. *Spinal Cord.* 2004;42(4): 235–239.
58. Tang V, Harvey D, Park Dorsay J, Jiang S, Rathbone MP. Prognostic indicators in metastatic spinal cord compression: using functional independence measure and Tokuhashi scale to optimize rehabilitation planning. *Spinal Cord.* 2007;45(10):671–677.
59. Raven RW. Rehabilitation of patients with paralyses caused by cancer. *Clin Oncol.* 1975;1(3):263–268.

CHAPTER 11

Rehabilitation of the Child with Brain and Spinal Cord Cancer

NAOMI KAPLAN, BSC (HONS), MBBS • COSMO KWOK, MD • RUTH E. ALEJANDRO, MD • HILARY BERLIN, MD

INTRODUCTION

Central nervous system (CNS) tumors account for 25% of all cancers in childhood.[1] Primary central nervous system tumors constitute the second most common tumor and most common solid tumor in children. Tumors of the CNS include both nonmalignant and malignant tumors of the brain and spinal cord and are the leading cause of pediatric cancer–related mortality, as well as significant morbidity.[1] Pediatric tumors of the brain and spinal cord differ from those occurring in adulthood in their relative incidences, histologic features, sites of origin, and responsiveness to therapy. Establishing accurate incidence rates for pediatric CNS tumors (PCNST) is a challenge not only because they are a very heterogeneous group with more than 100 distinct pathologic entities but also because of the variations in cancer registry requirements, classification changes, and improvements in diagnostic techniques over time. Brain metastases in children occur in 1%–20% of cases of pediatric cancer, compared with 20%–40% in adults.[2]

The Central Brain Tumor Registry of the United States (CBTRUS) estimates that approximately 4300 US children are diagnosed yearly.[3] Primary brain tumors are significantly more common and account for 98%–99% of childhood CNS tumors, whereas primary spinal cord tumors account for the remaining 1%–2%. Classification of primary CNS tumors is based on histopathology, although tumor location and extent of spread are important to consider for treatment and prognosis.[4]

This chapter will highlight aspects of CNS cancer in the pediatric population. The chapter will not detail emerging and experimental treatments, although this knowledge is also important when planning a pediatric cancer rehabilitation program.

Primary malignant CNS tumors are the second most common childhood malignancies, after hematologic malignancies, and they are the most common pediatric solid organ tumor. Although significant progress has been made with earlier tumor diagnosis and more effective therapies in the treatment of childhood cancers, significant mortality and morbidity are still associated with malignant brain tumors, more so than with leukemia. Incidence rates were initially increasing due to improvement in diagnostics after the introduction of computerized tomography (CT) and magnetic resonance imaging (MRI) in the 1970s and 1980s. This was followed by a decrease in incidence rates in all age groups by approximately 0.2% annually over the past 15 years due to advanced technologies and better treatment.

Overall, childhood cancers are rare, but their importance in the pediatric population is highlighted by the fact that PCNST are now the leading cause of cancer-related death in individuals between 1 and 19 years of age in the United States. Acknowledging the differences between pediatric and adult CNS cancer patients is important due to the important implications on future research, treatment, and prognostic factors. For example, specific histologic types are more common in children than in adults; significant differences exist in the molecular biology and tumor behavior of pediatric and adult glial tumors. A higher percentage of pediatric primary brain tumors are malignant. Owing to multimodal treatment regimens with chemotherapy, radiation therapy, and neurosurgery, coupled with aggressive supportive care regimens, overall pediatric survival rates continue to rise. Cure from cancer, however, is not without its complications. Every organ system can be affected by previous cancer therapy. Therefore, comprehensive long-term follow-up (LTFU) care is essential for this high-risk pediatric population, especially during their developmental maturation and as adult survivors. Pediatric cancer survivorship is associated with neurocognitive, musculoskeletal, and endocrine disorders, as well as a decreased quality of life (QoL) and quality of survivorship. The *Children's Oncology Group* (COG, https://www.survivorshipguidelines.org)[5] has developed evidence-based screening recommendations based on previous therapeutic exposure to be followed in LTFU care of physical late effects for pediatric survivors in survivorship care plans (SCPs). SCPs are used to guide optimal, individualized interdisciplinary care in oncology clinic settings and for transitioning to a primary care physician after young adulthood. SCPs include essential surveillance and screening recommendations to prevent and reduce late effects from exposure to cancer treatment. Based on a 2003 Institute of Medicine report entitled, *"Childhood Cancer Survivorship: Improving Care and Quality of Life,"* approximately 25% of survivors will experience a late effect that is life-threatening or severe.[6] It is essential for pediatric cancer survivors to receive annual, comprehensive LTFU care throughout childhood and into adulthood. LTFU care should be interdisciplinary in approach to ensure that patient-family-centered care is delivered.

TUMORS

Most cases of brain tumors in children are sporadic, although 5% are associated with hereditary syndrome with increased risk of various cancers. In neurofibromatosis type 1, neurofibromas predominantly affect the peripheral nervous system. In neurofibromatosis type 2, the associated tumors are schwannomas, meningiomas, and glial hamartomas. Children affected by tuberous sclerosis complex can have CNS tumors, including cortical hamartomas, subcortical glioneuronal hamartomas, subependymal glial nodules, and subependymal giant cell astrocytomas (most common). Cowden disease is associated with dysplastic gangliocytoma of the cerebellum, a benign tumor. Von Hippel-Lindau disease has associated hemangioblastomas of the nervous system and retina. Turcot syndrome is associated with glioblastoma. Li-Fraumeni syndrome is characterized by multiple primary neoplasms in children and young adults, including low-grade astrocytomas, anaplastic astrocytomas, and glioblastomas, medulloblastomas, and primitive neuroectodermal tumor. Nevoid basal-cell carcinoma syndrome is also associated with medulloblastoma. In rhabdoid tumor predisposition syndrome, atypical teratoid rhabdoid tumor is a highly malignant CNS tumor.[7]

Environmental exposure from ionizing radiation, such as previous radiotherapy (due to recurrent diagnostic imaging or treatment), has been implicated in meningiomas, gliomas, and nerve sheath tumors. No convincing evidence has demonstrated a link with trauma, diet, or electromagnetic fields.

Histologically benign tumors can be life-threatening because of the space-occupying effects within the skull, local infiltration, and for some, a risk for malignant transformation. Significant morbidity from both the disease and treatment results in decreased health-related quality of life (HRQoL).

Primary brain tumors arise from one of many different cell types in the CNS. Diagnosis, treatment, and prognosis depend on the tumor cell of origin, pattern of growth, and location.

Brain tumors are categorized as hemispheric tumors, middle fossa tumors, or posterior fossa tumors. Spinal cord tumors are classified as intradural or extradural. Intradural tumors can be intramedullary or, more commonly, extramedullary.

Astrocytomas can arise anywhere in the CNS. Presenting symptoms depend on tumor location, rate of tumor growth, tumor size, and chronologic/developmental age of the child. Low-grade astrocytomas presenting in the hypothalamus may result in diencephalic syndrome, which results in failure to thrive in an emaciated and seemingly euphoric child with little other neurologic findings.[8] Diagnosis is often limited to MRI of the brain or spine. Classification is based on World Health Organization (WHO) histologic grade (grade I and II are low, whereas grade III and IV are high). More than 80% of astrocytomas located in the cerebellum are low grade; malignant tumors are rare in this location.[4,9] High-grade astrocytomas are locally invasive, extensive, and tend to occur above the tentorium in the cerebrum.[10,11] Astrocytomas arising in the brainstem may be of any grade, although tumors exclusively involving the pons tend to be high grade, and those outside the pons tend to be low grade.[12,13]

Prognosis for low-grade astrocytomas is generally favorable. Unfavorable prognostic features include young age, diencephalic syndrome, inability to obtain complete resection, intracranial hypertension at initial presentation, certain oncomutations, and presence of metastases.[14] High-grade astrocytomas carry a poor prognosis.

About two-thirds of childhood ependymomas arise in the posterior fossa. The most common subtype is EPN-PFA. EPN-PFA has a high rate of disease recurrence

(33% progression-free survival at 5 years) and low survival rates compared with other subtypes (68% at 5 years). The EPN-PFB subtype is less common but carries a more favorable prognosis: 73% progression-free survival at 5 years and 100% overall survival at 5 years.[15] Spinal cord ependymomas make up about 13% of all ependymomas, 30% of which occur in the cervical spinal cord.[16]

Infratentorial (posterior fossa) ependymomas may present with signs and symptoms of obstructive hydrocephalus (due to obstruction of the fourth ventricle), ataxia, neck pain, or cranial nerve palsies. Supratentorial ependymomas may present with seizures, headaches, or focal neurologic deficits based on location of the tumor. Spinal cord ependymomas may present with back pain, lower extremity weakness, or bowel/bladder dysfunction. MRI and cerebrospinal fluid (CSF) cytology are useful for diagnostic evaluation. Treatment generally involves surgery with or without adjuvant radiation therapy. Chemotherapy does not play a role in treatment,[17] except in some cases for children under 3 years of age.[18]

Embryonal tumors comprise 20%–25% of primary CNS tumors in children, clustered early in life (11 cases per million at the ages under 5, 7 cases per million at ages 5–9, and 3–4 cases per million at ages 10–19).[19] Medulloblastomas comprise the majority of pediatric embryonal tumors; these arise in the posterior fossa and account for 40% of all posterior fossa tumors. Other forms of embryonal tumors each make up 2% (or less) of all childhood brain tumors.

Clinical features depend on tumor location and age at the time of diagnosis. These tumors are fast growing and usually diagnosed within 3 months of symptom onset.[20] In about 80% of children, medulloblastomas arise in the fourth ventricle, with symptoms related to CSF blockage (hydrocephalus): headaches, nausea, vomiting, lethargy, ataxia, nystagmus, or papilledema.[21] A total of 20% of patients will not have symptoms of hydrocephalus initially and may instead present with cerebellar deficits.

Nonmedulloblastoma embryonal tumors generally present rapidly. Supratentorial embryonal tumors can result in focal neurologic deficits, and pineoblastomas can result in Parinaud syndrome. Diagnosis is made by MRI or CT (MRI preferred), with CSF evaluation if safe. Treatment includes surgery with adjuvant chemo- and radiation therapy.

Atypical teratoid/rhabdoid tumor (AT/RT) is a clinically aggressive and rare tumor that most often affects children 3 years of age or younger. One half of AT/RT tumors arise in the posterior fossa. Diagnosis is made with MRI of the brain/spine and CSF evaluation. There is no current standard of treatment; multimodal management with chemo- and radiation therapy, as well as surgery, is under current evaluation. Exact incidence is unknown, as this tumor has been widely recognized only in the last two decades. The Austrian Brain Tumor Registry (1996–2006) has shown that AT/RTs represent the sixth most common malignant brain tumor, with a peak incidence during the first 2 years of life.[22] Clinical presentation typically includes only a short history (days to weeks) due to rapid growth of the tumor. Signs and symptoms are dependent on tumor location, typically the posterior fossa. Patients often present with symptoms related to hydrocephalus, such as vomiting, lethargy, and early morning headaches.

Prognostic factors are not fully delineated at this time. Factors associated with poor outcome include age under 2 years, metastases at time of diagnosis, subtotal resection of tumor, and germline mutation.

Craniopharyngiomas are relatively uncommon, accounting for up to 10% of all intracranial tumors in children.[23] They occur in the region of the pituitary gland, so endocrine function can be affected. Proximity to the optic chiasm can result in visual deficits. Obstructive hydrocephalus due to tumor growth can also occur.[24] Diagnosis is made based on CT or MRI findings. Prognosis is good, with a long-term event-free survival of ~65% in children, with 5- and 10-year survival rates over 90%.[25]

CNS germ cell tumors (GCTs) are a heterogeneous group that make up 0.5% of all primary brain tumors; 90% of all cases are diagnosed before the patient's 20th birthday. CNS GCTs arise twice as frequently in the pineal region compared with the suprasellar region of the brain. A total of 5%–10% of patients have involvement of both regions at the time of diagnosis.[26] Tumors arising in the pineal region have a shorter history of signs and symptoms (weeks to months) that include raised intracranial pressure, diplopia, Parinaud syndrome, headache, nausea, and vomiting. Tumors arising in the suprasellar region present subtly with symptoms spanning months to years, including diabetes insipidus, visual deficits, and hormonal symptoms.[27,28] Diagnosis is made using clinical signs and symptoms, tumor markers (AFP and β-HCG), neuroimaging (MRI brain and spine with gadolinium), and lumbar CSF.

TREATMENT

The general goal of treatment mirrors that of adults. Surgical resection is often first-line treatment, although location of tumor can restrict success. Often, with low-grade tumors, removal of tumor and observation is sufficient. Adjuvant treatment (chemotherapy and radiation therapy) is usually reserved for higher grade and recurrent tumors. Owing to the well-known debilitating effects of radiation on growth and neurologic development, especially in younger children, chemotherapy may play a larger role than radiation therapy for children, depending on type of tumor.[29]

For low-grade gliomas/astrocytomas, surgical resection is primary treatment, although observation has played a role in some incidentally found cases or asymptomatic masses.[30] Lesions in the cerebellum, cerebrum, optic nerve, hypothalamus, thalamus, brainstem, and spinal cord are generally well resected, but optic nerve lesions may result in blindness and the midline structures may result in more significant neurologic sequelae. About 50% of cases that have less than gross total resection remain progression free at 5–8 years.[31] Chemotherapy for low-grade gliomas include carboplatin with or without vincristine[32] or a combination of thioguanine, procarbazine, lomustine, and vincristine.[33] In optic pathway gliomas, targeted therapy with bevacizumab plus irinotecan can result in visual improvement.[34]

For high-grade gliomas/astrocytomas, the extent of tumor resection correlates with prognosis.[35] Chemotherapy should be considered first as an adjuvant therapy, which can obviate the need for radiation therapy. Commonly used chemotherapy agents include lomustine, vincristine, and temozolomide.[36] For AT/RT tumors, surgical resection with or without adjuvant therapy is also the primary treatment. However, in AT/RT tumors, radiation therapy is more effective and can play a more prominent role.[37] For CNS GCTs, surgical resection with or without adjuvant therapy is the primary treatment protocol for teratomas, although chemoradiation therapy can avoid the need for surgery in germinomas as they are highly sensitive to chemoradiation.[38] Craniopharyngiomas treated with surgery alone or with adjuvant radiation therapy carry an excellent survival rate without the need for chemotherapy.[39] Treatment of ependymomas generally involves surgery with or without adjuvant radiation therapy; chemotherapy does not play a role in treatment[17] except in some cases for children under 3 years of age.[18] In embryonal tumors, treatment consists of surgery with or without adjuvant chemotherapy and radiation therapy; for children age 3 years or younger, radiation therapy is avoided.[40] Chemotherapy regimens include the combination of cisplatin, lomustine, and vincristine or the combination of cisplatin, cyclophosphamide, and vincristine; additionally, etoposide, methotrexate, mafosfamide may also be used for high-risk medulloblastomas.[41,42]

OUTCOMES AND PROGNOSIS

Overall prognosis depends on the likelihood of a cure. Functional outcomes depend on many factors including type and location of cancer, age at the time of diagnosis, function/deficits at the time of diagnosis, expected neurologic recovery or deterioration, and treatment. Deficits from treatment, including those related to surgery, chemotherapy, and radiation, will vary depending on type of tumor, location, extent of resection, type of chemotherapy, and RT. Intraoperative monitoring with somatosensory evoked potentials and transcranial motor evoked potentials can help predict postoperative deficits.[43] Brain mapping improves outcomes by aiding in surgical planning and reducing surgery-related morbidity.[44] Boys have higher cancer mortality than girls.[45]

More than 50% of PCNST are in the posterior fossa.[46] Following surgery, the incidence of posterior fossa syndrome has been reported as 28%.[47] Children may present with cerebellar mutism, dysarthria, slow speech, stuttering, or nasal-sounding speech. Swallow and feeding may also be impacted. Other findings may include neurobehavioral and emotional problems, as well as decreased initiation of voluntary movements. Factors related to the development of cerebellar mutism may include tumor type, with a higher incidence in children with medulloblastoma, midline location, and brainstem involvement.

Other CNS deficits, as seen in children with brain injury, include dysphagia, auditory impairment, hemiplegia (in up to 21% of survivors),[48] weakness, cognitive impairment, vision deficits, and cranial nerve palsies.

Surgical resection is often recommended for pediatric intramedullary spinal cord tumors and is associated with significant morbidity, including weakness/paralysis, bowel and bladder dysfunction, spinal instability, and spinal deformity.

Short-term side effects of radiation therapy depend on age of the child, location, and dose. Radiation over the spinal cord or the vertebral column can lead to bony effects and radiation myelopathy.

Short-term impairments from chemotherapy include neuropathy, bowel and bladder dysfunction, fatigue, myositis, swallowing difficulties, hearing loss, memory loss, and impairment of executive function.

Late effects are "health problems caused by cancer disease or treatment... [They] can occur during treatment or even decades after treatment is completed."[49] Over time, the prevalence of late effects increases.[50,51] The severity of late effects is variable, from chronic conditions to life-threatening health problems.[51] Survivors may not be aware of the risk for late effects[49] and may not have any symptoms at the time of transition to long-term care.[52] It is important that these patients are not lost to follow-up.[52] The risk of late effects can be minimized by long-term care from a provider who has detailed knowledge of the patient's cancer history and understanding of appropriate screening and surveillance.[53]

Discussion about late effects should be initiated early,[54] delivered in a balanced and patient-centered manner, and include discussion of physical and psychosocial late effects, routine screening schedule, and lifestyle education.[49] Physical late effects can be grouped into various categories: problems with growth and development, organ dysfunction, reproductive health, and risk of secondary cancers.[51] Late effects can be particularly challenging to pediatric cancer survivors, who may still be young and find it difficult to conceptualize future risk when they currently have no symptoms.[49] Some centers provide survivors and their families with educational "portfolios" that include information about late effects, long-term risks, and necessary follow-up care. This can help greatly with transition to LTFU care and patient self-advocacy.[52] Although late effects can be anticipated, and risks minimized, the prevalence and manifestation of these effects can vary, depending on patient factors (age, genetics, lifestyle, comorbidities), follow-up times, and means of risk assessment.[51]

There has been an overall decrease in pediatric cancer mortality; however, compared with matched cohorts, survivors have increased morbidity and mortality beyond their 40s, with females undergoing a steeper age-dependent decline than males.[51] Pediatric cancer survivors have higher rates of late onset health problems than their siblings or the age-matched general population.[55]

Specific late effects that will be discussed in more detail are neurocognitive deficits, hearing loss, endocrine morbidity, reproductive dysfunction, and fatigue. St Jude Lifetime Cohort (SJLIFE) should be mentioned by name as generating significant research regarding outcomes for pediatric cancer survivors.[56]

Platinum-based chemotherapy increases the risk of developing sensorineural hearing loss.[57] This risk is increased in patients who received platinum-based chemotherapy aged less than 5 years and/or those who received high-dose treatment (>400 mg/m^2).[57] Hearing loss can also present after a latent period in patients who received cranial irradiation.[57] Survivors associate serious hearing loss with negative impact on education and vocation. Although not statistically significant, survivors affected by hearing loss also report deleterious impact on their social functioning.[57]

Alkylating chemotherapy is associated with ovarian dysfunction.[50] Pediatric cancer survivors are at 13 × higher risk of undergoing premature menopause than their siblings.[50] Infertility as a late effect is associated with reduced QoL in survivors.[50,53]

Chemotherapy and radiotherapy are both gonadotoxic. Patients may have mild early puberty (due to premature GnRH activation) and then experience premature ovarian failure or azoospermia.[58] In other patients, surgery and irradiation may lead to arrest of pubertal development. Pituitary growth hormone (GH) deficit can be due to brain injury from cancer or from treatment such as surgery, chemotherapy, and/or radiotherapy.[58] GH deficit can be treated with replacement, although skeletal damage is only partially reversible.[55]

Pediatric brain tumor survivors (PBTS) are at risk of academic/intellectual deficits. They are less likely to graduate from high school than their unaffected classmates,[59] which can have a major impact on life trajectory. They have lower achievement in spelling, reading, and arithmetic.[59] Difficulties with reading and arithmetic are associated with chemotherapy and whole brain irradiation.[59] Difficulties with reading and spelling are more likely to be seen in PBTS who were diagnosed with cancer at a younger age.[59] Over time, PBTS will experience age-referenced intellectual and academic decline. Reading deficits in PBTS may be improved with remedial training and emphasis on phonologic skills.[59]

Other areas of neurocognitive deficit in PBTS include reduced attention, processing speed, and executive function.[60] Deficits can be seen in children who have had surgery only, even without chemo- or radiotherapy.[60] Survivors of CNS tumor are at greater risk than pediatric leukemia survivors.[60] Cognitive training programs are safe interventions that carry no adverse effects.[60] The literature has shown that attention is a good target for cognitive remediation.[60] Working memory and mathematics also show potential. Executive function can be more difficult to target for intervention. Exercise is also a low-risk intervention which can have benefits for cognition, as it may help to promote neuroplasticity.[60] The size and/or severity of the cancer insult is not always proportional to the neurocognitive deficits; some neural circuitry can be more resilient than other networks.[60] There is ongoing research looking at modafinil for brain tumor survivors, and metformin for cognition in pediatric populations.[60] Overall, PBTS should be assessed for neurocognitive deficits, if patient, family, caregivers, or educators express concerns. Tools include NIH Toolbox (<2 h to administer) and a brief computer-based battery Cogstate.[60] A multi-approach intervention plan may be of most benefit.

Fatigue is a prevalent late effect in pediatric cancer survivors, which can be very distressing. It is important to address pain management, sleep hygiene, and mood when trying to reduce fatigue.[55] Behavioral strategies (e.g., relaxation and lifestyle changes) and psychosocial interventions (e.g., cognitive behavioral therapy and self-coping strategies) can both be used to manage fatigue.[55] The literature shows that exercise provides moderate improvement in cancer-related fatigue [55] and should be encouraged.

Pain can be vague and nonspecific, especially in pediatric patients; however, it is important to manage to improve QoL. Of note, pain is the most common presenting symptom of spinal cord tumors.[61] When CNS tumors are treated, pain often improves; however, certain types of pain may persist, e.g., neuropathic pain.[62] Nociceptive pain can be managed as per the WHO analgesic ladder, starting with simple analgesics and escalating accordingly.[62] Neuropathic pain may respond to certain anticonvulsant or antidepressant medications.[62] In the pediatric population, attention must be paid to weight-adjusted dosing. If pain is difficult to control, it is beneficial to consult a pain team or pediatric palliative care (PPC) team.[62]

Other symptoms that may need management in pediatric CNS cancer cases include agitation, insomnia, spasms, seizures, vomiting, constipation, dyspnea, and respiratory secretions.[63] Complementary care for pain and symptom management can include music therapy, mind/body therapy (including meditation), dance and movement therapy, yoga, and touch/massage therapy.[64,65]

REHABILITATION AND THE PHYSIATRIST'S ROLE

A total of 500,000 adult survivors of childhood cancer are expected to be living in the United States by 2020.[66] A 5-year relative survival rate for children with cancer of the CNS varies between 20% (glioblastoma) up to 95% (low-grade astrocytoma).[67] Along with increased survival comes the impact of persistent disability, QoL impact, and premature mortality. The interdisciplinary approach to cancer care should include rehabilitation to optimize function, along with support services to include QoL and pain management. The multidisciplinary approach in the rehabilitation of a child with brain and spinal cord cancer includes the child and family, physicians, physical, occupational, and speech therapists, along with psychosocial support and involvement of the school. Goals of rehabilitation for a child with cancer of the brain or spinal cord, like those of brain or spinal cord injury, can include regaining skills that were affected by the tumor or because of treatment, improving and maintaining function to the maximum extent possible, developing new, age-appropriate skills, and optimizing QoL. Motor deficits and mobility impairment, deficits in cognition (memory, thinking, attention, problem-solving, reasoning), ADLs, speech, feeding, and play skills all need to be addressed, as well as management of learning, behavior, and emotional wellbeing.

Various approaches have been reported to address the provision of rehabilitation to cancer patients throughout the continuum from diagnosis through end of life. Dietz [68] defined four categories of rehabilitation intervention: preventive to lessen effects, restorative to return to prior level of function, supportive to accommodate change, and palliative for increasing level of disability and advanced disease. The cancer care trajectory [69] created a framework to integrate palliative, psychosocial, and rehabilitative care across the continuum through cancer-directed treatment, survivorship, and end of life.

Rehabilitation should start once the child is well enough and stabilized in the acute care setting, and it can continue through survivorship or end of life. The specific goals are determined based on individual needs and expected deficits/outcomes and should incorporate the family and child's plan. The rehabilitation team provides communication and management of expectations at initial consult and throughout provision of services, continued review of the treatment plan, updating of goals and level of service based on medical condition (fatigue, treatment effects, disease progression), and support to family and child.

Pediatric physiatrists play an important role as experts in implementing and coordinating cancer rehabilitation programs via an interdisciplinary team approach. They can optimize the rehabilitation of a cancer patient by identifying and treating neuromusculoskeletal impairments, spasticity, pain, fatigue, bladder/bowel dysfunction, neuro-arousal, and sleep hygiene. Pediatric physiatrists can address barriers in therapy for better participation, coordinate therapies with appropriate dissemination of medical histories to therapists, and define medical therapy precautions and appropriate modalities based on individualized clinical status. In addition, they can prescribe prosthetics, orthotics, and equipment as needed and coordinate an interdisciplinary team approach with a patient- and family-centered focus.

Depending on the needs of the child and other factors, therapy can be provided in the acute hospital setting, an inpatient rehabilitation setting (either acute or subacute), outpatient, or home. School-age children will have access to educationally based rehabilitation services in the home or school setting.

In the period after diagnosis and during early treatment, the rehabilitation specialist can formulate a program to address bed mobility, ADLs, maintenance of strength, and prevention of effects of immobility related to prolonged bed rest or cancer-related motor deficits. Specific attention is paid to pain management, skin integrity, and family education. Based on the treatment plan, functional deficits, and child/family plan, the appropriate venue for ongoing service provision, whether restorative or supportive, can be determined. The child may require further assessment and intervention for deficits related to surgery, chemotherapy, or RT, as well evaluation of the home for modifications, equipment needs, and need for support services.

During outpatient cancer treatment, the physiatrist can aid in anticipating further weakness or deconditioning from ongoing treatment, treat neuropathy, manage cognitive impairments, spasticity, ataxia, and pain, as well as determine the need for equipment, bracing, and educational support. Support of the child and their family should take into consideration their own views of rehabilitation needs.

With advancing delivery models of care for childhood cancer survivors, there will be an increasing need for pediatric physiatry specialists as part of the medical team to use their neuromusculoskeletal expertise and interdisciplinary team skills approach in SCPs. Lifetime surveillance of these high-risk survivors is needed to monitor late effects and their impact on affected organ systems. Pediatric physiatrists are uniquely placed to coordinate comprehensive LTFU with various other pediatric specialists, such as oncologists, cardiologists, gastroenterologists, neurosurgeons, endocrinologists, neurologists, and neuropsychologists.

In children who have entered surveillance, it is necessary to monitor for signs of recurrence and late effects and to provide physician input for appropriate rehabilitation, education, and social services. For progressive or recurrent cancer, review of the palliative care plan of child and family will assist with a shift in rehabilitation goals.

Pediatric rehabilitation specialists play an important role in palliation, especially in progressive or recurrent cancer cases. Goals are set to maintain mobility and function where possible, provide comfort care and pain management, manage new onset conditions from tumor or treatment, review and adjust equipment and home needs, provide anticipatory guidance, optimize fall/injury prevention, and maintain skin integrity.

Rehabilitation treatment modalities can be applied to pediatric CNS cancer patients. Exercise interventions have been studied in adult cancer patients. There is limited literature on exercise interventions in the pediatric oncology population, most of which is conducted with acute lymphoblastic leukemia patients. A systematic review found exercise to be feasible with benefits in managing disease and treatment-related side effects of strength, fatigue, and QoL.[70,71] Small studies and case reports for treatment of deficits in children with PCNST include constraint-induced movement therapy (CIMT) and treadmill training. A pilot study of CIMT in children with hemiplegia resulting from brain tumors, 1–10 years out from diagnosis, showed improved quality and use of the affected upper extremity, while maintaining HRQoL.[72] Treadmill training can be incorporated into a rehabilitation program after resection of spinal cord tumors.[73]

SCHOOL REINTEGRATION

The diagnosis and treatment of pediatric CNS cancer occurs at a time of life which is extremely disruptive to a child's academic career and their learning. As the survival rate of pediatric CNS cancer increases, so does the number of children returning to school.

Children with CNS cancer are more likely to repeat a grade and have reduced academic achievement compared with their healthy siblings.[74] Late effects, particularly those related to chemo- and radiation therapy exposure can worsen academic outcomes, which in turn has a negative impact on QoL.[74]

School reintegration for pediatric cancer survivors is crucial and requires careful coordination between family, physicians, and educators. Children and their families can receive services very early in the pediatric cancer journey; therefore school reintegration planning should start at the time of diagnosis.

Physiatrists should have knowledge of educational services available to children undergoing cancer treatment, as they can provide crucial documentation that allows children and families to access the services they need. Letters should be provided if children are missing class due to clinic appointments, medical treatment, or inpatient rehabilitation so that they are not taken off their school register due to absences.[74] In certain cases, children who are homebound can receive instruction in the home through the public school system, provided that their physician documents how the illness and disability affect "major life activities" and how the child's physical and cognitive deficits impact their needs.[74] It is gold standard care for students with pediatric brain cancer to be assessed by a neuropsychologist, and if not provided, parents can have their child independently assessed with costs covered by the school district.

Pediatric rehabilitation specialists can be involved in the process of children obtaining special education through the Individuals with Disabilities Education Act. Children who are not yet of school age (even those as young as 3 years old) are still entitled to educational services through their local school district. A child receiving *medically* relevant therapies from outside school is still entitled to *academically* relevant therapies from their school district should they need them.[74]

Pediatric cancer survivors frequently have ongoing medical needs. An individual healthcare plan is a physician formulated plan, which outlines a student's medical needs, treatment history, medications, and side effects, as well as an action plan for specific emergencies.[74] This plan can be executed at school by the school nurse.

For students with pediatric CNS cancer, it may be necessary to build up their class schedule gradually, starting with half days and scheduled downtime. School reintegration can be best achieved when there is clear communication of a child's medical and functional condition, as well as their educational and health-related needs.[74] Physiatrists can play a major role in providing documentation for pediatric CNS cancer survivors to access resources to facilitate school reintegration.

TRANSITION

Pediatric CNS cancer survivors will age out of pediatric care and must transition to adult, LTFU care. Transition can be defined as "purposeful, planned movement of adolescents with chronic health conditions from child-centered to adult-oriented health systems."[52] At the time of transition, survivors start to assume full responsibility for their healthcare needs. It cannot be emphasized enough that a smooth and comprehensive transition from pediatric oncology care to LTFU care is critical to reducing morbidity and mortality from late effects and increasing QoL in pediatric CNS cancer survivors.[52] LTFU care should be provided by skilled physicians who know the patient's cancer history in depth and understand the specific late effects associated with the type of cancer and its treatment, which may require long-term screening and surveillance.[52]

A significant contributor to a successful transition to LTFU care is the survivor's readiness to transition. This can be perceived within a SMART framework: "social-ecological model of adolescent and young adult readiness for transition."[75] There are reversible and irreversible factors that contribute to readiness to transition. These include (1) patient worry, (2) self-management skills (SMSs), and (3) expectations of adult LTFU care.[52,75]

Worry can work both to facilitate and block successful transition to LTFU care. Cancer worry can be measured and followed during this transitional period.[52] Patient expectations should be discussed, as adolescents and young adults (AYAs) may be unfamiliar with the differences between pediatric care and adult follow-up.

SMSs allow a patient to manage their healthcare needs and navigate the transitional period. SMSs include, but are not limited to, booking appointments, taking medications, and attending relevant screening and surveillance testing.[75] Work and school obligations are frequent reasons given for missed appointments.[52] A lack of SMSs can lead to ongoing dependence on parents and caregivers, which is a barrier to transition. SMS interventions are associated with improved healthcare outcomes.[75] These interventions should take place ideally before the transition to LTFU care. Better SMSs are seen in older, female patients. Leukemia survivors have more SMSs than CNS tumor survivors. Therefore, interventions for improving SMSs may be of most benefit if they are targeted at younger, male, CNS tumor survivors.[75]

There is evidence to show that AYAs may use complementary or alternative medicine during the transition period.[76] There is qualitative data describing spirituality and faith as an important coping mechanism when moving through the journey of diagnosis to survivorship.[54]

Unfortunately, the social transition for pediatric CNS cancer survivors to adulthood is often unsuccessful. In CNS cancer survivors over the age of 18 years who are 10 years out from diagnosis, as much as 69% are not living independently, 79% are not married, and 61% never graduated high school.[57] The underlying etiology of these statistics is likely multifactorial, relating to physical and cognitive deficits, late effects, and disruption of milestones at a formative time of life.

AYA CNS cancer survivors have lower health literacy than adult cancer survivors, which can lead to poorer health status.[55] Cancer health literacy is even more complex. It is important to cater to the needs of AYA cancer survivors with information in plain language, online resources, and a "wellness-centered approach."[55] There are cancer rehabilitation and survivorship programs that already exist, which are interdisciplinary, age specific, and promote self-management. It is beneficial to both the patient and healthcare provider to have a standardized approach to LTFU care to accurately and comprehensively address issues relating to cancer survivorship such as fertility, sexuality, mental health, and late effects.[55]

Support of both pediatric CNS cancer survivors and their families comes in different guises, with the goals of improving qualitative and quantitative long-term outcomes.

Improving survivors' SMSs helps them to successfully transition from pediatric to adult LTFU care.[75] Group social skills interventions have been devised to improve social problem-solving and performance for brain tumor survivors.[77]

Family factors have been shown to play a role in academic achievement in pediatric brain tumor survivors.[59] A supportive environment with reduced conflict is associated with less academic impairment in pediatric CNS brain tumor survivors (PBTS). Higher socioeconomic status is associated with reduced reading score discrepancy between PBTS and unaffected individuals. Families with more social needs may benefit from more intensive support services.

There is qualitative data to show that pediatric cancer survivors have more difficulty dating and forming romantic relationships as well as sexual dysfunction.[53] This may be due to reduced social competence and changes in body image post cancer treatment. These difficulties can have a negative impact on day-to-day life. Parents have their own specific worries about cancer survivorship negatively impacting their children's ability to form future relationships.[53] Support in this area should be age appropriate both in content and means of delivery, for example, adolescent survivors may prefer to seek support from peer advisors or from the Internet.[53] Female pediatric cancer survivors have specific anxiety about fertility and may benefit from focused psychologic support.[11]

Interventions to improve coping skills during diagnosis and treatment can improve quality of future survivorship. Family, friends, and spiritual/faith counselors are often reported by survivors as being important sources of support throughout the journey of treatment, recovery, and survivorship.[54]

Complementary and alternative medicine (CAM, or integrative medicine) is often used by pediatric cancers survivors, more so in brain tumor survivors than in leukemia/lymphoma patients.[76] CAM can aid wellness and sometimes address specific symptoms, but given that there is insufficient research and evidence for these treatments, providers should support patients in making the most informed decisions possible.[76]

Certified Child Life Specialists (CCLSs) are professionals who work with infants, children, youth, and families.[78] They have an evidence-based grounding in child development, therapeutic play, stress and coping mechanisms, as well as family dynamics, which allows them to provide psychosocial support in the healthcare setting.[78] Child Life interventions can facilitate healing, coping, problem-solving, and good communication for children and their families. Pediatric cancer is an all-consuming journey for patient and family, and the CCLS can play an integral role in the young patient's support team.

Pediatric cancer patients must often undergo extensive imaging as part of the oncologic workup, treatment, and subsequent surveillance. A randomized control trial demonstrated significantly better experiential outcomes for parents, children, and radiology staff when a CCLS was assigned to the patient during imaging.[79] Benefits were seen in parent and staff satisfaction, as well as the child's overall experience and fear levels.[79] Further research has shown that employing a CCLS reduces the frequency of daily anesthesia for children undergoing radiation therapy, and subsequently can provide significant cost savings to health systems, in addition to providing support to children and families.[80]

A CCLS in a pediatric oncology center can help a child adjust to the hospital environment, while ensuring that the patient's and family's wishes are being respected.[81] Children can emotionally and psychologically prepare for blood tests, chemotherapy, and other treatments through medical play with a doll, also known as their "hospital buddy."[81] Other activities that Child Life specialists can facilitate are milestones (such as birthdays and end-of-chemotherapy parties), creative outlets such as crafts, and entertainment (for example, specially trained clowns for hospitalized children).[81] Through the Child Life experience, the young patient is learning about their illness and medicosurgical treatment and how to express their feelings and emotions throughout the cancer journey.[81]

MEASURE OF QUALITY

In the realm of pediatric CNS cancer rehabilitation, it may be better to measure "quality of survival" (QoS), instead of QoL.[58] QoL is a subjective measurement, reported by the survivor. QoS captures not only more than just survivorship statistics but also more than the qualitative data gleaned from QoL measures.[58] QoS focuses on long-term sequelae, including but not limited to, neurocognitive, endocrine, medical, and functional. As survival rates in pediatric CNS cancer are increasing due to aggressive treatments and their associated toxicities, QoS has become even more important to consider. Moreover, QoS can then be used in clinical trials to look at the benefit versus burden of certain treatment and management regimens.[58]

When looking at QoS measures, it is important to frame questions of survival using the social model for disability, as opposed to the biomedical model.[58] The former emphasizes society's role in the disability etiology and the removal of barriers to reduce disability.

There are three areas to focus on in QoS measurements. First, there is direct testing of survivors, for example, using the Wechsler Intelligence Scale for Children.[58] Next, there is indirect measurement, using questionnaires that focus on health, QoL, behavior, executive function, and demographics, which are summarized below:

Health	Health Utilities Index (HUI)
QoL	Pediatric Quality of Life Inventory (PedsQL)
Behavior	Strength and Difficulties Questionnaire (SDQ)
Executive function	Behavior Rating Inventory of Executive Function (BRIEF)
Demographics	Medical, Educational, Employment

Finally, specific add-on measurements may be used, for example, looking at adaptive behavior using the Vineland Adaptive Behavior Scale (VABS). This is important, as pediatric cancer survivors have low rates of independence, education/employment, and relationship stability in adulthood. There are also specific endocrine assessments that can be completed, which are crucial, given that endocrine dysfunction plays a significant role in QoS and QoL.[58]

More research needs to be done in the field of QoS, which is an important measure of outcome in pediatric cancer and a tool which can be fed back in the system to help make decisions for treatment regimens in clinical trials.

PEDIATRIC PALLIATIVE CARE

Pediatric palliative care (PPC) can be beneficial to many patients and their families. Most patients with pediatric CNS cancer will experience suffering at some point in their journey and could benefit from PPC.[69] PPC is a holistic philosophy and framework for care delivery for children with life-threatening/limiting illness that can be offered at any age, any stage of cancer, and even in conjunction with curative treatment.[64] PPC is provided by an increasing number of hospitals, mostly on an inpatient basis,[63] although can be delivered at home as well.[69] PPC can improve QoL through pain reduction, symptom management,[64] and relief of physical suffering.[63] Goals of PPC also include relief of emotional and psychologic suffering, reduction in spiritual distress and social isolation, coordination of care (including complex home care), facilitation of decision-making, and assistance during the transition from curative treatment to comfort care (if necessary).[63] Most oncology teams provide "primary" palliative care by managing pain and initiating goal-directed communication. If further assistance is needed, they may consult a specialist PPC team. A PPC team may comprise of a physician, nurse, social worker, chaplain, psychologist, and various other allied healthcare professionals.[69]

Barriers exist to good PPC. Parents may have different expectations, a different understanding of the prognosis, and a hesitancy to delve into such a difficult discussion. Providers, in turn, do not want to take away hope and can be uncertain when to initiate the discussion.[63] Pain and symptom identification can be challenging in young and/or nonverbal children.[63] Contrary to popular opinion, PPC does not reduce hope or cause distress to families.[63] In cases where PPC is used, children undergo less aggressive interventions during end of life (which are often of minimal benefit) and are more likely to die in a preferred location.[63] This may in turn decrease the duration of hospital stays. When parents can choose the place of death, the child is more likely to die at home, and the family is less likely to express regrets over the location.

Patient- and family-centered care is a way of delivering PPC.[64] It stresses the importance of the family as the child's greatest advocate. Four guiding principles include dignity and respect for patient and family, seamless information sharing, parental involvement in decision-making, and use of family feedback to develop new policy and programs.

Parents report that preferred time for PPC is at diagnosis or during a period of medical stability, but often discussions only happen during critical illness or end of life.[63] Few providers feel that advanced care decisions are addressed with appropriate timing.[63] In some countries, it is national policy to have an end-of-life plan for every child with a life-limiting illness.[61] This can be a hard copy document that can be photocopied if a patient is moving between home, the emergency department, or multiple hospital locations. The document can be initiated around the time of diagnosis and filled in over time. It may be helpful for the document to be introduced by a provider that the patient and family trusts. It may be beneficial to discuss each topic with a view of hope and benefit, as well as discussion of, and preparation for, harm.[63] The document can be divided according to time periods: wishes during life, plans for when the child is unwell, plans for life-threatening complications, and wishes at end of life as well as after death.[61] The document should be shaped by the medical, psychosocial, spiritual, and cultural needs of the family. As the child gets older, they may contribute more of their own opinions and preferences to the document. Important medical decisions that may be documented include decisions about invasive/noninvasive respiratory support, use of feeding tubes, use of antibiotics, when/if to go to the ICU, and preferences regarding organ donation.

Pediatric patients can have different end-of-life symptoms and neurologic deterioration depending on tumor location: supratentorial versus infratentorial versus brainstem.[82] This will influence decisions regarding pain and symptom management. Complementary care can reduce pain, calm breathing, and manage symptoms such as anxiety, fatigue, and nausea.[64] It can be taught to family members and provide a peaceful transition during end of life.

For clinicians who would like formal training in facilitating palliative discussion, there are several tools available: VITALtalk, Center to Advance Palliative Care, ELNEC curricula, and Textbook of Palliative Care Communication.[69]

CONCLUSION

Pediatric CNS cancer survivors are at risk for a myriad of potential long-term and late effects of cancer treatment. Surviving and thriving after childhood CNS cancer requires follow-up care by an integrated team including primary caregivers, specialists, and subspecialists. These teams deliver survivorship care plans (SCPs) with a risk-based approach, following a systematic plan for lifelong screening, surveillance, and prevention that incorporates risks based on cancer type, cancer therapy, genetic predispositions, lifestyle behaviors, and comorbid health conditions.

Pediatric CNS cancer is viewed as a catastrophic disease in children, resulting in physical and psychologic changes from their disease and treatment that increasingly challenges their ability to function during developmental maturation. As such, cancer is now being viewed more as a chronic illness, requiring us to focus on patient function rather than merely their disease process.

Planning a pediatric rehabilitation program that provides restoration and maintenance of functional abilities throughout disease and treatment management, in conjunction with, or followed by, SCPs is increasingly emphasized. Owing to increased survival and increasing demand for follow-up care of cancer survivors, pediatric cancer survivorship plans must address management of late effects related to recurrent disease and/or treatment effects.

Pediatric physiatrists are medically trained and responsible for coordinating cancer rehabilitation programs in acute and subacute inpatient settings, as well as on an outpatient and home services basis. They address optimum rehabilitation of the pediatric cancer patient via physiatric interventions and coordinate an interdisciplinary team with a patient- and family-centered focus.

Pediatric CNS cancer patients face unacceptably high mortality rates. While other areas of oncologic research have made great strides in recent years, pediatric CNS cancer research needs to generate more advances with translation into clinical benefit for these most vulnerable pediatric patients.

In pediatric CNS cancer rehabilitation, the patient-family-centered approach allows rehabilitation specialists and allied health professionals to coordinate efforts to maximize short-term and long-term medical, rehabilitation, and survivorship outcomes.

REFERENCES

1. Arora RS, Alston RD, Eden TOB, Estlin EJ, Moran A, Birch JM. Age–incidence patterns of primary CNS tumors in children, adolescents, and adults in England. *Neuro Oncol.* 2009l;11(4):403–413.
2. Keller DM. Children's solid tumors rarely metastasize to the brain. *J Spinal Cord Med.* 2007;30(suppl 1):S15–S20.
3. Ostrom QT, Gittleman H, Farah P, et al. CBTRUS statistical report: primary brain and central nervous system tumors diagnosed in the United States in 2006–2010. *Neuro Oncol.* 2013;15(suppl 2):ii1–ii56.

4. Louis DN, Perry A, Reifenberger G, et al. The 2016 World Health Organization Classification of Tumors of the Central Nervous System: a summary. *Acta Neuropathol.* 2016;131(6):803–820.
5. Children's Oncology Group (COG, https://www.survivorshipguidelines.org).
6. Hewitt M, Weiner SL, Simone JV, eds. *Childhood Cancer Survivorship: Improving Care and Quality of Life. Institute of Medicine (US) and National Research Council (US) National Cancer Policy Board.* Washington (DC): National Academies Press (US); 2003.
7. Stefanaki K, Alexiou GA, Stefanaki C, Prodromou N. Tumors of central and peripheral nervous system associated with inherited genetic syndromes. *Pediatr Neurosurg.* 2012;48(5):271–285.
8. Kilday JP, Bartels U, Huang A, et al. Favorable survival and metabolic outcome for children with diencephalic syndrome using a radiation-sparing approach. *J Neurooncol.* 2014;116(1):195–204.
9. Louis DN, Ohgaki H, Wiestler OD, et al., eds. *WHO Classification of Tumours of the Central Nervous System.* 4th ed. Lyon, France: IARC Press; 2007.
10. Pollack IF. Brain tumors in children. *N Engl J Med.* 1994; 331(22):1500–1507.
11. Pfister S, Witt O. Pediatric gliomas. *Recent Results Cancer Res.* 2009;171:67–81.
12. Fried I, Hawkins C, Scheinemann K, et al. Favorable outcome with conservative treatment for children with low grade brainstem tumors. *Pediatr Blood Cancer.* 2012; 58(4):556–560.
13. Fisher PG, Breiter SN, Carson BS, et al. A clinicopathologic reappraisal of brain stem tumor classification. Identification of pilocystic astrocytoma and fibrillary astrocytoma as distinct entities. *Cancer.* 2000;89(7):1569–1576.
14. Stokland T, Liu JF, Ironside JW, et al. A multivariate analysis of factors determining tumor progression in childhood low-grade glioma: a population-based cohort study (CCLG CNS9702). *Neuro Oncol.* 2010;12(12): 1257–1268.
15. Pajtler KW, Witt H, Sill M, et al. Molecular classification of ependymal tumors across all CNS compartments, histopathological grades, and age groups. *Cancer Cell.* 2015; 27(5):728–743.
16. Oh MC, Sayegh ET, Safaee M, et al. Prognosis by tumor location for pediatric spinal cord ependymomas. *Neurosurg Pediatr.* 2013;11(3):282–288.
17. Bouffet E, Capra M, Bartels U. Salvage chemotherapy for metastatic and recurrent ependymoma of childhood. *Childs Nerv Syst.* 2009;25(10):1293–1301.
18. Duffner PK, Horowitz ME, Krischer JP, et al. The treatment of malignant brain tumors in infants and very young children: an update of the Pediatric Oncology Group experience. *Neuro Oncol.* 1999;1(2):152–161.
19. Smoll NR, Drummond KJ. The incidence of medulloblastomas and primitive neurectodermal tumours in adults and children. *J Clin Neurosci.* 2012;19(11):1541–1544.
20. Chintagumpala MM, Paulino A, Panigrahy A, et al. Embryonal and pineal region tumors. In: Pizzo PA, Poplack DG, eds. *Principles and Practice of Pediatric Oncology.* 7th ed. Philadelphia, Pa: Lippincott Williams and Wilkins; 2015: 671–699.
21. Ramaswamy V, Remke M, Shih D, et al. Duration of the pre-diagnostic interval in medulloblastoma is subgroup dependent. *Pediatr Blood Cancer.* 2014;61(7):1190–1194.
22. Woehrer A, Slavc I, Waldhoer T, et al. Incidence of atypical teratoid/rhabdoid tumors in children: a population-based study by the Austrian Brain Tumor Registry, 1996–2006. *Cancer.* 2010;116(24):5725–5732.
23. Jane Jr JA, Laws ER. Craniopharyngioma. *Pituitary.* 2006; 9(4):323.
24. Zhou L, Luo L, Xu J, et al. Craniopharyngiomas in the posterior fossa: a rare subgroup, diagnosis, management and outcomes. *J Neurol Neurosurg Psychiatry.* 2009;80(10): 1150–1154.
25. Zacharia BE, Bruce SS, Goldstein H, et al. Incidence, treatment and survival of patients with craniopharyngioma in the surveillance, epidemiology and end results program. *Neuro Oncol.* 2012;14(8):1070–1078.
26. Weksberg DC, Shibamoto Y, Paulino AC. Bifocal intracranial germinoma: a retrospective analysis of treatment outcomes in 20 patients and review of the literature. *Int J Radiat Oncol Biol Phys.* 2012;82(4):1341–1351.
27. Hoffman HJ, Otsubo H, Hendrick EB, et al. Intracranial germ-cell tumors in children. *J Neurosurg.* 1991;74(4): 545–551.
28. Afzal S, Wherrett D, Bartels U, et al. Challenges in management of patients with intracranial germ cell tumor and diabetes insipidus treated with cisplatin and/or ifosfamide based chemotherapy. *J Neurooncol.* 2010;97(3):393–399.
29. Packer RJ, Sutton LN, Atkins TE, et al. A prospective study of cognitive function in children receiving whole-brain radiotherapy and chemotherapy: 2-year results. *J Neurosurg.* 1989;70(5):707–713.
30. Listernick R, Ferner RE, Liu GT, et al. Optic pathway gliomas in neurofibromatosis-1: controversies and recommendations. *Ann Neurol.* 2007;61(3):189–198.
31. Wisoff JH, Sanford RA, Heier LA, et al. Primary neurosurgery for pediatric low-grade gliomas: a prospective multi-institutional study from the Children's Oncology Group. *Neurosurgery.* 2011;68(6):1548–1554; discussion 1554–1555.
32. Dodgshun AJ, Maixner WJ, Heath JA, et al. Single agent carboplatin for pediatric low-grade glioma: a retrospective analysis shows equivalent efficacy to multiagent chemotherapy. *Int J Cancer.* 2016;138(2):481–488.
33. Ater JL, Zhou T, Holmes E, et al. Randomized study of two chemotherapy regimens for treatment of low-grade glioma in young children: a report from the Children's Oncology Group. *J Clin Oncol.* 2012;30(21):2641–2647.
34. Avery RA, Hwang EI, Jakacki RI, et al. Marked recovery of vision in children with optic pathway gliomas treated with bevacizumab. *JAMA Ophthalmol.* 2014;132(1):111–114.

35. Yang T, Temkin N, Barber J, et al. Gross total resection correlates with long-term survival in pediatric patients with glioblastoma. *World Neurosurg*. 2013;79(3–4):537–544.
36. Espinoza JC, Haley K, Patel N, et al. Outcome of young children with high-grade glioma treated with irradiation-avoiding intensive chemotherapy regimens: final report of the Head Start II and III trials. *Pediatr Blood Cancer*. 2016;63(10):1806–1813.
37. Hilden JM, Meerbaum S, Burger P, et al. Central nervous system atypical teratoid/rhabdoid tumor: results of therapy in children enrolled in a registry. *J Clin Oncol*. 2014; 22(14):2877–2884.
38. Joo JH, Park JH, Ra YS, et al. Treatment outcome of radiation therapy for intracranial germinoma: adaptive radiation field in relation to response to chemotherapy. *Anticancer Res*. 2014;34(10):5715–5721.
39. Winkfield KM, Tsai HK, Yao X, et al. Long-term clinical outcomes following treatment of childhood craniopharyngioma. *Pediatr Blood Cancer*. 2011;56(7): 1120–1126.
40. Rutkowski S, Gerber NU, von Hoff K, et al. Treatment of early childhood medulloblastoma by postoperative chemotherapy and deferred radiotherapy. *Neuro Oncol*. 2009;11(2):201–210.
41. Nageswara Rao AA, Wallace DJ, Billups C, et al. Cumulative cisplatin dose is not associated with event-free or overall survival in children with newly diagnosed average-risk medulloblastoma treated with cisplatin based adjuvant chemotherapy: report from the Children's Oncology Group. *Pediatr Blood Cancer*. 2014;61(1):102–106.
42. Grundy RG, Wilne SH, Robinson KJ, et al. Primary postoperative chemotherapy without radiotherapy for treatment of brain tumours other than ependymoma in children under 3 years: results of the first UKCCSG/SIOP CNS 9204 trial. *Eur J Cancer*. 2010;46(1):120–133.
43. Cheng JS, Ivan ME, Stapleton CJ, et al. Intraoperative changes in transcranial motor evoked potentials and somatosensory evoked potentials predicting outcome in children with intramedullary spinal cord tumors. *J Neurosurg Pediatr*. 2014;12:591–599.
44. Rutka JT, Kuo JS. Pediatric surgical neuro-oncology: current best care practices and strategies. *J Neuro-Oncol*. 2004;69:139–150.
45. Ward E, DeSantis C, Robbins A Kohler B, Jemal A. *Childhood and Adolescent Cancer Statistics, 2014*. 31 January 2014.
46. Wibroe M, Cappelen J, Castor C, et al. Cerebellar mutism syndrome in children with brain tumours of the posterior fossa. *BMC Cancer*. 2017;17:439–445. https://doi.org/10.1186/s12885-017-3416-0.
47. Catsman-Berrevoets CE, Aarsen FK. The spectrum of neurobehavioral deficits in the posterior fossa syndrome in children after cerebellar tumour surgery. *Cortex*. 2010; 46(7):933–946.
48. Pietila S, Korpela R, Lenko HL, et al. Neurological outcome of childhood brain tumor survivors. *J Neurooncol*. 2012; 108(1):153–161.
49. Mellblom AV, Korsvold L, Finset A, Loge J, Ruud E, Lie HC. Providing information about late effects during routine follow-up consultations between pediatric oncologists and adolescent survivors: a video-based, observational study. *J Adolesc Young Adult Oncol*. 2015;4(4):200–208. https://doi.org/10.1089/jayao.2015.0037.
50. Tomioka A, Maru M, Kashimada K, Sakakibara H. Physical and social characteristics and support needs of adult female childhood cancer survivors who underwent hormone replacement therapy. *Int J Clin Oncol*. 2017. https://doi.org/10.1007/s10147-017-1120-3.
51. NIH: National Cancer Institute. *Late Effects of Treatment for Childhood Cancer (PDQ) – Health Professional Version*. NIH; 2017.
52. Klassen AF, Rosenberg-Yunger ZRS, D'Agostino NM, et al. The development of scales to measure childhood cancer survivors' readiness for transition to long-term follow-up care as adults. *Health Expect*. 2014;18:1941–1955. https://doi.org/10.1111/hex.12241.
53. Stinson JN, Jibb LA, Greenberg M, et al. A qualitative study of the impact of cancer on romantic relationships, sexual relationships, and fertility: perspectives of Canadian adolescents and parents during and after treatment. *J Adolesc Young Adult Oncol*. 2015;4:84–90. https://doi.org/10.1089/jayao.2014.0036.
54. Foster RH, Brouwer AM, Dillon R, Bitsko MJ, Godder K, Stern M. "Cancer was a speed bump in my path to enlightenment:" a qualitative analysis of situational coping experiences among young adult survivors of childhood cancer. *J Psychosoc Oncol*. 2017. https://doi.org/10.1080/07347332.2017.1292575.
55. Gupta AA, Papadakos JK, Jones JM, et al. Reimagining care for adolescent and young adult cancer programs: moving with the times. *Cancer*. 2016:1038–1046. https://doi.org/10.1002/cncr.29834.
56. Hudson MM, Ehrhradt MJ, Bhakta N, et al. Approach for classification and severity grading of long-term and late-onset health events among childhood cancer survivors in the St. Jude lifetime cohort. *Cancer Epidemiol Biomarkers Prev*. 2017;26(5):666–674. https://doi.org/10.1158/1055-9965.EPI-16-0812.
57. Brinkman TM, Bass JK, Li Z, et al. Treatment-induced hearing loss and adult social outcomes in survivors of childhood CNS and non-CNS solid tumors: results from the St. Jude lifetime cohort study. *Cancer*. 2015. https://doi.org/10.1002/cncr.29604.
58. Limond JA, Bull KS, Calaminus G, Kennedy CR, Spoudeas HA, Chevignard MP. On behalf of the brain tumour quality of survival group, international society of pediatric oncology (Europe) (SIOP-E). Quality of survival assessment in European childhood brain tumour trials, for children aged 5 years and over. *Eur J Paediatr Neurol*. 2015; 19:202–210. https://doi.org/10/1016/j.ejpn.2014.12.003.
59. Ach E, Gerhardt CA, Barrera M, et al. Family factors associated with academic achievement deficits in pediatric brain tumor survivors. *Psycho-Oncology*. 2013;22(8): 1731–1737.

60. Olson K, Sands SA. Cognitive training programs for childhood cancer patients and survivors: a critical review and future directions. *Child Neuropsychol.* 2016;22(5):509–536. https://doi.org/10.1080/09297049.2015.1049941.
61. Fraser J, Harris N, Berringer AJ, Prescott H, Finlay F. Advanced care planning in children with life-limiting conditions- the wishes document. *Arch Dis Child.* 2010;95: 79–82. https://doi.org/10.1136/adc.2009.160051.
62. Wilne S, Walker D. Spine and spinal cord tumours in children: a diagnostic and therapeutic challenge for healthcare systems. *Arch Dis Child Educ Pract Ed.* 2010;95:47–54. https://doi.org/10.1136/adc.2008.143214.
63. Hauer JM, Wolfe J. Supportive and palliative care of children with metabolic and neurological diseases. *Curr Opin Support Palliat Care.* 2014;8:296–302. https://doi.org/10.1097/SPC.0000000000000063.
64. St. Jude Children's Research Hospital. *What Is Patient and Family-centered Care? [Internet]*. Memphis: St. Jude; 2018. Available at: https://www.stjude.org/treatment/patient-resources/family-centered-care.html.
65. Memorial Sloan Kettering. *Integrative Medicine & Complementary Services [Internet]*; 2018. Available from: https://www.mskcc.org/pediatrics/cancer-care/treatments/managing-symptoms-side-effects/integrative-medicine-complementary-services.
66. Armstrong GT, Kawashima T, Leisenring W, et al. Aging and risk of severe, disabling, life threatening, and fatal events in the childhood cancer survivor study. *J Clin Oncol.* 2014;32:1218–1227.
67. Survival rates for selected childhood brain and spinal cord tumors. https://www.cancer.org/cancer/brain-spinal-cord-tumors-children/detection-diagnosis-staging/survival-rates.html
68. Diez Jr JH. Rehabilitation of the cancer patient. *Med Clin North Am.* 1969;53(3):607–624.
69. Kirch R, Reaman G, Feudtner C, et al. Advancing a comprehensive cancer care agenda for children and their families: institute of medicine workshop highlights and next steps. *CA Cancer J Clin.* 2016;66:398–407.
70. Baumann FT, Bloch W, Beulertz J. Clinical exercise interventions in pediatric oncology: a systematic review. *Pediatr Res.* 2013;74(4):366–374.
71. Braam KI, van der Torre P, Takken T, et al. Physical exercise training interventions for children and young adults during and after treatment for childhood cancer. *Cochrane Database Syst Rev.* 2016;3.
72. Sparrow J, Zhu L, Gajjar A, et al. Constraint-induced movement therapy for children with brain tumors. *Pediatr Phys Ther.* 2017;29:55–61.
73. Heathcock JC, Christianson C, Bush K, et al. Treadmill training after surgical removal of a spinal tumor in infancy. *Phys Ther.* 2014;94:1176–1185.
74. Grandinette S. Supporting students with brain tumors in obtaining school intervention services: the clinician's role from and educator's perspective. *J Pediatr Rehabil Med.* 2014;7:307–321. https://doi.org/10.3233/PRM-140301.
75. Syed IA, Nathan PC, et al. Examining factors associated with self management skills in teenage survivors of cancer. *J Cancer Surviv.* 2016;10:686–691.
76. Ndao DH, Ladas EJ, Bao Y, et al. Use of complementary and alternative medicine among children, adolescent, and young adult cancer survivors: a survey study. *J Pediatr Hematol Oncol.* 2013;35:281–288.
77. Schulte F, Vannatta K, Barrer M. Social problem solving and social performance after a group social skills intervention for childhood brain tumor survivors. *Psycho-Oncology.* 2014;23:183–189. https://doi.org/10.1002/pon.3387.
78. Association of Child Life Professionals. *Mission, Values, Vision [Internet]. ACLP*; 2018. Available from: https://www.childlife.org/child-life-profession/mission-values-vision.
79. Tyson ME, Bohl DD, Blickman JG. A randomized control trial: child life services in pediatric imaging. *Pediatr Radiol.* 2014;44(11):1426–1432.
80. Scott MT, Todd KE, Oakley H, et al. Reducing anesthesia and health care cost through utilization of child life specialists in pediatric radiation oncology. *Int J Radiat Oncol Biol Phys.* 2016;96(2):401–405.
81. Johns Hopkins Medicine. Pediatric oncology child life [Internet]. Pediatric Oncology. Available from: https://www.hopkinsmedicine.org/kimmel_cancer_center/centers/pediatric_oncology/becoming_our_patient/patient_information/pediatric_child_life.html.
82. Kuhlen M, Hoell J, Balzer S, Borkhardt A, Janssen G. Symptoms and management of pediatric patients with incurable brain tumors in palliative home care. *Eur J Paediatr Neurol.* 2016;20(2):261–269.

CHAPTER 12

Cancer-Related Fatigue

VISHWA S. RAJ, MD • JOANNA EDEKAR, DPT • TERRENCE MACARTHUR PUGH, MD

Cancer-related fatigue (CRF) is defined as:

> *... a distressing, persistent, subjective sense of physical, emotional, and/or cognitive tiredness or exhaustion related to cancer or cancer treatment that is not proportional to recent activity and interferes with usual functioning.*

Unlike fatigue for individuals without cancer, CRF is more severe and distressing, and less likely to be relieved by rest. Patients describe a general sense of tiredness associated with functional deficits.[1]

EPIDEMIOLOGY

Demographic and Prevalence

CRF is a common condition, and its prevalence can range from 50% to 100% based on the clinical status of the cancer.[2] The presence of CRF varies according to diagnosis. For instance, individuals with lung cancer experience CRF in 37%–78% of cases, whereas those with breast cancer range from 28% to 91% and prostate can be as low as 15%.[3] However, for some population the presence of CRF can improve over time (Fig. 12.1).[4] For patients receiving active oncologic treatment, moderate to severe fatigue was reported by 45% of individuals and associated with several variables (Table 12.1). In cases for individuals not currently receiving cancer treatment, who are either in complete remission or have no evidence of disease, severe fatigue was noted for 29%. Moderate to severe fatigue was also associated with poor performance status and history of depression.[5]

Individuals with central nervous system (CNS) tumors may also experience symptoms. Between 89% and 94% of patients with recurrent malignant gliomas experience fatigue.[6] For primary brain tumors, severity is associated with difficulty sleeping, distress, drowsiness, pain, and weakness. Strong predictors of fatigue include disease status, female gender, and poor Karnofsky performance status. Disease status is closely associated with severity in women, whereas for men, stronger associations are noted with antidepressant use, opioid utilization, and performance status.[7] In advanced cancer, risk factors may include brain metastases, poor performance status and quality of life (QOL), and reduced ability to perform activities. Prior radiation therapy was associated with less fatigue. However, severity was independently predicted by the presence of brain metastases and poor QOL.[8] CRF can also be present before, during, and after intervention for spinal cord tumors.[9]

ETIOLOGY

Pathophysiology

CRF is a multifactorial condition, and variables that influence its development can be both microscopic and macroscopic. At the cellular level, fatigue may originate within the muscle or neuromuscular junction. Factors such as decreased pH, accumulation of lactate, and changes in intra- and extracellular ion concentrations can influence membrane excitability in the muscle, thus causing weakness and fatigue at the synaptic level. Fatigue originating at this level is termed peripheral fatigue. Prevalence for peripheral fatigue may range from 19% to 39%.[10]

However, fatigue may also be the result of ineffectiveness of the CNS to deliver appropriate responses. This central activation failure is also known as central fatigue and may originate from the brain, spinal cord, and nerves. Central fatigue had a greater association with CRF, compared with peripheral fatigue. Causes may include systemic treatments with chemotherapy or focal effects from radiation. Interestingly, between 70% and 96% of individuals who receive either chemotherapy and/or radiation experienced fatigue, whereas those who received surgery alone are at less risk.[10] However, at the molecular level, several other factors can influence the CNS (Table 12.2). Disruptions in the cortical and spinal sensorimotor centers, energy metabolism, and process muscle activation may all lead to reduced physical performance.[11] Many of these may be the result of the tumor itself, as opposed to treatment effects.

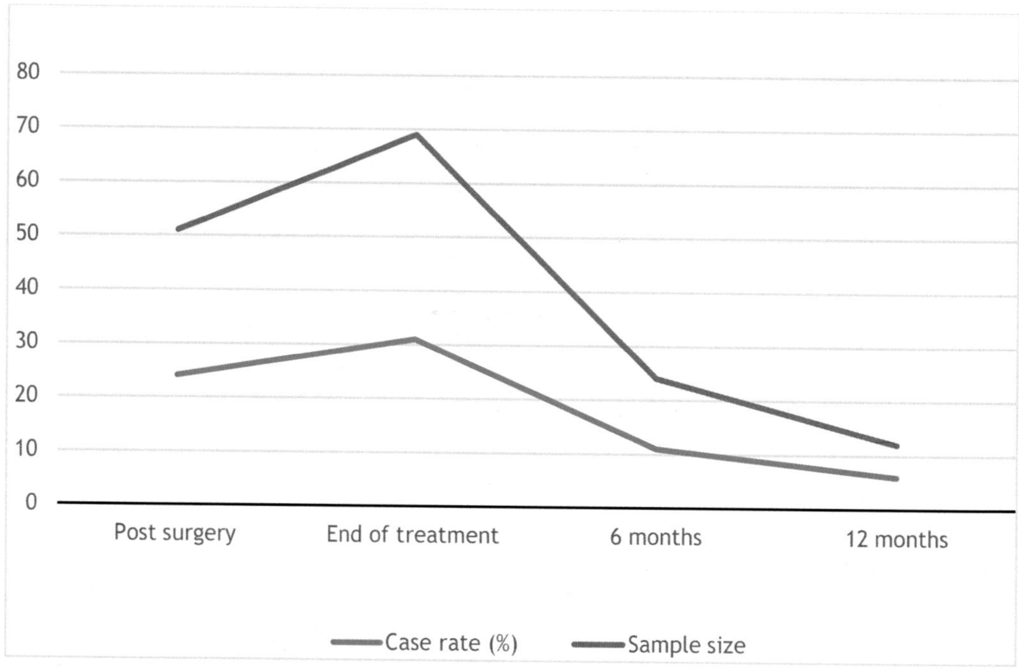

FIG. 12.1 Rates of CRF for breast cancer patients. CRF, cancer-related fatigue.

TABLE 12.1
Characteristics Associated With Moderate to Severe Fatigue in Cancer Patients and Survivors

Risk Factor	Odds Ratio
Strong opioid use	3.00
Poor Eastern Cooperative Oncology Group (ECOG) performance status	2.00
Greater than 5% weight loss within 6 months	1.60
Greater than 10 concurrent medications	1.58
Lung cancer	1.55
History of depression	1.42

Medical Comorbidities

Several conditions may lead to fatigue in cancer patients. Disturbances in sleep-wake cycles are a common occurrence for the cancer patient.[12] For individuals with breast cancer, poor sleep correlates with high levels of fatigue and delayed circadian rhythms result in increased daily dysfunction due to fatigue.[13] Factors that affect circadian rhythms may include disruptions in biologic rhythmicity, mitotic processes of cancer cells, oncologic treatments and their time of day for administration, and QOL. Other factors that lead to insomnia or daytime sleepiness include chemotherapy, pain, psychiatric disturbances, and radiation. Specific consideration should be given to whether an individual has difficulty falling asleep versus staying asleep.[14]

Anemia is often a comorbidity associated with cancer and is found in 40% of cancer patients as well as 90% of those receiving chemotherapy.[15] The causes of anemia may be multifactorial and related to cancer and its treatment, in addition to organ dysfunction (Table 12.3).[16] Cancer patients with lower hemoglobin concentrations may experience decreased ability to work, greater fatigue, and poorer QOL.[17] Improvement in hemoglobin levels correlate with decreased fatigue and better physical functioning.[18]

Endocrinology disorders can be associated with CRF. Specifically, hypothyroidism is the primary factor associated with fatigue.[19] Cytotoxic agents delivered in the treatment of breast cancer can influence thyroid function, which subsequently contributes to both fatigue and decreased physical activity.[20] Considerations should be made for structural abnormalities in the thyroid, incidental thyroid cancer, medications associated with hormone abnormalities, and history of neck or brain radiation.[21] Thyroid dysfunction can also result from radioactive iodine therapy and newer antineoplastic agents used to treat various malignancies.[22]

TABLE 12.2
Molecular Risk Factors for Central Fatigue

Molecular Factors
Alterations of circadian melatonin secretions
Changes in the central nervous system serotoninergic system
Disturbances of hypothalamic regulatory circuits
Dysregulation of inflammatory cytokines produced by the body or tumors
Expression of proinflammatory cytokines used for treatment of cancer
Gene polymorphisms for regulatory proteins of oxidative phosphorylation
Metabolism of catecholamines
Transduction signals in B cells

TABLE 12.3
Causes of Anemia in Cancer Patients

Etiology of Anemia
Blood loss
Chemotherapy-induced myelosuppression
Erythropoietin deficiencies due to renal disease
Functional iron deficiency
Marrow involvement of tumor

Dietary intake during and after treatment may play a significant role in fatigue. Nutritional components have an effect at the cellular level (Table 12.4).[23] Poor nutrition may lead to cancer cachexia, which is a form of malnutrition characterized by progressive and involuntary weight loss. Associated with cachexia is depletion of lean body mass and muscle wasting, which can result in fatigue.[24] Patient-specific nutritional programs can reduce or reverse deficiencies and lead to improved performance status.[25] Nutritional interventions may also significantly contribute to QOL improvements.[26]

MEDICATION EFFECTS

When considering the treatment of cancer and its associated symptoms, several medication classes have been used to improve functionality and QOL. However, utilization of these agents may have the unintended

TABLE 12.4
Nutritional Molecules and Their Cellular Roles

Molecule	Cellular Function
Carbohydrates and fats	Energy production
Proteins	Cellular construction and structural maintenance
Water	Muscle turgor and medium for anabolic and catabolic products

consequence of fatigue as a side effect. Although pain itself may be a cause, several analgesics can lead to fatigue and drowsiness.[27] Similar proportions of patients with moderate to severe pain had symptoms of moderate to severe fatigue. Both pain and fatigue have been also shown to negatively correlate with emotional functioning, and both along with depression tend to present as a symptom cluster with cancer diagnoses.[28] Unfortunately many of the medications used to treat this cluster can also cause fatigue. Opioid-induced sedation is common and can be managed with additional medications such as methylphenidate and donepezil. Tricyclic antidepressants have been helpful for anxiety and depression but are commonly associated with lethargy and drowsiness. Antihistamines are used for allergic reactions; however, first-generation H_1-antihistamines readily caused sedation, drowsiness, and fatigue. Newer second-generation H_1-antihistamines cause less sedation and have improved efficacy.[29] Furthermore, antiepileptic medications, such as gabapentin or levetiracetam, are often used in the brain tumor population to prevent or treat seizures but can cause lethargy and fatigue.[30]

Psychologic Considerations

Fatigue in cancer patients is associated with both anxiety and depression.[31] Depression can subsequently lead to physical and cognitive impairments in brain tumor populations.[32] For individuals with glioma, who have received concurrent radiation, clinical depression commonly presented within the first 6 months of the radiation treatment. Patients with greater functional impairment were at greater risk.[33] The relationship between fatigue and depression is unclear. Depression may be the result of fatigue, or vice versa. Both may also be the result of an alternate but common pathway. However, depression has been shown to be moderately associated with cancer fatigue, as has, to a lesser but consistent extent, anxiety.[31] Benzodiazepines are well known to cause lethargy and fatigue.[34] As noted earlier, fatigue may also result from administration of antidepressant medications, such as tricyclic antidepressants.[35] Careful attention to the emotional status of cancer patients is also important, as fatigue can result from emotional pain and coping mechanisms.[36]

Treatment Effects

Although CRF may be multifactorial in nature, it is important to understand how the treatments directed toward cancer itself may lead to worsening symptoms of fatigue. Surgery can cause physiologic responses contributing to worsening energy levels (Table 12.5). Preoperative levels of fatigue have also been showed to predict the postoperative severity and should be considered during clinical evaluations. Malaise is common after chemotherapy, as well as anemia and neurotoxicity. For patients receiving radiation, anemia, anorexia, chronic pain, diarrhea, and weight loss may result and can negatively influence physical and psychologic components.[37]

DIAGNOSIS

Patient-Reported Symptoms

As cancer survivorship evolves as a major focus of cancer care, so too does CRF. The National Comprehensive Cancer Network (NCCN) recommends that clinicians evaluate for CRF during initial consultation and at all subsequent visits with associated cancer treatments for advanced diseases.[38] Typically, CRF presents with a noticeable decrease in QOL due to physical and psychosocial impairments. Symptoms are disproportionate to levels of exertion and not relieved by rest or sleep. It is often more severe than other forms of fatigue and may persist far after cancer treatment. As a subjective experience, observable behavioral and physiologic levels may be influenced by the individual's personal understanding and experiences. Further complicating assessment of CRF is that cancer patients may have difficulty reporting the presence and absence of symptoms, as well as severity. Levels of fatigue may fluctuate throughout the day, as well as longitudinally throughout the oncologic spectrum.[39]

TABLE 12.5
Sources of Fatigue From Surgery

Causes of Physiologic Stressors
Analgesia
Anesthesia
Immobilization
Infection
Mood

Screening

The primary method by which individuals are identified with CRF is screening. Several organizations, including the NCCN, Oncology Nursing Society (ONS), Collaborative Partnership between the Canadian Partnership Against Cancer and the Canadian Association of Psychological Oncology (CPAC/CAPO), and the American Society of Clinical Oncology (ASCO), have published guidelines related to screening and management of CRF. All consistently recommend frequent assessments. Although CPAC/CAPO uses the Edmonton Symptom Assessment Systems (ESAS) as their recommended tool, each organization has other tools that are similarly scaled.[40] The ESAS specifically uses a 0 to 10 scale and rates fatigue as mild, moderate, and severe.[41]

Self-reported measures are being used with more frequency to identify CRF. However, consistency is variable between different tools as it relates to measurements and areas of assessment. Specifically, some tools may evaluate severity, impact on daily functioning combined with severity, or various manifestations of CRF.[40] Unidimensional tools screen for single items that may detect the presence or absence of CRF but may not focus on symptom severity or the personal effects of CRF on the individual. For example, the Visual Analog Fatigue Scale assesses fatigue severity, and the Brief Fatigue Inventory measures severity over 24 h. Multidimensional tools evaluate CRF in a more comprehensive manner, specifically focusing on behavior, cognition, somatic complaints, and affective domains of function. The Multidimensional Fatigue Inventory is a validated tool that emphasizes subjective experiences of fatigue and captures changes over five domains (general, physical, activity, motivation, and mental).[39] The Patient Reported Outcomes Measurement Information System (PROMIS) tool is a new method for screening based on a fatigue questionnaire and short form. With the use of Item Response Theory and computer adaptive testing, the evaluation process can be made both more efficient and precise.[40] Consensus has yet to be achieved regarding which tools may be most efficient and effective. Unidimensional approaches provide quicker but superficial assessments, whereas multidimensional methods are comprehensive but time consuming.

Clinical Evaluation

When evaluating CRF, a focused clinical and physical history is necessary to understand symptoms and their effects on functionality and QOL. Important considerations include disease status, type and length of oncologic treatment, capacity to induce fatigue, and response to interventions. Understanding whether CRF is related to disease progression versus recurrence may affect short- and long-term clinical decision-making. Assessment of current medications and their potential side effects may provide further insight into potential etiologies. Several medical comorbidities may also contribute to fatigue, including anemia, cardiopulmonary issues, endocrine dysfunction, gastrointestinal and hepatic disorders, infection, neurologic impairments, and renal dysfunction. Hypothyroidism may result from certain types of radiation and systemic therapies. In addition to hypothyroidism, endocrinologic conditions such as hot flashes, hypogonadism from advanced cancers, and adrenal insufficiency can contribute to fatigue.[1] Primary evaluation of hypothyroidism includes thyroid-stimulating hormone (TSH) and free T_4 levels. Subclinical hypothyroidism is possible if TSH is normal or mildly elevated while T_4 levels are normal and may be amenable to hormone supplementation.[42] If there is concern for anemia, initial workup would include a complete blood count to evaluate hemoglobin levels and mean corpuscular volume of red blood cells. Microcytic anemia may suggest iron deficiency, and ferritin levels can be ordered to assess iron stores. Low transferrin saturation and increased total iron-binding capacity also indicate iron deficient states.[43] Macrocytic anemias can be due to B12 and folate deficiencies. Serum folate and B12 levels can be assessed, and if low, can be treated with supplementation. Recommendations may also be made to avoid alcohol, which has been known to contribute to these vitamin deficiencies.[44]

A more global review of the physical, emotional, and cognitive status is necessary to understand how these may impair activities of daily living, function, and overall QOL. Several additional factors can contribute to fatigue (Table 12.6). Sleep disturbances may result from mood disorders, and sleep apnea is a possibility, given potential anatomic changes from cancer and its treatment. Evaluation of appropriate sleep hygiene may provide further insights. An understanding of the sleep environment can provide more information into potentially reversible causes. Examples that can be addressed include daytime napping; individual habits; ingestion of foods high in sugar, caffeine or alcohol; deviation from regularly scheduled sleep; and stimulating activities prior to bedtime. Anxiety and depression may also have a role in sleep irregularities.[45]

TABLE 12.6
Nonmedical Contributors to Fatigue

Additional Considerations for Fatigue
Activity level
Alcohol and substance use
Emotional status
Hygiene
Nutrition
Pain
Sleep disturbances

TABLE 12.7
Exercise Prescription

Exercise Prescription Using Frequency, Intensity, Type, and Time Principles

- Frequency: 3–5 times per week
- Intensity: 4–7/10 RPE
- Type/mode: aerobic, strength training and stretching
- Time:
    - Aerobic: 20–60 min/day, 3–5 days/week
    - Strength training: 1–3 sets of 8–12 reps, 2–3 days/week
    - Stretching: major muscle groups performed on same day of exercising those muscles

A comprehensive nutritional assessment may provide insight regarding the development of fatigue. For cancer patients, changes in oral intake may lead to weight loss or gain and changes in lean body mass. These in turn can lead to fluid and electrolyte imbalances which may subsequently affect performance status. Several medical issues can cause difficulties with oral diet, including nausea, vomiting, odynophagia, bowel irregularity, and mucositis. Interest in food may decrease for these reasons, which may then lead to loss of appetite and decreased caloric consumption.[45]

Although currently used in a research capacity, imaging may provide novel methods to understand the neurobiology of CRF. Current studies are using noninvasive techniques to evaluate altered neural networks. Functional connectivity magnetic resonance imaging (fcMRI) has identified aberrant brain connectivity patterns for pain, depression, and insomnia. Using either a seed-based approach or independent component analysis, blood oxygen level dependence signals can be used to display further resting-state connectivity.[46]

MANAGEMENT

Physical and Functional Interventions

QOL is strongly associated with both CRF and fitness levels in cancer survivors. By improving mobility and thus fatigue, exercise provides a ripple effect, which has been shown to improve QOL.[45] Other benefits of exercise may include positive effects for anxiety, body composition, functionality, lab values, mood, and strength.[47,48] Research confirms that exercise is one of the most effective treatments for CRF,[49,50] and exercise and psychologic interventions can be more beneficial than pharmacologic options.[51]

Current recommendations for exercise vary according to mode, intensity, and frequency, and maybe influenced by type and stage of cancer, prior functionality and fitness level, length of exercise program, and phase of cancer treatment (Table 12.7). Although the magnitude of benefits may fluctuate, different forms of exercise, such as aerobic, strength training, and multimodal, are inversely related to fatigue and can attenuate CRF.[47,48,50,52–56] Aerobic exercise for 6 weeks has shown improvements in symptoms.[55] Enhanced intervention effects are seen early during multimodal programs, continue through follow-up appointments, and are maintained after completion of exercise programs.[53] Multimodal exercise programs, including aerobic exercise and strength training, demonstrate improvements in CRF for various cancer diagnoses.[48,52–54] Group aquatic therapy, focusing on aerobic and endurance training, can also play a role in mitigating fatigue.[56] Initiation of some type of exercise program, regardless of potential variables and lack of standard protocols, can still play a significant role.[47,48,52–54]

The Department of Health and Human Services recommends avoidance of inactivity, as it can be linked with carcinogenic processes.[55,57] They suggest that some physical activity is better than none.[57] Initiation of an exercise program as early as possible is beneficial and ideal.[58] Exercise is not only safe but also positively impacts the course of fatigue and should be performed throughout the continuum of care.[59] It has been shown during radiation therapy to positively influence CRF.[48] Low-, moderate-, and high-intensity programs have shown improved fatigue after radiation treatment.[47] Even in advanced cancer and for those nearing the end of life, physical activity can have positive effects[50] and may be beneficial in decreasing fatigue.[60] For the geriatric oncology population, CRF correlates with functional dependence, and improvements can lead to greater independence.[61] Adherence, however, remains a barrier to exercising, and survivors are slightly less committed to exercise programs compared with other patient populations.[62]

The American College of Sports Medicine (ACSM) has published guidelines related to exercise in cancer, but prescriptions should be individualized based on age, gender, type of cancer, and physical fitness level.[63,64] Exercise testing is not required for low-intensity aerobic exercise, stretching, or resistance training, but it is recommended for higher intensity aerobic activities.[65] Considerations for programs include current fitness level, cancer treatment, fatigue levels, and medical comorbidities, such as abnormal blood counts and severe anemia, as well as fracture risk. Incorporating goals of the individual and modifying program based on current condition are important components to successful implementation.[64]

The individualized exercise program should begin with lower levels of intensity and duration and progress slowly in terms of frequency, intensity, type, and time. Duration should be increased first, followed by frequency, and then intensity. Cancer survivors, who participate in 3–5 h of moderate intensity exercise a week, are more likely to reap the benefits of exercise. The weekly recommended minimum is 150 min of moderate to vigorous activities, or 75 min of vigorous intensity activities.[66] Energy conservation should also be factored into the exercise program. Teaching survivors to conserve energy and simplify tasks allows completion of activities and fulfillment of survivor's goals. Energy conservation strategies help patients plan and prioritize, prevent burn-out before completion of task, and avoid inactivity due to feelings of being overwhelmed (Table 12.8). Integration of energy conservation techniques with the oncology population can improve fatigue.[66]

Medical Management

A multifaceted approach for medication management is necessary to address all potential sources for fatigue. In the case of hypothyroidism, thyroid hormone supplementation with levothyroxine and similar agents may provide a rapid reversal of fatigue symptoms.[65] Iron supplementation or erythropoiesis-stimulating agents, such as epoetin or darbepoetin-α, can be used to address iron deficiency anemia. However, caution is necessary with erythropoiesis-stimulating agents as

TABLE 12.8
Energy Conservation

Methods for Energy Conservation
• Plan day ahead and prioritize tasks • Eat small, more frequent meals and snacks throughout the day, rather than eating three large meals. • Take short rest breaks between activities. Sit when performing activities longer than 10 min. • Avoid sitting in low chairs. • Simplify tasks and avoid unnecessary tasks. • Space self-care and other activities out. • Alternate light and heavy activities. • Consider using bath bench or shower chair. • Avoid extreme temperatures. • Use proper breathing techniques. • Wear loose fitting clothing. • Consider a portable telephone. • Use light-weight pots and pans. • Slide heavy objects instead of lifting them. • Consider use of utility cart on wheels. • Avoid unnecessary bending, reaching, stooping. • Keep items within reach. • Get enough sleep at night. • Reduce distractions. • Pace.

they are sometimes contraindicated for specific cancer diagnoses.[67] Increases in hemoglobin for individuals with stable disease who have responded to chemotherapy have reflected improved energy levels and QOL.[68]

In cases of CRF that persists after more conservative measures, other medications have been used to address symptomatic complaints. Methylphenidate is a medication commonly used for fatigue, drowsiness, and lethargy, and has been used in the treatment of CRF. Its primary mechanism of action is to increase dopamine levels in the CNS and has been effective in treating opioid-induced sedation, depression, and fatigue. With a prolonged duration of treatment, its therapeutic effects and efficacy seem to improve. Individuals who suffered from more severe fatigue with advanced disease have shown improved fatigue levels. Potential negative reactions associated with methylphenidate dosing include vertigo, anxiety, nausea, or anorexia.[69] Modafinil has been shown to control CRF in patients with severe fatigue.[70] It may also have a role in improving alertness and cognitive skills in patients with cancer pain.[71]

Although other agents have been used for CRF, efficacy of treatment has not been established. For example, therapeutic effects for CRF are not conclusive for dexamphetamine, paroxetine, or testosterone. The evidence supporting amantadine, pemoline, modafinil, donepezil, and carnitine in CRF is weak and inconclusive. Further work is necessary to understand how dexamethasone, methylprednisolone, acetylsalicylic acid, and armodafinil may affect CRF. With larger and more comprehensive clinical trials, an evidence basis may be developed that supports other agents in the treatment of symptomatic fatigue.[72]

Supportive Management

Several supportive measures can be implemented in a multifaceted approach for CRF. Nutritional insufficiencies are common due to the cancer, the body's response to its diagnosis, and treatment effects. For improved homeostasis, cells require appropriate nutrients for efficient function, including carbohydrates, fats, protein, vitamins, minerals, and water.[23] Medical management of conditions such as nausea, vomiting, mucositis, and diarrhea may allow for improved intake. Agents can also be used for malabsorption to help with dysmotility.

Dietary counseling is an intervention that can influence nutritional management.[73] In the breast cancer population, survivors with better quality diets had lower total fatigue levels.[74] Although several different options are available to optimize nutrition, considerations may include higher levels of dietary fiber, fruits, and vegetables, and decreased saturated fats, as these have potential to improve overall levels of fatigue. Protein supplementation may be valuable as low protein intake correlates with higher degrees of CRF in patients with advanced cancer who received chemotherapy.[75] Antioxidants may be of some benefit given the inflammatory component of malnutrition as they have been shown in select populations to improve CRF.[76] Assessment for obesity should be considered as it is a modifiable risk factor in the development of CRF.[77] With appropriate dietary consultation, nutritional intake can be optimized to improve fatigue levels.[78]

Disorders in mood can be managed both with medications and psychosocial interventions. Paroxetine is a selective serotonin reuptake inhibitor and has shown to be of benefit for fatigue when it is a symptom of clinical depression. Similarly, the mechanism of action of bupropion is reuptake inhibition of both norepinephrine and dopamine, which may provide a stimulatory effect for CRF.[79] Data for newer agents as it relates to CRF are limited, but with further research other medications may be determined effective in the amelioration of symptoms. Current evidence also suggests that psychosocial interventions can reduce fatigue in patients

TABLE 12.9
Options for Psychosocial Intervention

Intervention
Behavioral interventions
Coping strategy training
Education
Group support intervention
Individual support intervention
Stress management

TABLE 12.10
Conditions Associated With Sleep Disruption

Conditions
Circadian rhythm sleep disorders
Hypersomnias
Insomnia
Parasomnias
Sleep-related breathing disorders
Sleep-related movement disorders

receiving cancer treatment (Table 12.9).[80] Patients may benefit from intervention during and at the completion of oncology care, but consensus has not been established as it relates to specific interventions based on technique, duration, and timing of psychosocial intervention.[75] Multimodal approaches may prove beneficial to address symptomatic complaints.[81]

Sleep hygiene is a reversible cause of fatigue, and several interventions can provide improvements in severity of symptoms. Several conditions may cause disruption to sleep, and referral to a sleep specialist may be warranted for further workup (Table 12.10). Management of the time for administration of medications, such as those for bowel and bladder or stimulants, may allow for appropriate efficacy with minimal disruption of sleep patterns. In addition, agents that cause daytime sleepiness may be given later in the day to allow for improved alertness during the day and rest at night. Although hypnotic medications, including benzodiazepines and antihistamines, may help induce and maintain sleep, residual fatigue after awakening may be a concern.[82] Stress reduction techniques, such as yoga or meditation, and cognitive behavioral therapies can be used at bedtime to ease hyperarousal responses.[45,68] An appropriate sleep environment should be dark, free of stimuli, and comfortable.[45]

PATIENT-CENTERED CONSIDERATIONS

Return to Work and Financial Impacts

Difficulties in physical functioning and performance of activities of daily living may preclude survivors from higher level activities, such as work. Several considerations can affect return into the work environment (Table 12.11). For patients with fatigue at 6 months, sick leave was predictably longer. However, at 18 months, 64% of patients evaluated did return to work. Fatigue scores closely correlated with age, gender, diagnosis, and treatment type, but fatigue levels did predict return to work.[83] For cancer patients, self-assessed work ability is an important factor for the return to work process and is independent of age and clinical factors. Ability to work at 6 months after the first day of sick leave is a strong predictor of actual return to work at 18 months.[84] Adjustments of work and support can be accomplished with occupational work assessments and interventions, which regularly assess working ability and hours.[85] Limiting fatigue can be a promising intervention to enhance earlier return to work.[86]

TABLE 12.11
Factors That May Influence Return to Work

Considerations
Age
Cancer diagnosis and type
Depression and depression scores
Fatigue
Gender
Oncologic treatment
Physical complaints

The financial and social consequences of cancer can be as significant as somatic and psychologic effects.[87] Cancer-related financial burden is associated with lower health-related QOL and increased risk of depressed mood.[88] Furthermore, increased financial burden due to cancer care costs is the strongest independent predictor of poor QOL among cancer survivors.[89] Individuals receiving cancer treatment have higher healthcare expenditures and are less likely to be employed full time. Future focus on these issues is necessary to ensure survivors will not be burdened by both high medical costs and impaired health status.[90]

CONCLUSIONS

CRF remains a significant component of cancer care. It is both severe and distressing, and not alleviated by rest. Individuals with CNS tumors are highly susceptible to fatigue. Although the etiology may be multifactorial, it may be influenced at the microscopic and macroscopic levels. Evaluation of medical comorbidities is important to assess reversible causes, including treatment effects from oncologic interventions. Careful review of medications and their side effect profiles, as well as mood, are essential to comprehensively address symptoms. Patient-reported symptom measures are the most common method for screening, which if sensitive should lead to a more sophisticated clinical evaluation. Treatment options include medications, exercise, and supportive measures. Consideration should be made regarding the impact of fatigue on daily functioning, as well as higher level activities such as work.

REFERENCES

1. Berger AM, Mooney K, Alvarez-Perez A, et al. Cancer-related fatigue, version 2.2015. *J Natl Compr Cancer Netw.* 2015;13(8):1012–1039.
2. Weis J. Cancer-related fatigue: prevalence, assessment and treatment strategies. *Expert Rev Pharmacoecon Outcomes Res.* 2011;11(4):441–446.
3. Hofman M, Ryan JL, Figueroa-Moseley CD, et al. Cancer-related fatigue: the scale of the problem. *Oncologist.* 2007;12(suppl 1):4–10.
4. Goldstein D, Bennett BK, Webber K, et al. Cancer-related fatigue in women with breast cancer: outcomes of a 5-year prospective cohort study. *J Clin Oncol.* 2012;30(15): 1805–1812.
5. Wang XS, Zhao F, Fisch MJ, et al. Prevalence and characteristics of moderate to severe fatigue: a multicenter study in cancer patients and survivors. *Cancer.* 2014;120(3): 425–432.
6. Liu R, Page M, Solheim K, et al. Quality of life in adults with brain tumors: current knowledge and future directions. *Neuro Oncol.* 2009;11(3):330–339.
7. Armstrong TS, Cron SG, Bolanos EV, et al. Risk factors for fatigue severity in primary brain tumor patients. *Cancer.* 2010;116(11):2707–2715.
8. Hauser K, Walsh D, Rybicki LA, et al. Fatigue in advanced cancer: a prospective study. *Am J Hosp Palliat Care.* 2008; 25(5):372–378.
9. Raj VS, Lofton L. Rehabilitation and treatment of spinal cord tumors. *J Spinal Cord Med.* 2013;36(1):4–11.
10. Prinsen H, Bleijenberg G, Zwarts MJ, et al. Physiological and neurophysiological determinants of postcancer fatigue: design of a randomized controlled trial. *BMC Cancer.* 2012;12:256.
11. Horneber M, Fischer I, Dimeo F, et al. Cancer-related fatigue: epidemiology, pathogenesis, diagnosis, and treatment. *Dtsch Arztebl Int.* 2012;109(9):161–171; quiz 172.
12. Berger AM, Parker KP, Young-McCaughan S, et al. Sleep wake disturbances in people with cancer and their caregivers: state of the science. *Oncol Nurs Forum.* 2005; 32(6):E98–E126.
13. Ancoli-Israel S, Liu L, Marler MR, et al. Fatigue, sleep, and circadian rhythms prior to chemotherapy for breast cancer. *Support Care Cancer.* 2006;14(3):201–209.
14. Ancoli-Israel S, Moore PJ, Jones V. The relationship between fatigue and sleep in cancer patients: a review. *Eur J Cancer Care.* 2001;10(4):245–255.
15. Dicato M, Plawny L, Diederich M. Anemia in cancer. *Ann Oncol.* 2010;21(suppl 7):vii167–vii172.
16. Gilreath JA, Stenehjem DD, Rodgers GM. Diagnosis and treatment of cancer-related anemia. *Am J Hematol.* 2014; 89(2):203–212.
17. Cella D. Factors influencing quality of life in cancer patients: anemia and fatigue. *Semin Oncol.* 1998;25(3 suppl 7):43–46.
18. Cella D, Kallich J, McDermott A, et al. The longitudinal relationship of hemoglobin, fatigue and quality of life in anemic cancer patients: results from five randomized clinical trials. *Ann Oncol.* 2004;15(6):979–986.
19. Mock V, Atkinson A, Barsevick A, et al. NCCN practice guidelines for cancer-related fatigue. *Oncology (Williston Park).* 2000;14(11A):151–161.
20. Kumar N, Allen KA, Riccardi D, et al. Fatigue, weight gain, lethargy and amenorrhea in breast cancer patients on chemotherapy: is subclinical hypothyroidism the culprit? *Breast Cancer Res Treat.* 2004;83(2):149–159.
21. Hartmann K. Thyroid disorders in the oncology patient. *J Adv Pract Oncol.* 2015;6(2):99–106.
22. Carter Y, Sippel RS, Chen H. Hypothyroidism after a cancer diagnosis: etiology, diagnosis, complications, and management. *Oncologist.* 2014;19(1):34–43. https://doi.org/10.1634/theoncologist.2013-0237.
23. Winningham ML. Strategies for managing cancer-related fatigue syndrome: a rehabilitation approach. *Cancer.* 2001;92(4 suppl):988–997.
24. Van Cutsem E, Arends J. The causes and consequences of cancer-associated malnutrition. *Eur J Oncol Nurs.* 2005; 9(suppl 2):S51–S63.
25. Marín Caro MM, Laviano A, Pichard C. Nutritional intervention and quality of life in adult oncology patients. *Clin Nutr.* 2007;26(3):289–301.
26. Caro MM, Laviano A, Pichard C, et al. Relationship between nutritional intervention and quality of life in cancer patients. *Nutr Hosp.* 2007;22(3):337–350.
27. Berger A. Treating fatigue in cancer patients. *Oncologist.* 2003;8(suppl 1):10–14.
28. Iwase S, Kawaguchi T, Tokoro A, et al. Assessment of cancer-related fatigue, pain, and quality of life in cancer patients at palliative care team referral: a multicenter observational study (JORTC PAL-09). *PLoS One.* 2015; 10(8):e0134022.

29. Church MK, Church DS. Pharmacology of antihistamines. *Indian J Dermatol.* 2013;58(3):219–224.
30. Siniscalchi A, Gallelli L, Russo E, et al. A review on antiepileptic drugs-dependent fatigue: pathophysiological mechanisms and incidence. *Eur J Pharmacol.* 2013;718(1–3):10–16.
31. Brown LF, Kroenke K. Cancer-related fatigue and its associations with depression and anxiety: a systematic review. *Psychosomatics.* 2009;50(5):440–447.
32. Schiff D, Lee EQ, Nayak L, et al. Medical management of brain tumors and the sequelae of treatment. *Neuro Oncol.* 2015;17(4):488–504.
33. Rooney AG, McNamara S, Mackinnon M, et al. Frequency, clinical associations, and longitudinal course of major depressive disorder in adults with cerebral glioma. *J Clin Oncol.* 2011;29(32):4307–4312.
34. Griffin CE, Kaye AM, Bueno FR, Kaye AD. Benzodiazepine pharmacology and central nervous system–mediated effects. *Ochsner J.* 2013;13(2):214–223.
35. Rooney A, Grant R. Pharmacological treatment of depression in patients with a primary brain tumour. *Cochrane Database Syst Rev.* 2013;(5):CD006932.
36. Corbett T, Devane D, Walsh JC, et al. Protocol for a systematic review of psychological interventions for cancer-related fatigue in post-treatment cancer survivors. *Syst Rev.* 2015;4:174.
37. Wang XS. Pathophysiology of cancer-related fatigue. *Clin J Oncol Nurs.* 2008;12(5 suppl):11–20.
38. Campos MP, Hassan BJ, Riechelmann R, et al. Cancer-related fatigue: a review. *Rev Assoc Med Bras (1992).* 2011;57(2):211–219.
39. Jean-Pierre P, Figueroa-Moseley CD, Kohli S, et al. Assessment of cancer-related fatigue: implications for clinical diagnosis and treatment. *Oncologist.* 2007;12(suppl 1):11–21.
40. Berger AM, Mitchell SA, Jacobsen PB, et al. Screening, evaluation, and management of cancer-related fatigue: ready for implementation to practice? *CA Cancer J Clin.* 2015;65(3):190–211.
41. Watanabe SM, Nekolaichuk C, Beaumont C, et al. A multicenter study comparing two numerical versions of the Edmonton Symptom Assessment System in palliative care patients. *J Pain Symptom Manage.* 2011;41(2):456–468.
42. Gaitonde DY, Rowley KD, Sweeney LB. Hypothyroidism: an update. *Am Fam Physician.* 2012;86(3):244–251.
43. Short MW, Domagalski JE. Iron deficiency anemia: evaluation and management. *Am Fam Physician.* 2013;87(2):98–104.
44. Aslinia F, Mazza JJ, Yale SH. Megaloblastic anemia and other causes of macrocytosis. *Clin Med Res.* 2006;4(3):236–241.
45. Buffart LM, De Backer IC, Schep G, Vreugdenhil A, et al. Fatigue mediates the relationship between physical fitness and quality of life in cancer survivors. *J Sci Med Sport.* 2013;16(2):99–104.
46. Hampson JP, Zick SM, Khabir T, et al. Altered resting brain connectivity in persistent cancer related fatigue. *NeuroImage Clin.* 2015;8:305–313.
47. Kampshoff CS, Chinapaw MM, Brug J, et al. Randomized controlled trial of the effects of high intensity and low-to-moderate intensity exercise on physical fitness and fatigue in cancer survivors: results of the Resistance and Endurance exercise after ChemoTherapy (REACT) study. *BMC Med.* 2015;13:275–287.
48. Windsor PM, Nicol KF, Potter J. A randomized, controlled trial of aerobic exercise for treatment-related fatigue in men receiving radical external beam radiotherapy for localized prostate carcinoma. *Cancer.* 2004;101:550–557.
49. Mitchell SA, Beck SL, Hood LE, et al. Putting evidence into practice: evidence-based interventions for fatigue during and following cancer and its treatment. *Clin J Oncol Nurs.* 2007;11:99–113.
50. Knols R, Aaronson NK, Uebelhart D, et al. Physical exercise in cancer patients during and after medical treatment: a systematic review of randomized and controlled clinical trials. *J Clin Oncol.* 2005;23:3830–3842.
51. Mustian KM, Alfano CM, Heckler C, Kleckner AS, et al. Comparison of pharmaceutical, psychological, and exercise treatments for cancer-related fatigue a meta-analysis. *JAMA Oncol.* 2017;3(7):961–968.
52. Huether K, Abbott L, Cullen L, et al. Energy through motion: an evidence-based exercise program to reduce cancer-related fatigue and improve quality of life. *Clin J Oncol Nurs.* 2016;20(3):60–70.
53. Santa MD, Au D, Howell D, et al. Effects of the community-based Wellspring Cancer Exercise Program on functional and psychosocial outcomes in cancer survivors. *Curr Oncol.* 2017;24(5):284–294.
54. Strong A, Karavatas G, Reicherter EA. Recommended exercise protocol to decrease cancer-related fatigue and muscle wasting in patients with multiple myeloma: an evidence-based systematic review. *Top Geriatr Rehabil.* 2006;22:172–186.
55. Patel JG, Bhise RA. Effect of aerobic exercise on cancer-related fatigue. *Indian J Palliat Care.* 2017;23:355–361.
56. Cantarero-Villanueva I, Fernandez-Lao C, Cuesta-Vargas AI, et al. The effectiveness of a deep water aquatic exercise program in cancer-related fatigue in breast cancer survivors: a randomized controlled trial. *Arch Phys Med Rehabil.* 2013;94:221–230.
57. Physical Activities Guidelines Advisory Committee. *Physical Activity Guidelines Advisory Committee Report.* Washington, DC: US Department of Health and Human Services; 2008. https://health.gov/paguidelines/guidelines/summary.aspx.
58. Courneya KS, Friedenreich CM. Physical activity and cancer control. *Semin Oncol Nurs.* 2007;23(4):242–252.
59. Cramp F, Byron-Daniel J. Exercise for the management of cancer-related fatigue in adults. *Cochrane Database Syst Rev.* 2012;11:CD006145.

60. Oldervoll LM, Loge JH, Paltiel H, et al. The effect of a physical exercise program in palliative care: a phase II study. *J Pain Symptom Manage.* 2006;31:421–430.
61. Luciani A, Jacobsen PB, Extermann M, et al. Fatigue and functional dependence in older cancer patients. *Am J Clin Oncol.* 2008;31:424–430.
62. Pickett M, Mock V, Ropka M, et al. Adherence to moderate-intensity exercise during breast cancer therapy. *Cancer Pract.* 2002;10:284–292.
63. Mock V, Frangakis C, Davidson NE, et al. Exercise manages fatigue during breast cancer treatment: a randomized controlled trial. *Psychooncology.* 2005;14:464–477.
64. Schmitz KH, Courneya KS, Matthews C, et al. American College of Sports Medicine roundtable on exercise guidelines for cancer survivors. *Med Sci Sports Exerc.* 2010; 42(7):1409–1426.
65. Chakera AJ, Pearce SH, Vaidya B. Treatment for primary hypothyroidism: current approaches and future possibilities. *Drug Des Devel Ther.* 2012;6:1–11.
66. Barsevick AM, Dudley W, Beck S, et al. A randomized clinical trial of energy conservation for patients with cancer-related fatigue. *Cancer.* 2004;100:1302–1310.
67. Camaschella C. Iron deficiency: new insights into diagnosis and treatment. *Hematol Am Soc Hematol Educ Program.* 2015;2015:8–13.
68. Carroll JK, Kohli S, Mustian KM, et al. Pharmacologic treatment of cancer-related fatigue. *Oncologist.* 2007;12(suppl 1):43–51.
69. Gong S, Sheng P, Jin H, et al. Effect of methylphenidate in patients with cancer-related fatigue: a systematic review and meta-analysis. *PLoS One.* 2014;9(1):e84391.
70. Jean-Pierre P, Morrow GR, Roscoe JA, et al. A phase 3 randomized, placebo-controlled, double-blind, clinical trial of the effect of modafinil on cancer-related fatigue among 631 patients receiving chemotherapy: a University of Rochester Cancer Center Community Clinical Oncology Program Research base study. *Cancer.* 2010;116(14): 3513–3520. https://doi.org/10.1002/cncr.25083.
71. Wirz S, Nadstawek J, Kühn KU, et al. Modafinil for the treatment of cancer-related fatigue : an intervention study. *Schmerz.* 2010;24(6):587–595.
72. Mücke M, Mochamat Cuhls H, et al. Pharmacological treatments for fatigue associated with palliative care. *Cochrane Database Syst Rev.* 2015;(5):CD006788.
73. Mustian KM, Morrow GR, Carroll JK, et al. Integrative nonpharmacologic behavioral interventions for the management of cancer-related fatigue. *Oncologist.* 2007; 12(suppl 1):52–67.
74. George SM, Alfano CM, Neuhouser ML, et al. Better post-diagnosis diet quality is associated with less cancer-related fatigue in breast cancer survivors. *J Cancer Surviv.* 2014; 8(4):680–687.
75. Stobäus N, Müller MJ, Küpferling S, et al. Low recent protein intake predicts cancer-related fatigue and increased mortality in patients with advanced tumor disease undergoing chemotherapy. *Nutr Cancer.* 2015;67(5):818–824.
76. Maschke J, Kruk U, Kastrati K, et al. Nutritional care of cancer patients: a survey on patients' needs and medical care in reality. *Int J Clin Oncol.* 2017;22(1):200–206.
77. Bower JE, Lamkin DM. Inflammation and cancer-related fatigue: mechanisms, contributing factors, and treatment implications. *Brain Behav Immun.* 2013;30(0):S48–S57.
78. Baguley BJ, Bolam KA, Wright ORL, Skinner TL. The effect of nutrition therapy and exercise on cancer-related fatigue and quality of life in men with prostate cancer: a systematic review. *Nutrients.* 2017;9(9):1003.
79. Breitbart W, Alici-Evcimen Y. Update on psychotropic medications for cancer-related fatigue. *J Natl Compr Cancer Netw.* 2007;5(10):1081–1091.
80. Goedendorp MM, Gielissen MF, Verhagen CA, et al. Psychosocial interventions for reducing fatigue during cancer treatment in adults. *Cochrane Database Syst Rev.* 2009;(1): CD006953.
81. Wang XS, Woodruff JF. Cancer-related and treatment-related fatigue. *Gynecol Oncol.* 2015;136(3):446–452.
82. Armstrong TS, Gilbert MR. Practical strategies for management of fatigue and sleep disorders in people with brain tumors. *Neuro Oncol.* 2012;14(suppl 4):iv65–iv72.
83. Spelten ER, Verbeek JH, Uitterhoeve AL, et al. Cancer, fatigue and the return of patients to work-a prospective cohort study. *Eur J Cancer.* 2003;39(11):1562–1567.
84. De Boer AGEM, Verbeek JHAM, Spelten ER, et al. Work ability and return-to-work in cancer patients. *Br J Cancer.* 2008;98(8):1342–1347.
85. Munir F, Yarker J, McDermott H. Employment and the common cancers: correlates of work ability during or following cancer treatment. *Occup Med (Lond).* 2009; 59(6):381–389.
86. Wolvers MDJ, Leensen MCJ, Groeneveld IF, et al. Predictors for earlier return to work of cancer patients. *J Cancer Surviv.* 2017;12 [Epub ahead of print].
87. Seifart U, Schmielau J. Return to work of cancer survivors. *Oncol Res Treat.* 2017;40(12):760–763.
88. Kale HP, Carroll NV. Self-reported financial burden of cancer care and its effect on physical and mental health-related quality of life among US cancer survivors. *Cancer.* 2016;122(8):283–289.
89. Fenn KM, Evans SB, McCorkle R, et al. Impact of financial burden of cancer on survivors' quality of life. *J Oncol Pract.* 2014;10(5):332–338.
90. Finkelstein EA, Tangka FK, Trogdon JG, et al. The personal financial burden of cancer for the working-aged population. *Am J Manag Care.* 2009;15(11):801–806.

CHAPTER 13

Spinal Imaging, Stability and Management of Spine Pain due to Cancer

T. LEFKOWITZ, DO, DABPMR • A. IANNICELLO, MD • N. OZURUMBA, MD

INTRODUCTION

As physiatrists continue to fill the role of *"gate keepers"* in many outpatient- and hospital-based orthopedic and neurosurgical practices, our surgical colleagues increasingly rely upon us to quickly identify those patients presenting with spinal pain, constitutional symptoms (i.e., red flags), and abnormal imaging findings indicative of metastatic spinal disease or primary spinal tumors. There is a need to further educate physiatrists practicing in these settings on the relevant patient histories, radiologic evaluations, management strategies, and disposition of patients presenting with cancer-induced back pain (CIBP). This chapter will review some of the more commonly seen benign and malignant spinal lesions that physiatrists may encounter in clinical practice by way of brief case histories and expected imaging findings. It is the authors' hope that the information provided within will lessen any anxieties surrounding these patients, especially related to their imaging and treatment.

HISTORY

The term *"red flag"* was first used by the Clinical Standards Advisory Group in 1994 to identify signs and symptoms associated with cancer or an active malignancy.[1] Red flags including age over 50, night pain, unexplained weight loss, fever or chills, progressive neurologic deficit, bladder dysfunction, saddle anesthesia or any history of cancer, immune suppression, or environmental or toxin exposure should be elicited in the patient's review of symptoms. Furthermore, the patient's smoking history and alcohol intake should be documented in the social history. A family history of cancer should be established, particularly in first-degree relatives, such as parents or siblings.

Constitutional or systemic symptoms are often nonspecific and may be encountered in a variety of disease states including certain infectious (i.e., pyogenic discitis or Pott's disease), hematologic (i.e., sickle cell or Gaucher's disease), rheumatologic (i.e., rheumatoid arthritis or systemic lupus erythematosus), and neurologic conditions (i.e., multiple sclerosis). It is therefore imperative for physiatrists to screen for them while developing an appropriate differential diagnosis.

Any unexplained weight loss of more than 5% within a 4-week period should alert the physiatrist to the possibility of an underlying malignancy and prompt further investigation.[1] Other nonspecific signs and symptoms associated with malignancy in a patient presenting with spinal pain include feeling generally unwell, malaise, loss of appetite, and decreased exercise tolerance.

The age of the patient presenting with back pain should be kept in mind as vertebral metastases are much more frequent in individuals older than 50 years.[1] Conversely, spinal pain in children, teenagers, and young adults should raise concern for more benign tumors such as osteoid osteomas or osteoblastomas. Certain malignant cancers, however, including sarcomas, lymphomas, and leukemias may be encountered in this patient population, and corroboration from the medical record should be sought.

Further in the review of systems, the physiatrist should query the patient on the quality and character of the pain experienced. Chronic cancer–related pain can arise from visceral or neural structures, but is most commonly related to bony metastases.[2] Pain that does not vary within a 24-h period; pain in the thoracic spine; severe, nonmechanical or night pain; or abdominal pain with a change in bowel habits should alert the physiatrist to the possibility of an underlying malignancy. A change is bowel habits is a red flag for metastases to the cauda equina in the appropriate clinical setting (i.e., invasion of the sacral roots by lymphoma).

Approximately 90% of all spinal (i.e., spinal cord + vertebral body) neoplasms are metastatic in origin and vertebral metastases are already present in 10% of newly diagnosed cancers.[3,4] Tumors that commonly metastasize to bone can be remembered using the mnemonic *"lead kettle"* spelled PBKTL (where lead is Pb on the Periodic Table of Elements) for prostate, breast, kidney, thyroid, and lung.[4] The axial skeleton (i.e., ribs, pelvis, and spine) is generally involved earlier than the appendicular skeleton (i.e., long bones) given the persistence of red bone marrow there. In women, breast and lung cancers represent nearly 80% of tumors metastasizing to the skeleton, whereas in males, prostate and lung cancers make up 80% of cancers metastasizing to bone.[5] The other 20% of tumors affecting both sexes include kidney, thyroid, and gastrointestinal (GI) tract cancers.

Historically, metastases to the spine were thought to occur primarily through Batson's venous plexus, a valveless plexus from the chest and pelvis, allowing malignant cells to enter the vertebral circulation without first passing through the lungs during periods of increased intra-abdominal pressure.[6] Malignant cell survival was favorable in this low-pressure venous system where repeated reversals of blood flow allowed cancer cells to lodge in the vertebral bodies. Alternatively, the *"seed and soil"* hypothesis was proposed whereby tumors were thought to metastasize through the arterial circulation rather than through venous routes.[7] Other malignancies including lymphomas and multiple myeloma may affect the spine leading to vertebral compression fractures (VCFs) and possibly spinal canal compromise.

In patients with an established cancer diagnosis, the appropriate medical records should be requested to ascertain the behavior of the cancer, its response to treatment, and any future planned medical or surgical interventions. In patients who are receiving or have undergone adjuvant chemotherapy (CTX) or radiation therapy (RTX), the physiatrist should perform a detailed medication reconciliation as various chemotherapeutic agents can cause myalgias and arthralgias (i.e., aromatase inhibitors), which may present as CIBP, in addition to the numbness, tingling, and burning sensations associated with chemotherapy-induced peripheral polyneuropathies. ISODOSE color wash maps can be requested to see how much of an individual's total radiation dose was given to nearby spinal structures which could predispose to painful VCFs. Any patient with a recent history of malignancy who presents with spinal pain to the office or clinic should raise a high suspicion for metastatic disease to the spine or iatrogenic injury from adjuvant therapies (i.e., RTX).

In reviewing the patient's past medical history, the physiatrist should also inquire about any history of immune suppression (i.e., HIV/AIDS), conditions requiring prolonged corticosteroid or immune modulating treatment (i.e., organ transplantation), or treatment of childhood cancers that may predispose to secondary cancers as an adult (i.e., leukemia).

PHYSICAL EXAMINATION

A complete physical examination should be performed with special attention paid to the neuromusculoskeletal examination. Specifically, focal motor deficits, asymmetric muscle stretch reflexes, and sensory loss should be looked for. Depending upon the location of the tumor, the patient may present with prominent upper motor neuron findings such as spastic weakness, hyperreflexia, and neurogenic bowel and bladder dysfunction. In these patients, a digital examination assessing for anal sphincter tone may be indicated. Caution is advised in patients who are neutropenic or severely thrombocytopenic from recent chemotherapy or who have undergone RTX to the pelvis as the rectal mucosa may be friable and prone to bleeding.

Further inspection of the patient can uncover areas of muscle atrophy, skin fibrosis, radiation burns or dermatitis, scars, joint contractures, and other deformities. Restricted spinal range of motion, pelvic muscle imbalance, or scoliosis should be noted if present.

In certain patients, percussion over the spinous processes of the thoracolumbar spine may elicit pain, which should alert the physiatrist to the possibility of a VCF with involvement of the posterior elements. Pain with passive lumbar extension may indicate involvement of the pars interarticularis (i.e., spondylolysis) or the zygapophyseal joints from tumor invasion. Bilateral pars defects, however, with resulting spondylolisthesis, are more commonly seen in younger patients without a history of malignancy.[8]

A positive dural tension test (i.e., seated slump test or Lasegue's test), normally implying nerve root impingement from a herniated nucleus pulposus (HNP), may also be positive in patients with nerve root sheath tumors (i.e., schwannomas or neurofibromas) as the mass lesion prevents sliding of the nerve root in its dural sleeve from compression against the pedicle. As the physical examination alone cannot differentiate between these two spinal pathologies, the physiatrist must rely upon the appropriate imaging studies to make the diagnosis.

A Lhermitte's sign may be elicited in patients who are myelopathic or those who have received radiation to the head and neck. It is thought to be caused by transient demyelination of the posterior columns of the spinal cord. Lhermitte's sign has been described as an electric shock-like sensation travelling down the spine when the examiner flexes the patient's neck.

Gait and balance testing should be included in the physical examination as loss of proprioception due to an underlying diabetic, carcinomatous, or chemotherapy-induced polyneuropathy can alter patients' postural stability and predisposition to falls. In patients with severe neoplastic spinal cord compression, one of the earliest presenting symptoms may be gait disturbance, which should prompt the physiatrist to refer for neurosurgical evaluation.

IMAGING

As the triaging spine physician, it is imperative that the physiatrist attempt to correlate the patient's physical examination findings with their imaging studies. If the patient's physical examination findings do not correlate well with their imaging, then an alternate diagnosis should be considered or a new imaging study requested to help clarify the diagnosis.

Despite recent guidelines recommending against the routine use of spinal radiographs for patients presenting with lower back pain, physiatrists often need to screen new patients with a suspicion or history of malignancy.[9] Plain radiographs are widely available and relatively low cost. X-rays are useful for evaluating large masses and pathologic fractures and detecting the presence of lytic or blastic lesions. Radiographs are, however, considered a relatively insensitive means of screening for asymptomatic metastases.[10] When evaluating for osteolytic lesions from patients with primary lung, GI, renal, or multiple myeloma, for example, 30%–50% of bone mineral loss needs to occur before these lesions become prominent on plain radiographic studies.[11] Other modalities, discussed later in the chapter, are able to detect these lesions earlier.

Our first case is of a middle-aged female with no significant past medical history who presents with a breast lump and thoracic back pain with the following radiograph (Fig. 13.1).

Anteroposterior X-ray of the thoracolumbar spine shows an absent left L1 pedicle with the so-called *"winking owl"* sign. Early destruction of a pedicle is a classic sign of metastatic disease (differentiating it from multiple myeloma, for example), but in the presence of extensive disease, tissue or laboratory diagnosis is often needed.[11]

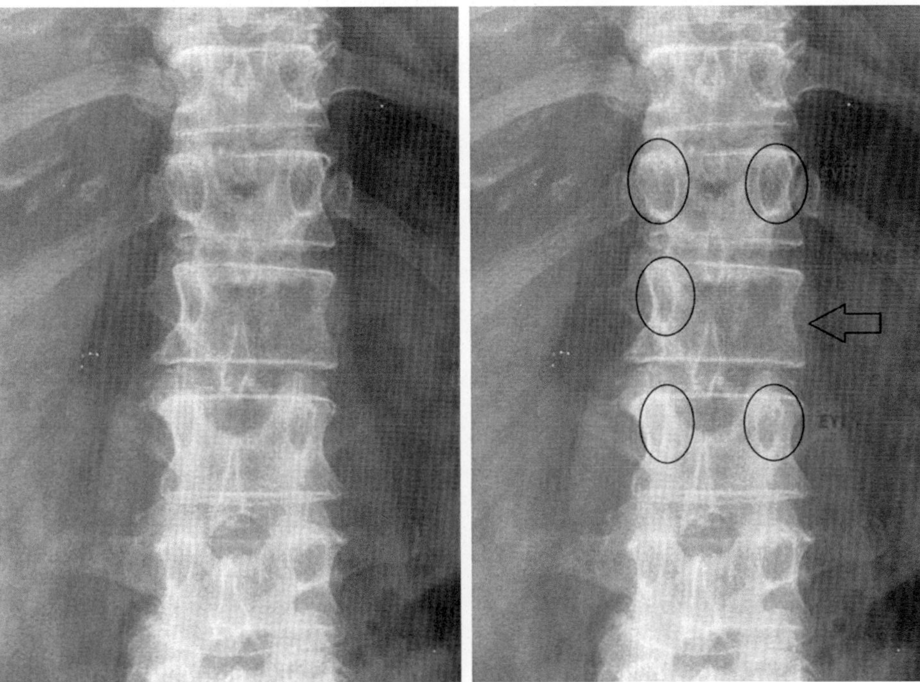

FIG. 13.1 (A) Anteroposterior radiograph thoracolumbar spine. (Case courtesy of Dr. Ian Bickle, Radiopaedia.org, rID: 21937.)

In anticipation of a metastatic workup, the physiatrist should obtain an MRI scan of the patient's thoracolumbar spine with and without contrast and discuss the findings with the patient's primary care physician.

An elderly patient referred by her primary care physician for worsening lower back pain for 6 months with a history of metastatic cancer presents with the below-mentioned MRI (Fig. 13.2). The images reveal multiple areas of abnormal signal involving the vertebral bodies and posterior elements along with prominent degenerative changes and spinal stenosis from L2-3 through L4-5. Incidentally, there is a left laminectomy defect at T11 (Fig. 13.2D). The areas of low signal on T1, high signal on T2 (excluding endplate regions), and contrast enhancement (excluding surgical bed) represent bony metastases to the spine with primary lung, prostate, renal, GI, and melanoma high on the differential. This case illustrates the difficulty differentiating tumor involvement from advanced degenerative disc disease given the latter's high prevalence in outpatient practice.[12] Similar difficulty is encountered when an infectious etiology is considered in the differential

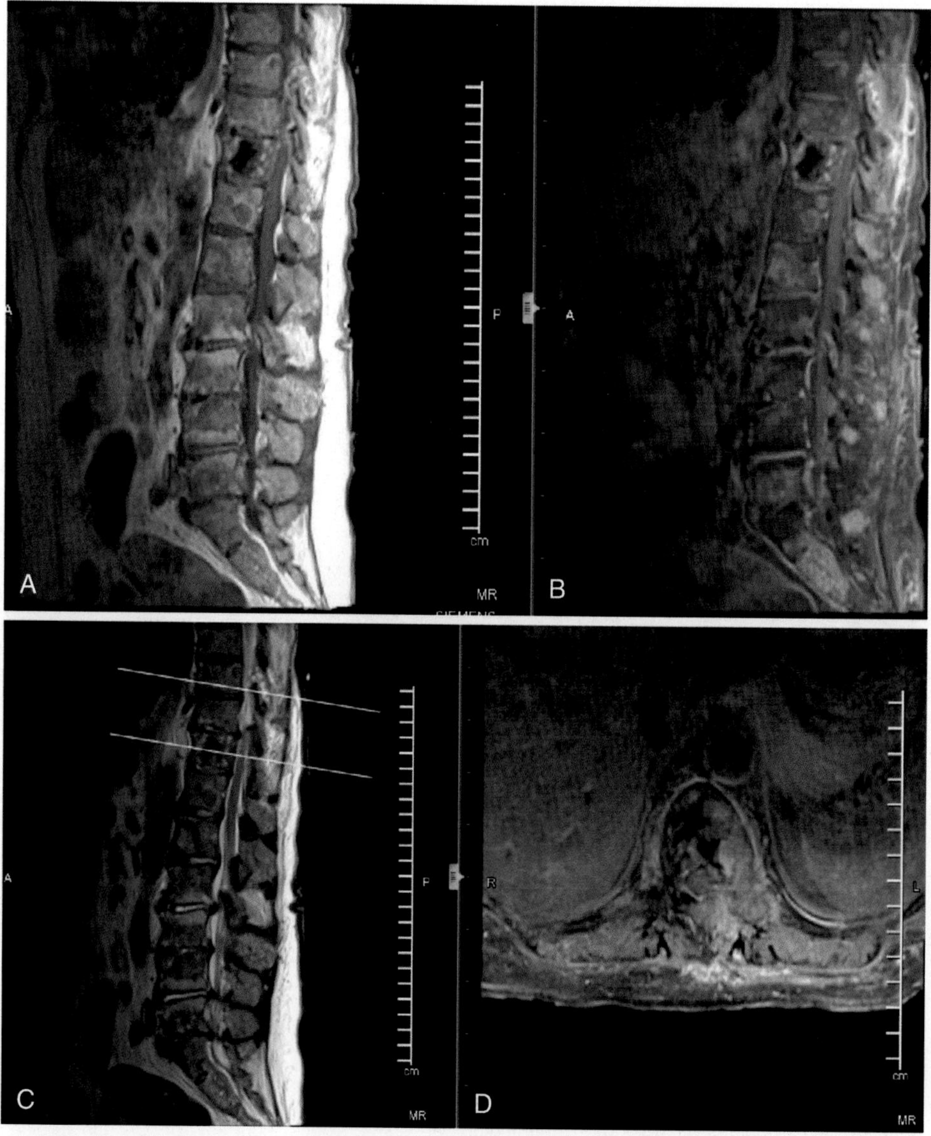

FIG. 13.2 (A) Sagittal T1-W, (B) T1-W+c, (C) T2-W, and (D) axial T1-W+c MRI lumbar spine.

diagnosis of patients with widespread degenerative disease; although, pyogenic discitis often crosses the involved disc space, whereas the signal change related to degenerative disc disease does not. Prompt discussion of the MRI findings with the patient's primary care physician is paramount to avoid further morbidity and mortality.

As a brief review of neuroimaging for the physiatrist, normal T1 imaging of bone marrow reveals high signal intensity due to its high fat content. Osseous metastases, on the other hand, have low T1 signal intensity due to remodeling and replacement of normal marrow fat with tumor.[5] On T2-weighted images, metastases appear hyperintense secondary to their elevated water content.[5] After gadolinium contrast administration, there is enhancement secondary to the increased vascularity associated with malignant cells.[5] Of note, gadolinium is a paramagnetic contrast agent that also crosses disrupted blood-brain and blood-nerve barriers. MRI does not show cortical bone very well, as such, bones with low marrow volume (i.e., ribs) are better evaluated with CT scan.

In patients with a history of cancer who present with new neurologic deficits, the physiatrist is obliged to image the entire neural axis from brain to sacrum with and without contrast. Fig. 13.3 is from a middle-aged male with metastatic prostate cancer. MRI findings are significant for diffuse predominantly low signal intensity osseous metastases on all pulse sequences typical for sclerotic metastases. At T5-6, there is high-grade

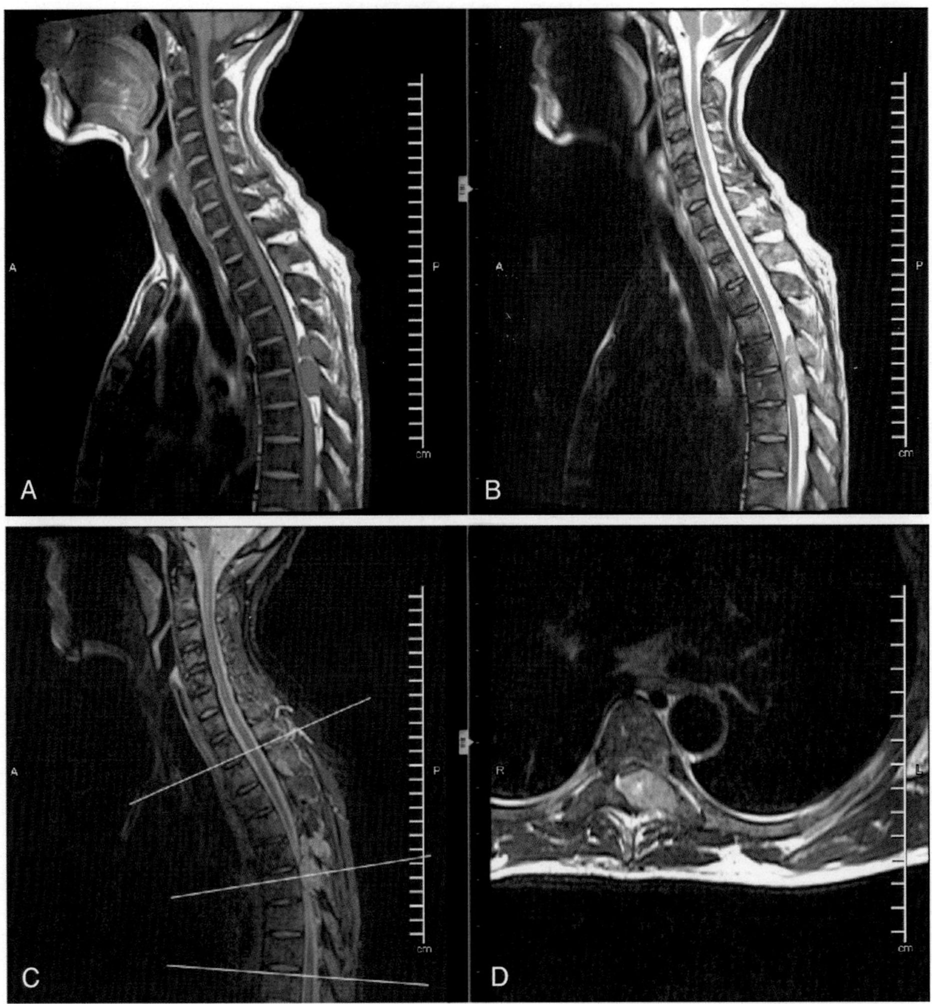

FIG. 13.3 (A) Sagittal T1-W, (B) sagittal T2-W, (C) sagittal STIR, (D) axial T2-W MRI C-spine.

epidural spinal cord compression (ESCC) arising from the left posterior elements. These findings could help explain the patient's leg weakness and bladder dysfunction.

The physiatrist may encounter the rare but concerning patient presenting with a combination of pain, weakness, sensory changes, gait disturbance, and bowel or bladder dysfunction. These individuals often report a gradual decline in physical functioning and a long history of symptoms prior to a proper diagnosis being made. The MRI in Fig. 13.4 is from a patient with an intramedullary spinal tumor extending from C2-3 to the midpoint of C4. Upon close inspection of the images, one sees low signal on T1 (with areas of high T1 signal consistent with hemorrhage), high signal on T2, and significant contrast enhancement on axial images. Vasogenic edema is seen extending above and below the lesion.

Intramedullary spinal tumors are relatively rare, representing 4%–10% of all central nervous system (CNS) tumors and less than 10% of all pediatric CNS neoplasms.[13,14] The differential diagnosis includes both glial and nonglial neoplasms, vascular lesions (i.e., cavernomas, arteriovenous fistulas), inflammatory lesions (i.e., multiple sclerosis, transverse myelitis), infectious lesions (i.e., spinal cord abscess), and spinal cord infarctions.[13,14] As the majority of intramedullary spinal tumors are of glial origin, the differential diagnosis

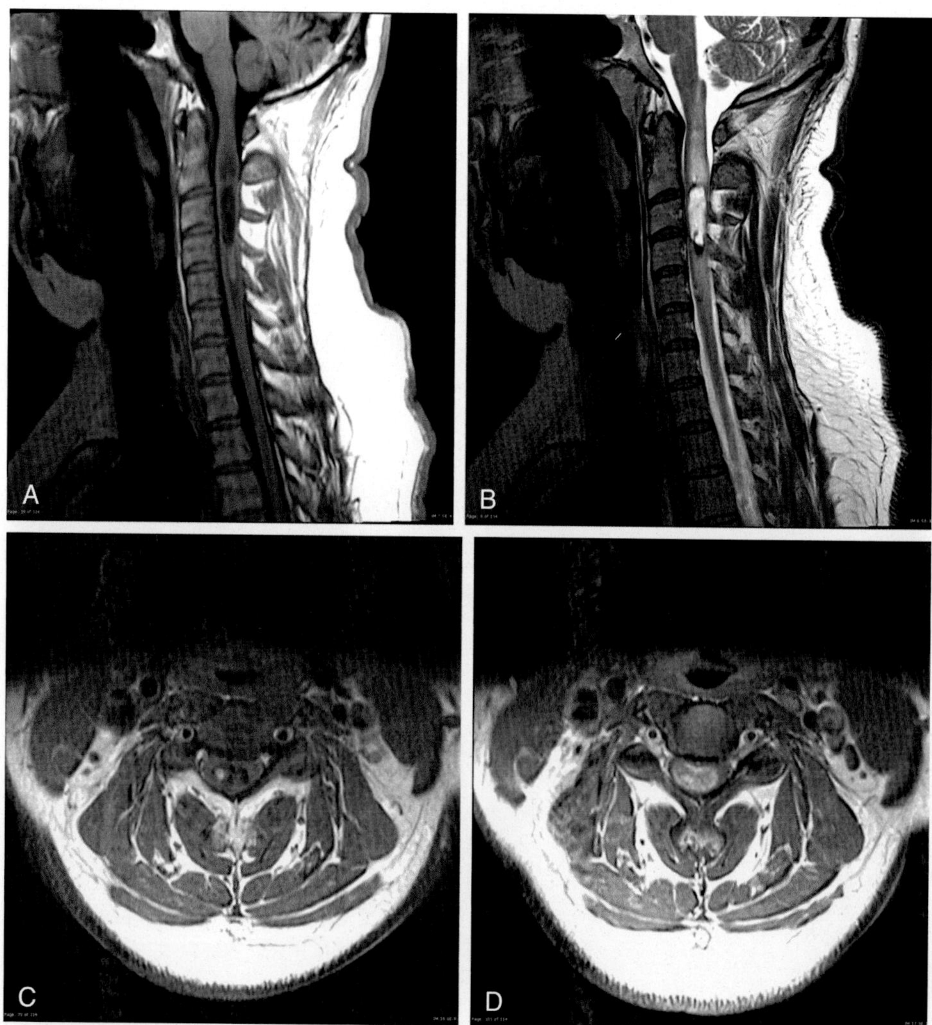

FIG. 13.4 (A) Sagittal T1-W, (B) T2-W, (C) axial T2-W, and (D) T1-W +c MRI cervical spine. (Case courtesy of Prof. Frank Gaillard, Radiopaedia.org, rID: 19319.)

shrinks to either an ependymoma (60%), astrocytoma (33%), or ganglioglioma (1%).[13,14]

The pathology and MRI characteristics in this case were most consistent with a spinal ependymoma. The physiatrist may recall the association of intramedullary spinal tumors with a history of neurofibromatosis, which may aid in making the correct diagnosis.[13]

In older patients with relapsing and remitting back pain who suffer exacerbations after minimal exertion or trauma, the physiatrist should have a lower trigger for ordering imaging studies. Fig. 13.5 is from an elderly patient whose X-ray reveals multiple thoracic VCFs causing an exaggeration of the thoracic kyphosis. These features are consistent with multiple myeloma; however, metastatic disease (i.e., breast and prostate), lymphoma, and leukemia remain in the differential as contiguous tumor involvement in the spine is common in these cancers.[15]

MRI is a more sensitive tool for detecting focal bone marrow lesions than CT or positron emission tomography (PET) scans. It is also superior when evaluating disease progression and can detect changes in lesions before they become lytic. If there is suspicion of extramedullary disease outside of the spine, whole body PET scanning is recommended as shown in Fig. 13.6.[5]

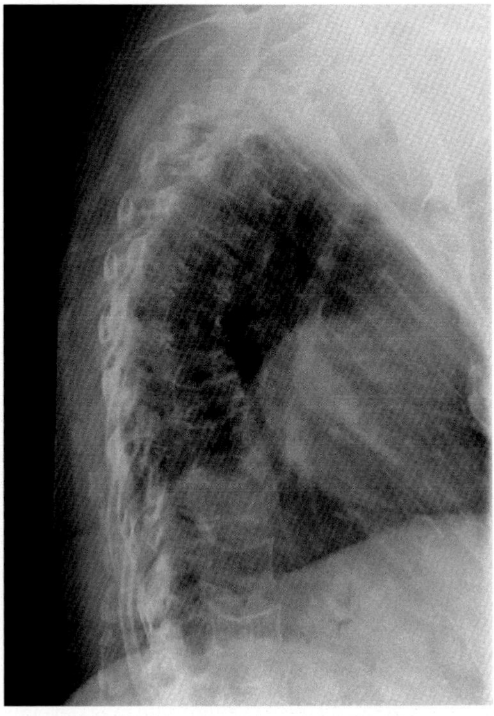

FIG. 13.5 Lateral X-ray thoracic spine.

It should be remembered that the distribution of multiple myeloma deposits mirrors that of red marrow in older individuals with the axial skeleton and proximal appendicular skeleton most commonly involved.[15] It is the most common bone neoplasm in adults, often presenting with pathologic fractures (i.e., VCFs, proximal long bone fractures), anemia, and renal failure.[15]

A 50-year-old male with a past medical history of biliary atresia and liver transplantation presents to the office with complaints of chronic lower back pain. Additional history reveals that the patient has been maintained on tacrolimus since 1998 without any episodes of rejection. The MRI scan in Fig. 13.7 was obtained revealing a pathologic crush fracture of L4 with complete replacement of the normal fatty marrow with low T1 signal soft tissue which enhances following contrast administration. At L4-5, there is moderate-to-severe central canal stenosis. An additional pathologic deposit is seen at T12. An old, nonpathologic crush fracture of L1 is also present with normal bone marrow signal.

The MRI findings are consistent with lymphoma, but multiple myeloma and metastatic disease are also in the differential. Pathology revealed diffuse large B cell lymphoma. This case illustrates the importance of taking a complete patient history and recognizing that chronic immune suppression may place patients at risk for the development of secondary cancers, which may preferentially affect the spine.

Another challenging problem arises when a patient presents without back pain but with predominantly painful radicular symptoms with a noncontrast-enhanced MRI. Fig. 13.8 is from a patient with a chronic right L4 radiculopathy. The images reveal an intradural, extramedullary mass. The differential at this point includes an HNP, schwannoma, neurofibroma, or a metastasis.

Without the administration of contrast, one may mistake this lesion for an atypical presentation of an HNP given its close proximity to the annular tear represented by the high-intensity zone seen along the posterior border of the L3-4 intervertebral disc.

Following the administration of contrast, however, as seen in Fig. 13.9, there is avid enhancement with small cystic areas of degeneration within, consistent with a schwannoma. Schwannomas are the most common intradural, extramedullary spinal tumors, accounting for 30% of such lesions.[16,17] They are most frequently seen in the cervical and lumbar spine, arising from the dorsal sensory nerve root sheaths.

In select cases, such as this, the physiatrist may request a peer-to-peer review with the medical director

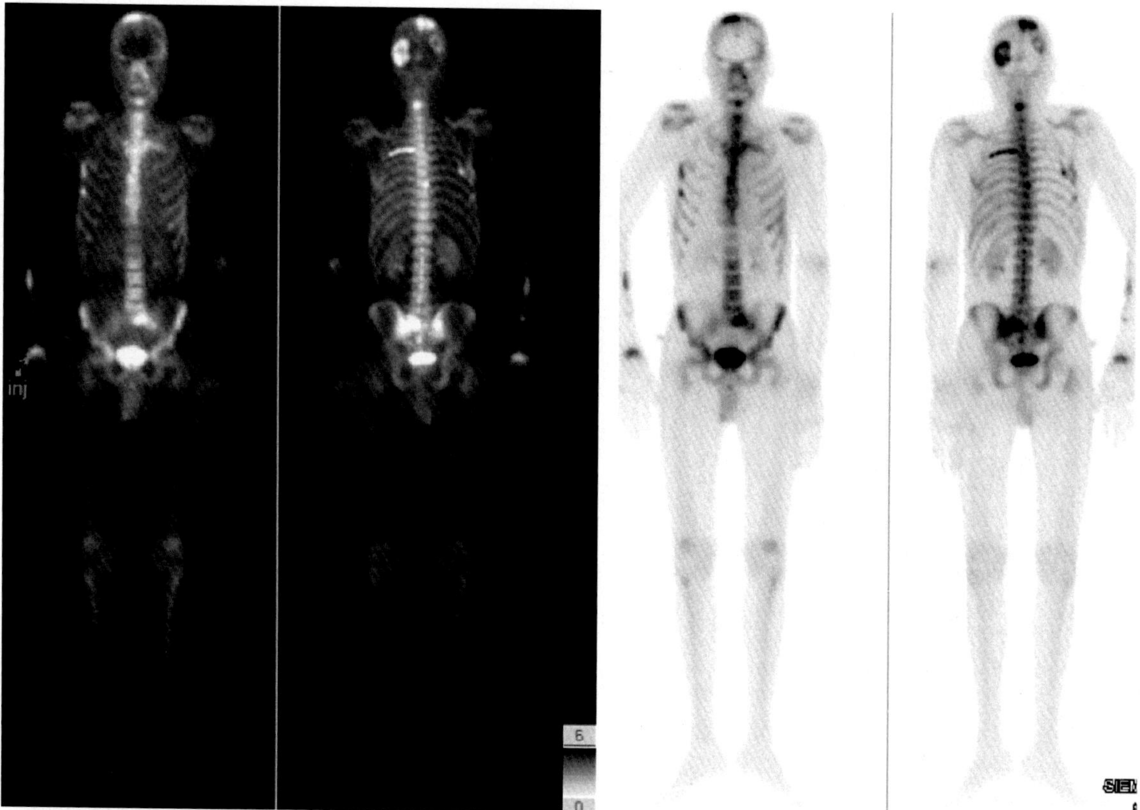

FIG. 13.6 Whole body nuclear medicine bone scan demonstrating osseous metastases within the calvarium, multiple vertebra, multiple ribs, and the sacrum.

of the patient's insurance company to help obtain authorization for an updated radiologic study to clarify the suspicious lesion seen on the prior nonenhanced MRI scan. As the mainstay of treatment for symptomatic nerve root sheath tumors remains surgical resection, this ensures that the consulting neurosurgeon has a complete MRI study for any planned surgical intervention. It is worth mentioning that the surgery to remove a presumed HNP (i.e., laminectomy and microdiscectomy) differs from that used to treat a symptomatic nerve root sheath tumor so it behooves the physiatrist to gather as much information about the lesion as early as possible.

Schwannomas and neurofibromas may occasionally compress the upper or middle trunk of the brachial plexus. Fig. 13.10 shows a well-circumscribed mass contiguous with the right C7 nerve root, which appears isointense on T1-W images, slightly hyperintense on T2-W images, and has homogeneous contrast enhancement. Compression by metastatic infiltration of axillary lymph nodes may affect the medial cord of the plexus and cause pain.[18] Workup often includes electrodiagnostic studies to rule out competing etiologies (i.e., cervical radiculopathy, entrapment neuropathy, or peripheral polyneuropathy) and MRI scans of the brachial plexus with contrast, preferably of each side, to compare any enhancing regions of the symptomatic plexus to the asymptomatic, normal plexus. Referral to a neurosurgeon specializing in peripheral nerve surgery may then be considered.

In patients presenting with shoulder and/or arm pain, paresthesias, or weakness in a predominantly lower trunk (i.e., C8/T1) distribution, the physiatrist should consider a Pancoast tumor in the differential diagnosis. Pancoast or superior sulcus tumors are relatively uncommon primary bronchogenic carcinomas typically located at the apical pleuropulmonary groove, adjacent to the subclavian vessels.[19] Weakness and atrophy of the intrinsic hand muscles may be prominent. Owing to the proximity to the paravertebral sympathetic chain and Stellate ganglion, a Horner's syndrome may develop with ipsilateral ptosis, miosis, enophthalmos, and

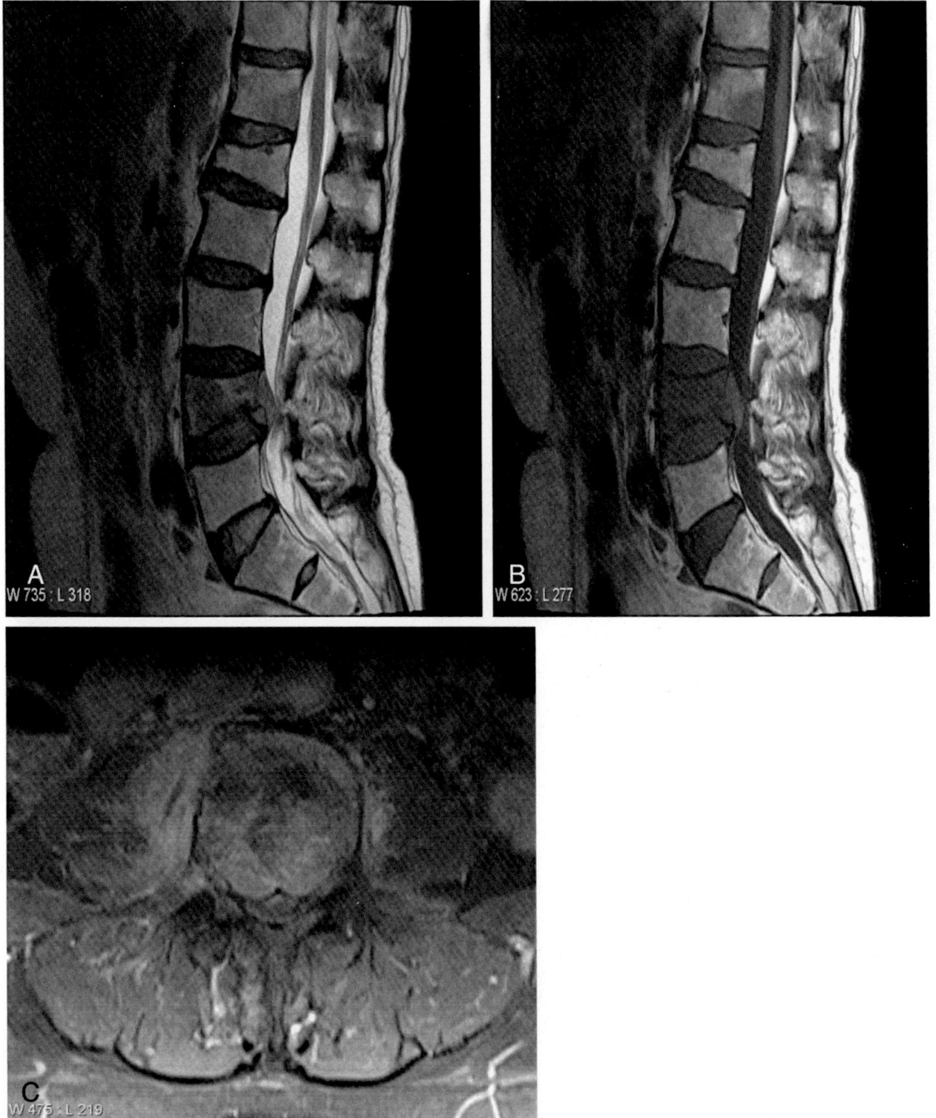

FIG. 13.7 (A) Sagittal T2-W, (B) T1-W+c, and (C) axial T1-W+c MRI lumbar spine. (Case courtesy of Prof. Frank Gaillard, Radiopaedia.org, rID: 14396.)

anhidrosis. Invasion of the intervertebral foramina may occur and cause spinal cord compression.

In younger patients, especially adolescents and young adults, complaining of back pain that cannot easily be explained by a heavy mechanical load (i.e., backpack use) or sporting injury, suspicion should be raised for neoplastic disease. Figs. 13.11 and 13.12 were obtained from a slightly older individual complaining of predominantly nocturnal lower back pain without a history of trauma, fever, or weight loss. Incidentally, the patient reported that his symptoms were relieved by the administration of aspirin.

The CT images show a sclerotic lesion within the left pedicle of L5. The MR images reveal a focal area of low T1 and T2 signal intensity. The T2 fat saturation sequence reveals bony edema within the pedicle. There is a central area of high signal intensity within the sclerotic area which enhances after contrast administration.

The clinical and radiologic findings are most consistent with an osteoid osteoma. Osteoid osteomas are

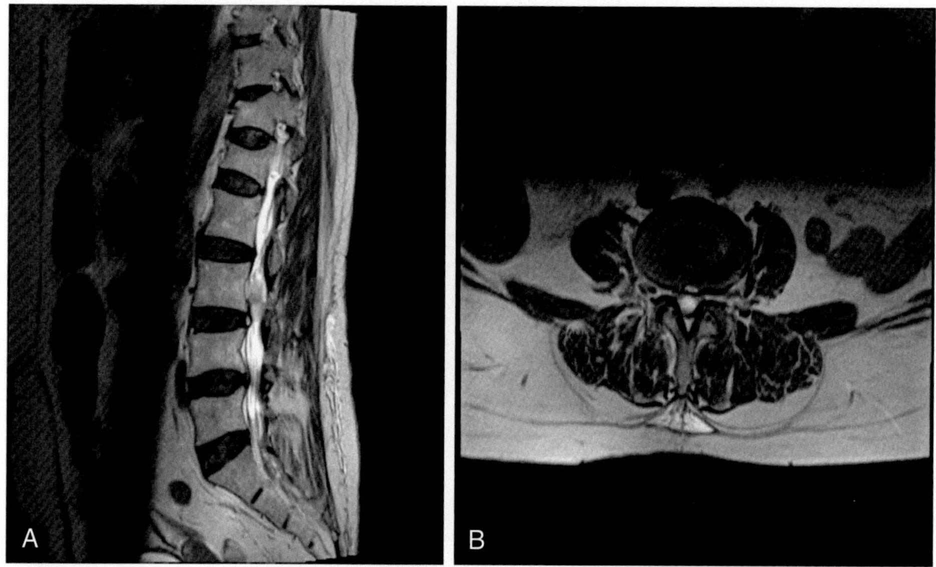

FIG. 13.8 (A) Sagittal T2-W and (B) axial T2-W MRI lumbar spine without contrast. (Case courtesy of Dr. Ian Bickle, Radiopaedia.org, rID: 25448.)

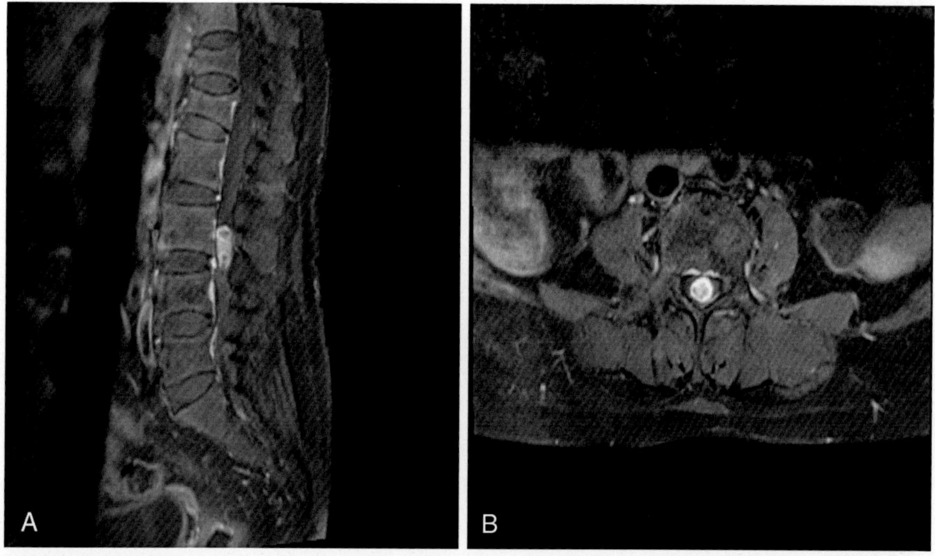

FIG. 13.9 (A) Sagittal T1-W +c and (B) axial T1-W MRI lumbar spine +c. (Case courtesy of Dr. Ian Bickle, Radiopaedia.org, rID: 25448.)

benign neoplasms which account for approximately 10% of all benign bone lesions.[20] Although they are predominantly found in long tubular bones of the limbs (i.e., proximal femur), when in the spine, a painful scoliosis, concave on the side of lesion, can develop. They are differentiated from osteoblastomas principally by size. Osteoid osteomas are typically 1 cm or less where osteoblastomas are 2 cm or larger.[20] The nidus releases prostaglandins which cause pain and are therefore exquisitely sensitive to the administration of aspirin or other NSAIDs.

It is not uncommon for patients presenting with back pain to ask the treating physician the significance of this incidental finding seen on routine spinal

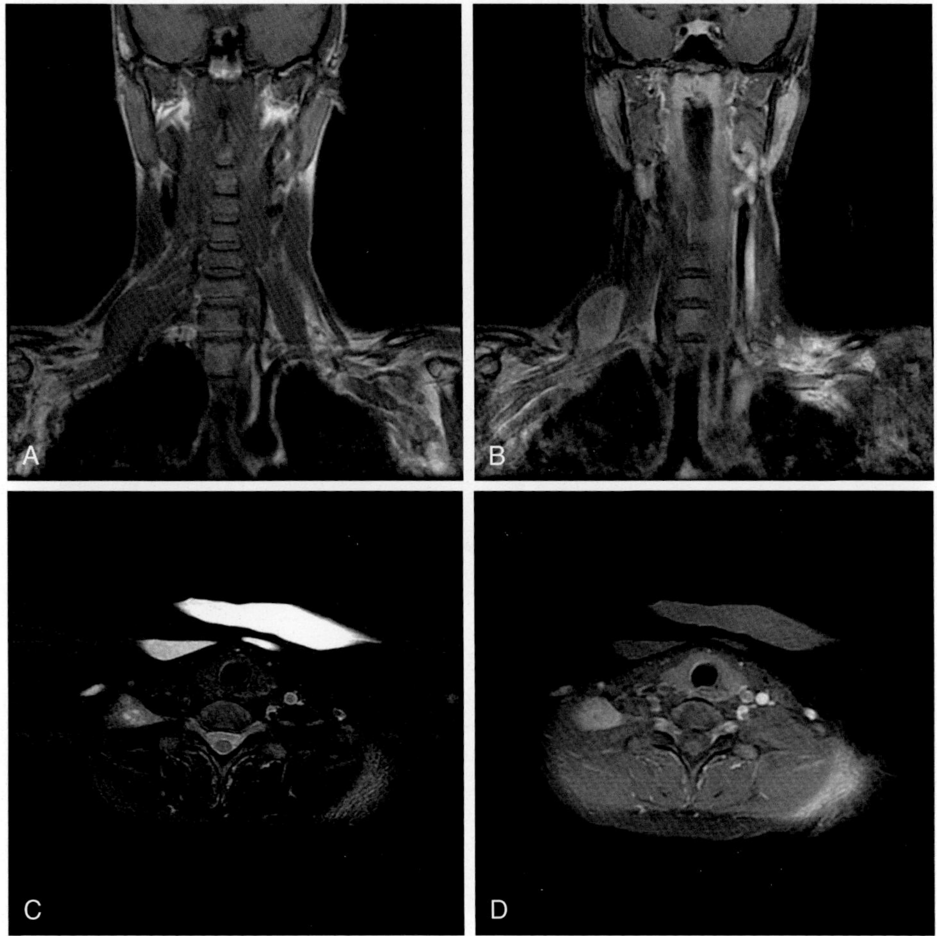

FIG. 13.10 (A) Coronal T1-W, (B) T1-W+C, (C) axial T2-W, (D) axial T1-W +C MRI brachial plexus. (Case courtesy of John Doe, Radiopaedia.org, rID: 30213.)

imaging (Fig. 13.13). Most of these lesions are found incidentally on routine radiographs or CT of the spine producing the so-called *"corduroy cloth"* appearance.[21] MRI typically shows a well-defined lesion characterized by increased T1-W and T2-W signal intensity.

The imaging findings are consistent with a hemangioma. Hemangiomas are the most common type of benign vertebral neoplasm.[21] Smaller hemangiomas not visualized on X-rays may be seen on MRI or CT. A majority of hemangiomas are asymptomatic and require no treatment but may cause pain if there is a sudden increase in vertebral loading or a collapse of the vertebral body. Invasion into the spinal canal is a relatively rare phenomenon.[22]

Although spinal metastases are part of the differential diagnosis, the physiatrist can reassure the patient of the benign nature of the lesion by remembering that metastases typically have decreased signal intensity on T1-W images and increased signal intensity on T2-W images. These lesions can also be differentiated from those of Paget's disease by the lack of cortical thickening.[21]

Another spinal neoplasm that should be considered in the differential diagnosis of patients presenting with spinal pain, particularly in the sacrococcygeal region, is a chordoma. Chordomas are relatively uncommon malignant tumors originating from the embryonic remnants of the primitive notochord.[23] They can be found in the spheno-occipital region, but are most commonly found in the sacrococcygeal spine, accounting for 30%–50% of all cases.[24] They may present as heterogeneously low signal intensity masses infiltrating the coccyx and extending into the perineum. Gross resection of the tumor is a considerable undertaking

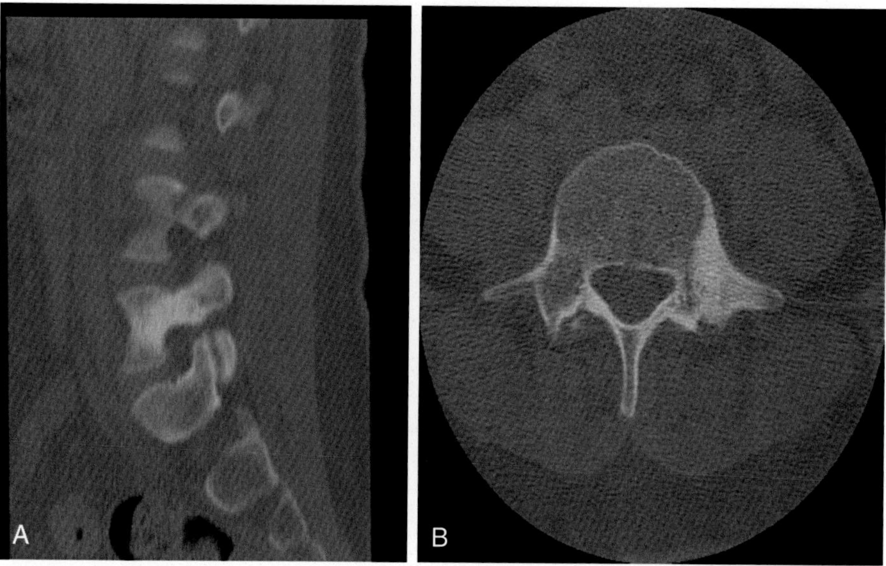

FIG. 13.11 (A) Sagittal and (B) axial bone windows CT lumbar spine. (Case courtesy of Dr. Ahmed Subaie, Radiopaedia.org, rID: 24216.)

with postoperative deficits in bladder and bowel functioning expected. Some authorities advocate for the combination of RTX and complete or subtotal surgical resection for selected patients.[25] Prognosis is generally poor due to the locally aggressive nature of these tumors, with a 10-year survival rate of approximately 40%.[24]

In patients who have undergone RTX to the spine, the physiatrist should familiarize him or herself with the MRI appearance of radiation changes to help differentiate between local tumor recurrence, progression of systemic disease and normal physiologic response to radiation. After the first 3 weeks of RTX, there is little change in signal intensity on spin echo sequences; however, Short Tau Inversion Recovery (STIR) may show increased signal intensity reflecting early marrow edema and necrosis.[26] Between 3 and 6 weeks, the marrow often shows a heterogeneous mottled appearance with prominence of MR signal from central marrow fat, best appreciated on T1-weighted images.[26] Late changes (6 weeks–14 months) vary in appearance, although homogenous fatty replacement predominantly surrounding the basivertebral veins is seen.[26] These MR changes may persist indefinitely. Fig. 13.14 is from a patient who underwent an L3 through L5 laminectomy followed by RTX from L2 to the sacrum with hyperintensity seen on the T1-weighted and long TR images reflecting post-RTX changes. The nerve roots of cauda equina demonstrate nodular thickening consistent with leptomeningeal involvement.

SPINAL STABILITY

For patients presenting with painful spinal metastases or primary spinal tumors, the physiatrist will often need to work in concert with the patient's primary medical oncologist, radiation oncologist, and spinal surgeon. One of the most important tasks for the treatment team is determining an individual's spinal stability as this will help inform operative or nonoperative treatment decisions. The Spine Oncology Study Group (SOSG) was formed prior to 2009 to establish evidence-based guidelines to aid in the assessment of spinal instability in the setting of neoplastic spinal disease.[27] The SOSG defines spinal instability as a loss of spinal integrity from a neoplastic process associated with movement-related pain, symptomatic or progressive deformity, and/or neural compromise under physiologic loads.[27] The authors developed the Spinal Instability Neoplastic Score (SINS) (Fig. 13.15), which encompasses tumor location, pain, type of bone lesion, radiographic spinal alignment, vertebral body collapse, and involvement of the posterolateral elements of the spine. A SINS score of 0–6 defines a stable spine, a score of 7–12 defines a potentially unstable spine, while a score of 13–18 defines true spinal instability.[27] Good interobserver agreement among both radiologists and radiation oncologists has been reported using the SINS score.[28]

A SINS of 7–18 is meant to warrant surgical spinal consultation to assess for instability prior to proceeding with RTX as it has been shown that patients with

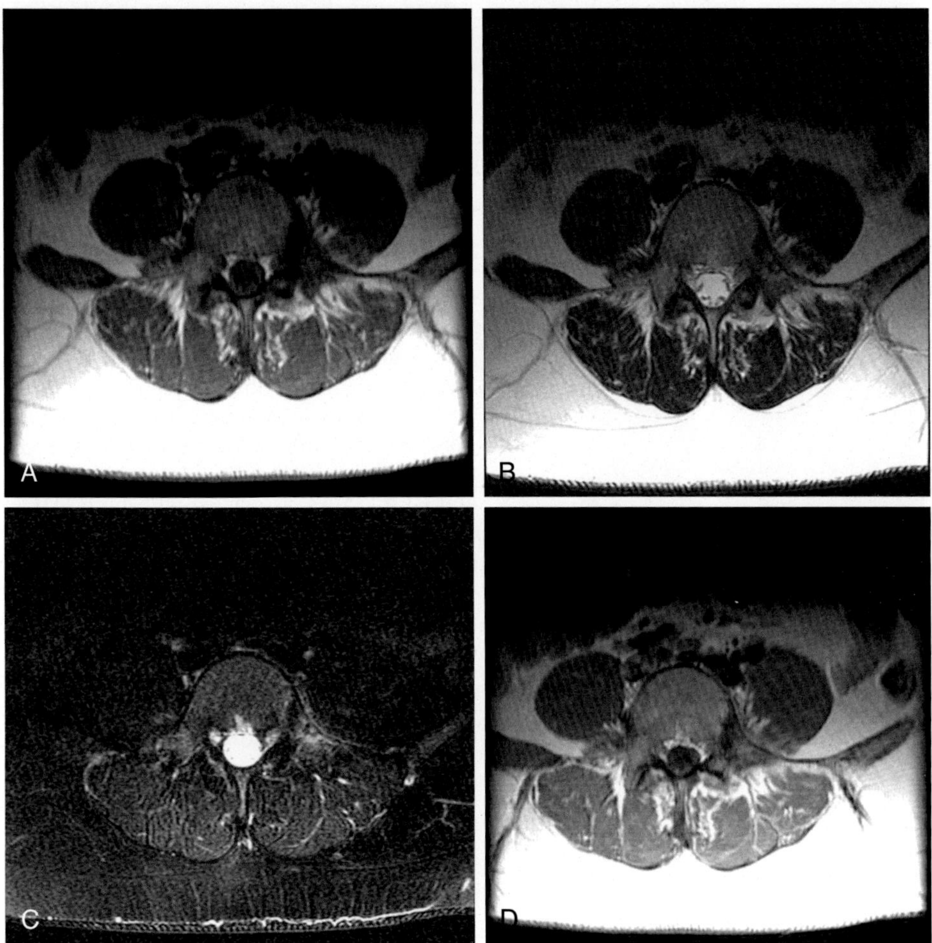

FIG. 13.12 (A) Axial T1-W, (B) T2-W, (C) T2 fat sat, and (D) T1-W+c MRI lumbar spine. (Case courtesy of Dr. Ahmed Subaie, Radiopaedia.org, rID: 24216.)

metastatic ESCC who undergo surgical decompression and reconstruction followed by radiation have superior outcomes compared with those who undergo RTX alone in terms of neurologic function, pain relief, and wound complications.[29,30] The physiatrist utilizing the SINS score may then act to prevent premature mobilization, thus preventing painful vertebral body collapse, neurologic compromise, and inappropriate treatment planning for patients with impending spinal instability.

A representative example of how the SINS score is used in physiatric and oncologic practice is that of the 60-year-old male with renal cell carcinoma who presents with back pain and right-sided T10 radiculopathy. The patient's pain is not relieved with recumbency and is not affected by thoracic rotation. He has a normal thoracic kyphosis and is neurologically intact on physical examination. The patient's imaging is shown in Fig. 13.16.

The SINS scoring for this patient is as follows: spine location—semirigid spine (T10) = 1; lack of mechanical pain, but presence of occasional nonspecific back pain = 1; bone lesion—lytic = 2; radiographic spinal alignment—normal = 0; vertebral body collapse/involvement—>50% involvement without collapse = 1; posterolateral involvement—unilateral = 1. Summing the component scores gives a total score of 6 out of a possible 18, suggesting a stable lesion. As with all metastatic spine tumors, however, surgical decision-making is not based on spinal stability alone. In practice, this patient was evaluated for surgery but surgical intervention was not pursued because of a shared

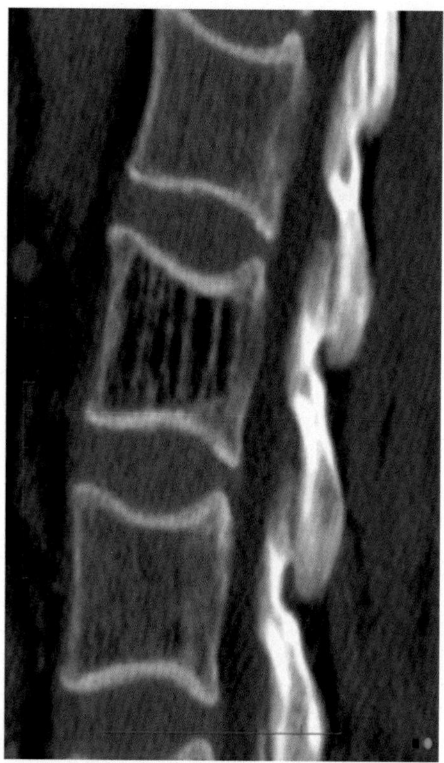

FIG. 13.13 Sagittal CT lumbar spine. (Case courtesy of Prof. Frank Gaillard, Radiopaedia.org, rID: 7483.)

blood supply of the tumor with the artery of Adamkiewicz.[27]

The physiatrist should also be aware of the existence of a validated MRI-based ESCC scoring system used to define the extent of spinal canal compromise in patients with metastatic spinal disease.[31] Utilizing the scoring system created by Bilsky and colleagues, the physiatrist can group patients into high-grade and low-grade ESCC groups to assist the multidisciplinary team in surgical decision-making.[32]

TREATMENT

Several pharmacologic therapies are available to treat the pain resulting from spinal metastases and VCFs. Acetaminophen and nonsteroidal anti-inflammatory drugs (NSAIDs) are still considered first-line treatment options for patients with mild-to-moderate CIBP as initially recommended by the World Health Organization (WHO) guidelines.[33,34] The WHO guidelines suggest that if acetaminophen and NSAIDs are not helpful enough, then the patient should be titrated on a weak opioid (i.e., codeine) followed by a stronger opioid (i.e., morphine). This three-tiered approach, however, is often too simplistic to treat the pain resulting from spinal malignancies, especially in patients with significant medical comorbidities (i.e., hypertension, diabetes, coronary atherosclerosis, chronic renal insufficiency, etc.) and more than one possible pain generator (i.e., bone, neuropathic, visceral).

Despite its popularity as a readily available over-the-counter (OTC) analgesic, acetaminophen has been shown to provide weak analgesia and has been associated with significant liver and renal toxicities.[35,36] With this in mind, physiatrists should inquire about any OTC pain remedies their patients are taking before prescribing a combination pain medication containing acetaminophen. Likewise, the cardiovascular, renal, and GI toxicities, associated with both OTC and prescription NSAIDs, complicate prescribing these medications in patients with a pre-existing history of cardiovascular disease, renal insufficiency, peptic ulcer disease, or those receiving renally excreted chemotherapies.

Nonselective NSAIDs (i.e., naproxen and ibuprofen) are thought to be the preferred NSAIDs for patients at high risk for cardiac toxicities.[37] High-dose diclofenac (i.e., 150 mg daily), and possibly ibuprofen (i.e., 2400 mg daily), have a comparable cardiovascular risk profile to the COX-2 inhibitors, whereas high-dose naproxen (i.e., 1000 mg daily) is associated with less vascular risk than the other NSAIDs.[38] Most recently, the COX-2 inhibitor, celecoxib, at moderate doses (i.e., 100 mg twice a day) was found to be noninferior to ibuprofen or naproxen in regard to its cardiovascular safety.[39]

Of particular importance to the physiatrist treating patients with CIBP and known cardiovascular disease is the interaction between the nonselective NSAIDs and cardioprotective doses of aspirin (i.e., doses <100 mg). It has previously been shown that ibuprofen competitively inhibits the binding of aspirin to its acetylation sites on the COX-1 isoenzyme of platelets such that the expected aspirin-mediated, irreversible inhibition of thromboxane A_2 production and, thus, inhibition of platelet aggregation is attenuated.[40,41] Theoretically, then, the coadministration of a nonselective NSAID with low-dose ASA may increase the risk of a second adverse cardiovascular event. It is now recommended that at least 8 hours elapse after ibuprofen dosing before giving aspirin to avoid this competitive inhibition.[41]

In opioid-naïve patients requiring stronger analgesics to control their CIBP, the physiatrist may consider

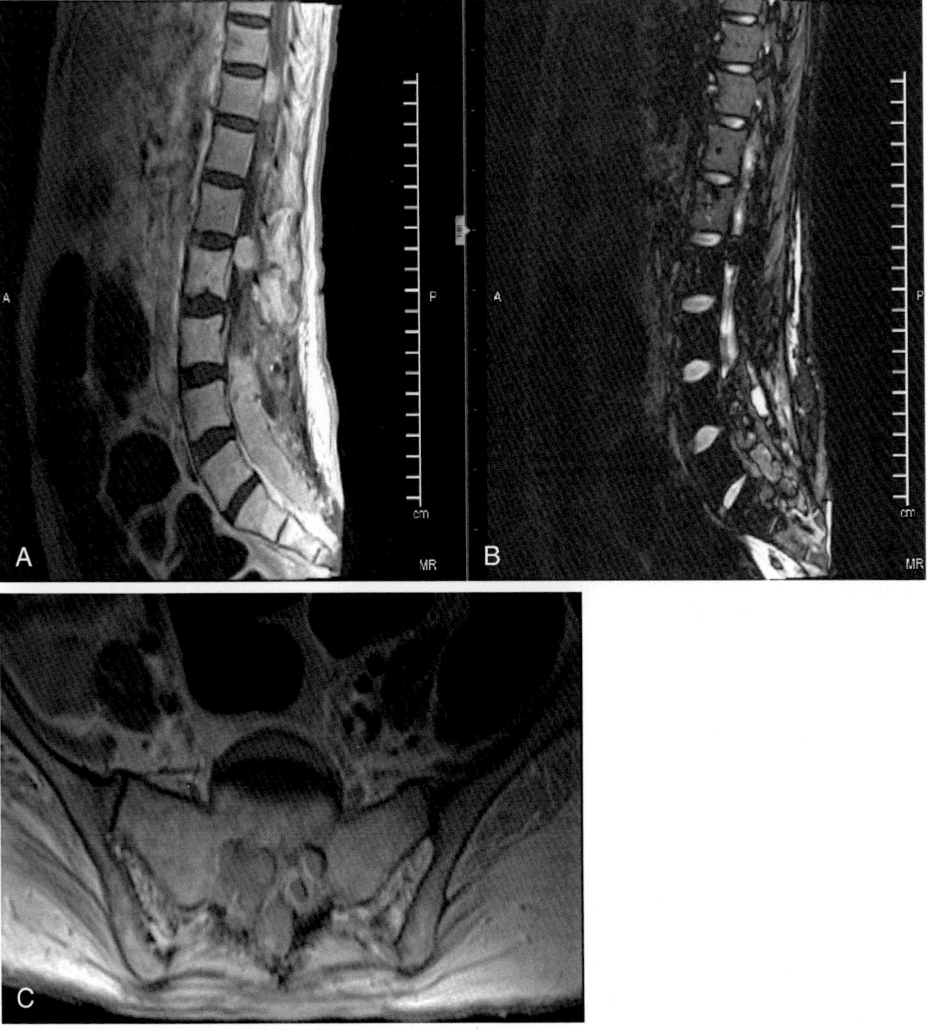

FIG. 13.14 (A) Sagittal T1-W, (B) sagittal STIR, (C) axial T1-W +c MRI lumbar spine.

titrating 5–15 mg of oral short-acting morphine sulfate or its equivalent while monitoring for adverse effects (i.e., sedation, pruritus, nausea, constipation, cognitive impairment, etc.).[37] Those patients who are opioid-tolerant (i.e., those taking at least 60 mg oral morphine/day, 25 mcg transdermal fentanyl/hour, 30 mg oral oxycodone/day, 8 mg oral hydromorphone/day, 25 mg oral oxymorphone/day, or an equianalgesic dose of another opioid for 1 week or longer) may require an additional 10%–20% of their total daily opioid dose taken in the previous 24 hours to control episodes of breakthrough pain.[37] It should be noted that cancer patients may require much higher doses of opioid analgesics than physiatrists are comfortable prescribing. The addition of NSAIDs to opioids, however, has the potential benefit of reducing the overall opioid dose when sedation or cognitive dysfunction stemming from opioid analgesic therapy becomes too burdensome for the patient.[37]

Care should be taken when prescribing long half-life analgesics such as methadone given its high potency and individual variations in pharmacokinetics. Methadone's half-life ranges from 8 to more than 120 hours, thus making its use difficult in patients with cancer-related pain.[37] Specific to methadone prescribing, the average dose needed to treat cancer-related pain seems to be much lower than that used for opioid dependency and chronic nonmalignant pain.[42] If the physiatrist is

Table 1. SINS

SINS Component	Score
Location	
Junctional (occiput-C2, C7-T2, T11-L1, L5-S1)	3
Mobile spine (C3-C6, L2-L4)	2
Semigrid (T3-T10)	1
Rigid (S2-S5)	0
Pain*	
Yes	3
Occasional pain but not mechanical	1
Pain-free lesion	0
Bone lesion	
Lytic	2
Mixed (lytic/blastic)	1
Blastic	0
Radiographic spinal alignment	
Subluxation/translation present	4
De novo deformity (kyphosis/scoliosis)	2
Normal alignment	0
Vertebral body collapse	
> 50% collapse	3
< 50% collapse	2
No collapse with > 50% body involved	1
None of the above	0
Posterolateral involvement of spinal elements↑	
Bilateral	3
Unilateral	1
None of the above	0

NOTE. Data adapted.[14]
Abbreviation: SINS, Spinal Instability Neoplastic Score.
*Pain improvement with recumbency and/or pain with movement/loading of spine.
↑Facet, pedicle, or costovertebral joint fracture or replacement with tumor.

FIG. 13.15 The spinal instability neoplastic score (SINS)[27].

not comfortable prescribing methadone, then a referral to a pain management specialist should be made.

In addition to NSAIDs and opioids, various adjuvant analgesics (i.e., anticonvulsants, antidepressants, corticosteroids, and topical anesthetics) are commonly prescribed by physiatrists and oncologists for the treatment of cancer-related pain.[37] It should be remembered that the most widely prescribed anticonvulsant drugs, gabapentin and pregabalin, as well as the tricyclic antidepressants (TCAs) were first studied in patients with nonmalignant neuropathic pain syndromes (i.e., postherpetic neuralgia and diabetic peripheral polyneuropathy) and that their effectiveness in cancer-related pain was extrapolated from these early reviews.[43–45]

A 2011 systematic review found that adjuvant analgesics provided additional cancer-related pain relief when added to patients' opioid regimens.[46] More recently, however, this finding was challenged after a new systematic review looking at patients with neuropathic cancer pain, cancer-related bone pain, and nonspecific cancer pain found that adding gabapentinoids to opioids did not significantly improve these cancer-related pain syndromes compared with opioids alone.[47] The heterogeneity of the patient populations studied, though, prevented the authors from looking at the benefits of gabapentinoids in patients with definite neuropathic cancer pain.

Certain drug-to-drug interactions need to be remembered by the physiatrist when treating patients with

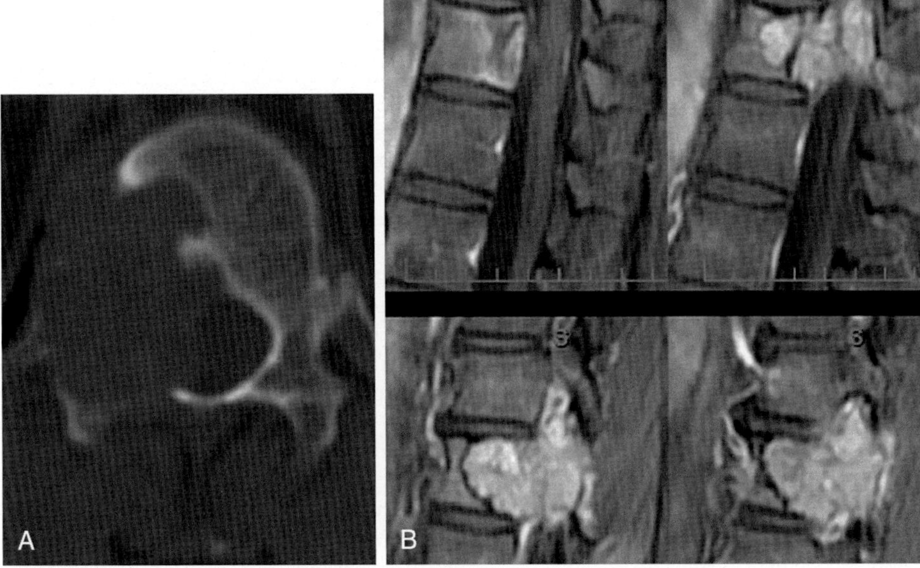

FIG. 13.16 (A) Axial CT showing lytic lesion of T10 with severe destruction right pedicle and (B) sequential sagittal MRI cuts showing T10 metastatic lesion.[27]

CIBP, other cancer-related pain syndromes (i.e., aromatase inhibitor musculoskeletal syndrome) or a concordant major depression. For example, in patients with hormone receptor-positive breast cancer being treated with tamoxifen, it is wise for the physiatrist to avoid certain selective serotonin reuptake inhibitors (SSRIs) (i.e., paroxetine or fluoxetine) and the selective serotonin norepinephrine reuptake inhibitors (i.e., bupropion or duloxetine) given their strong inhibition of cytochrome P450 enzymes (i.e., CYP2D6). Inhibition of CYP2D6 decreases production of tamoxifen's active metabolites, potentially increasing the risk of breast cancer recurrence.[48,49]

Tramadol, a popular drug among physiatrists and pain specialists treating pain in the outpatient setting, as a weak opioid receptor agonist with some norepinephrine and serotonin reuptake inhibition, should be avoided in cancer patients on stable doses of SSRIs, SNRIs, or TCAs for fear of inducing serotonergic toxicity. Tramadol has also been associated with more adverse effects including vomiting, weakness, and dizziness when compared w hydrocodone and codeine.[50] It is a poor drug for cancer-related pain as it is approximately one-tenth as potent as morphine.[51]

Corticosteroids (i.e., dexamethasone) may be indicated for certain patients with neuropathic pain syndromes, painful bony metastases, or for relieving the pain associated with malignant intestinal obstruction. The mechanism of action of corticosteroid-induced analgesia is not clear but is likely related to its anti-inflammatory effects via inhibition of prostaglandin and leukotriene synthesis and subsequent decrease in tumor-related edema.[52]

Bone-modifying agents (i.e., bisphosphonates and denosumab) have been used alongside other anticancer treatments to limit skeletal breakdown and relieve bone pain. Zoledronic acid has previously been shown to have the best efficacy among the bisphosphonates and was approved based on its ability to prolong the time to symptomatic skeletal-related events (SREs) defined as bone fracture, need for surgery, need for RTX, spinal cord compression, or hypercalcemia of malignancy, in patients with metastatic prostate cancer.[53] It did not, however, show an improvement in overall median survival time when compared with placebo.[53] For women with bone metastases from breast cancer, bisphosphonates reduced the risk of developing SREs, delayed the median time to an SRE, and appeared to reduce bone pain compared with placebo or no bisphosphonate.[54]

While interacting with the multidisciplinary treatment team, the physiatrist should familiarize him or herself with the RTX protocols used for primary and metastatic spinal disease. Conventional external beam RTX, administered as either a single dose or performed by dose fractionation, has been shown to provide partial pain relief of approximately 60% with only 24% of patients reporting complete pain relief.[55] The pain relief obtained was often delayed by 2–6 weeks.

Spine stereotactic body radiation therapy (SBRT) is an emerging treatment option for solitary and oligometastatic spinal tumors which may offer better rates of local control and pain relief compared with conventional RTX.[56] SBRT is typically performed in 1–5 fractions utilizing ablative radiation doses. Image-guided, intensity-modulated radiation therapy and volumetric modulated arc therapy (VMAT) are two techniques used to generate steep dose gradients a few millimeters away (≤2 mm) from the target lesion while protecting the adjacent spinal cord.[56] Fig. 13.17 demonstrates the dosimetry for an upper thoracic spine lesion treated with VMAT, highlighting the steep dose gradient generated between the vertebral body lesion and the surrounding spinal tissues. Any form of RTX, however, is deleterious to the cellular components of bone, which is then compounded by the harmful effects from vascular injury, ultimately predisposing these patients to pathologic VCFs.[56,57] One study found that a lytic lesion involving more than 40% of the vertebral body at or below the level of T10 confers a heightened risk of VCF.[58]

In one recent retrospective analysis, the cumulative incidence of symptomatic VCFs 5 years after ablative single-fraction stereotactic radiosurgery (SRS) was 7.2%.[59] Higher SINSs at the time of SRS correlated with earlier fractures.[59]

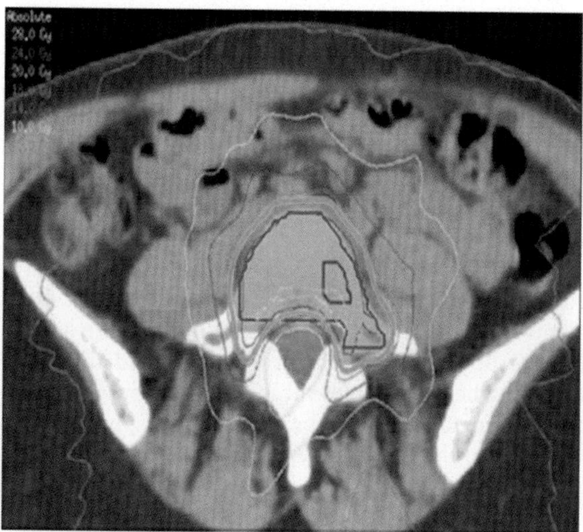

FIG. 13.17 Axial CT lumbar spine demonstrating dosimetry for lumbar spine lesion treated with volumetric modulated arc therapy.[57]

Treatment of painful VCFs without neurologic compromise may involve bracing with a thoracolumbosacral orthosis followed by progressive mobilization in physical therapy. Anecdotally, the application of a topical lidocaine patch to the skin overlying the VCF or the application of a transcutaneous electrical nerve stimulation unit may provide additional pain relief but studies in this population are lacking.[60]

If immobilization, topical, and oral analgesics are not effective or tolerated, several minimally invasive surgical options are available to treat painful VCFs in patients with metastatic spinal disease or multiple myeloma. Percutaneous vertebroplasty (PVP), percutaneous kyphoplasty (PKP), and radiofrequency ablation (RFA) are useful palliative treatments for cancer patients who are not candidates for open surgical procedures.[61] PVP is an injection of polymethylmethacrylate (PMMA) cement into a VCF under high pressure in an attempt to restore vertebral body height. Pain relief is thought to be due to the exothermic reaction caused by the bone cement hardening, which destroys afferent pain fibers in the fractured vertebral body.[61] PKP is similar to PVP but uses an inflatable balloon to control the PMMA cement extravasation into the vertebral body. Both PVP and PKP are effective in relieving the pain associated with malignant VCFs, but there is currently no consensus on which procedure to recommend first.[61,62] PKP was shown to have fewer cement leakages and a trend toward longer fracture-free survival.[63] RFA uses alternating currents to generate heat, which is thought to reduce pain from malignant VCFs by causing cancer cell death, reducing inflammatory cytokine release, decreasing bone lesion size, destroying pain fibers, and inhibiting osteoclastogenesis.[61,64]

CONCLUSION

Physiatrists are increasingly being recognized as integral members of the cancer patient's multidisciplinary treatment team. Earlier diagnoses and improved treatment algorithms are leading to longer periods of disease-free survival, but at the expense of an increase in neuromusculoskeletal pain complaints. Treating cancer patients requires a certain amount of *"due diligence"* performed by the physiatrist to ensure that subtle clinical signs and symptoms are not missed, radiologic findings are interpreted correctly in the right clinical context, and the treatment decisions made have appropriate medical evidence behind them.

REFERENCES

1. Higginson G. Clinical Standards Advisory Group. *Qual Health Care*. 1994;3(suppl):12–15.
2. Levy MH. Pharmacologic treatment of cancer pain. *N Engl J Med*. 1996;335:1124–1132.
3. Bell DJ, Dawes L, et al. Vertebral metastases. Radiopedia.
4. Kang O, Soares Zambon JD, et al. Tumours that metastasise to bone (mnemonic). Radiopedia.
5. Singh H, Neutze JA, eds. *Radiology Fundamentals: Introduction to Imaging & Technology*. 2012.
6. Batson OV. The function of the vertebral veins and their role in the spread of metastases. *Ann Surg*. 1940;112:138–149.
7. Arguello F, Baggs RB, Duerst RE, et al. Pathogenesis of vertebral metastasis and epidural spinal cord compression. *Cancer*. 1990;65:98–106.
8. De Mesmaeker M, Vokshoor A, et al. *Spondylolisthesis, Spondylolysis, and Spondylosis*. Medscape; 2014.
9. Chou R, Qaseem A, Owens DK, et al. Diagnostic imaging for low back pain: advice for high-value health care from the American College of Physicians. Clinical guidelines Committee of the American College of physicians. *Ann Intern Med*. 2011;154(3):181–189.
10. Heindel W, Gübitz R, Vieth V, et al. The diagnostic imaging of bone metastases. *Dtsch Arztebl Int*. 2014;111(44):741–747.
11. Salvo N, Christakis M, Rubenstein J, et al. The role of plain radiographs in management of bone metastases. *J Palliat Med*. 2009;12(2):195–198.
12. Bressler HB, Keyes WJ, Rochon PA, Badley E. The prevalence of low back pain in the elderly. A systematic review of the literature. *Spine*. 1999;24(17):1813–1819.
13. Koeller KK, Rosenblum RS, Morrison AL. Neoplasms of the spinal cord and filum terminale: radiologic-pathologic correlation. *Radiographics*. 2000;20(6):1721–1749.
14. Dähnert WF. *Radiology Review Manual*. 2007.
15. Thurston M, Yap K, et al. Multiple myeloma. Radiopedia.
16. Di Muzio B, Gaillard F, et al. Spinal schwannoma. Radiopedia.
17. Friedman DP, Tartaglino LM, Flanders AE. Intradural schwannomas of the spine: MR findings with emphasis on contrast-enhancement characteristics. *AJR Am J Roentgenol*. 1992;158(6):1347–1350.
18. Khadilkar SV, Khade SS. Brachial plexopathy. *Ann Indian Acad Neurol*. 2013;16(1):12–18.
19. Alifano M, D'aiuto M, Magdeleinat P, et al. Surgical treatment of superior sulcus tumors: results and prognostic factors. *Chest*. 2003;124(3):996–1003.
20. Greenspan A, Jundt G, Remagen W. *Differential Diagnosis in Orthopaedic Oncology*. Lippincott Williams & Wilkins; 2006.
21. Ibrahim D, Mapes M, et al. Vertebral haemangioma. Radiopedia.
22. Acosta Jr FL, Sanai N, Chi JH, et al. Comprehensive management of symptomatic and aggressive vertebral hemangiomas. *Neurosurg Clin N Am*. 2008;19(1):17–29.
23. Murphey MD, Andrews CL, Flemming DJ, et al. From the archives of the AFIP. Primary tumors of the spine: radiologic pathologic correlation. *Radiographics*. 1996;16(5):1131–1158.
24. Gaillard F, et al. Chordoma. Radiopedia.
25. Muro K, Das S, Raizer JJ. Chordomas of the craniospinal axis: multimodality surgical, radiation and medical management strategies. *Expert Rev Neurother*. 2007;7(10):1295–1312.
26. Stevens SK, Moore SG, Kaplan ID. Early and late bone-marrow changes after irradiation: MR evaluation. *AJR Am J Roentgenol*. 1990;154(4):745–750.
27. Fisher CG, DiPaola CP, Ryken TC, Bilsky MH, et al. A novel classification system for spinal instability in neoplastic disease: an evidence-based approach and expert consensus from the Spine Oncology Study Group. *Spine*. 2010;35(22):E1221–E1229.
28. Fourney DR, Frangou EM, Ryken TC, DiPaola CP, et al. Spinal instability neoplastic score: an analysis of reliability and validity from the spine Oncology study group. *J Clin Oncol*. 2011;29:3072–3077.
29. Patchell RA, Tibbs PA, Regine WF, et al. Direct decompressive surgical resection in the treatment of spinal cord compression caused by metastatic cancer: a randomised trial. *Lancet*. 2005;366:643–648.
30. Ghogawala Z, Mansfield FL, Borges LF. Spinal radiation before surgical decompression adversely affects outcomes of surgery for symptomatic metastatic spinal cord compression. *Spine*. 2001;26:818–824.
31. Bilsky MH, Laufer I, Fourney DR, et al. Reliability analysis of the epidural spinal cord compression scale. *J Neurosurg Spine*. 2010;13:324–328.
32. Barzilai O, Laufer I, Yamada Y, et al. Integrating evidence-based medicine for treatment of spinal metastases into a decision framework: neurologic, oncologic, mechanicals stability, and systemic disease. *J Clin Oncol*. 2017;35:2419–2427.
33. Stjernsward J. WHO cancer pain relief programme. *Cancer Surv*. 1988;7:195–208.
34. Stjernsward J, Colleau SM, Ventafridda V. The World Health Organization cancer pain and palliative care program. Past, present, and future. *J Pain Symptom Manage*. 1996;12:65–72.
35. Pharmacological management of persistent pain in older persons. *J Am Geriatr Soc*. 2009;57:1331–1346.
36. Israel FJ, Parker G, Charles M, et al. Lack of benefit from paracetamol (acetaminophen) for palliative cancer patients requiring high-dose strong opioids: a randomized, double-blind, placebo-controlled, crossover trial. *J Pain Symptom Manage*. 2010;39:548–554.
37. Adult cancer pain: clinical practice guidelines in Oncology. *JNCCN*. 2013;11:992–1022.
38. Coxib, traditional NSAID Trialists' (CNT) Collaboration. Vascular and upper gastrointestinal effects of non-steroidal anti-inflammatory drugs: meta-analyses of individual participant data from randomised trials. *Lancet*. 2013;382:769–779.
39. Nissen SE, Yeomans ND, Solomon DH, et al. *Cardiovascular Safety of Celecoxib, Naproxen, or Ibuprofen for Arthritis*; 2016. Available from: NEJM.org.

40. Catella-Lawson F, Reilly MP, Kapoor SC, et al. Cyclooxygenase inhibitors and the antiplatelet effects of aspirin. *N Engl J Med.* 2001;345:1809–1817.
41. Baigent C, Patrono C. Selective cyclooxygenase 2 inhibitors, aspirin, and cardiovascular disease: a reappraisal. *Arthritis Rheum.* 2003;48(1):12–20.
42. Parsons HA, de la Cruz M, El Osta B, et al. Methadone initiation and rotation in the outpatient setting for patients with cancer pain. *Cancer.* 2010;116:520–528.
43. Baron R, Brunnmuller U, Brasser M, et al. Efficacy and safety of pregabalin in patients with diabetic peripheral neuropathy or postherpetic neuralgia: open-label, non-comparative, flexible-dose study. *Eur J Pain.* 2008;12:850–858.
44. Saarto T, Wiffen PJ. Antidepressants for neuropathic pain. *Cochrane Database Syst Rev.* 2007;4:CD005454.
45. Saarto T, Wiffen PJ. Antidepressants for neuropathic pain: a Cochrane review. *J Neurol Neurosurg Psychiatry.* 2010;81: 1372–1373.
46. Bennett MI. Effectiveness of antiepileptic or antidepressant drugs when added to opioids for cancer pain: systematic review. *Palliat Med.* 2011;25:553–559.
47. Kane CM, Mulvey MR, Wright S, et al. Opioids combined with antidepressants or antiepileptic drugs for cancer pain: systematic review and meta-analysis. *Palliat Med.* 2017. https://doi.org/10.1177/0269216317711826.
48. Aubert R, Stanek EJ, Yao J, et al. Risk of breast cancer recurrence in women initiating tamoxifen with CYP2D6 inhibitors [abstract]. *J Clin Oncol.* 2009;27(suppl): Abstract CRA508.
49. Dezentje V, Van Blijderveen NJ, Gelderblom H, et al. Concomitant CYP2D6 inhibitor use and tamoxifen adherence in early-stage breast cancer: a pharmacoepidemiologic study [abstract]. *J Clin Oncol.* 2009;27(suppl): Abstract CRA509.
50. Rodriguez RF, Bravo LE, Castro F, et al. Incidence of weak opioids adverse events in the management of cancer pain: a double-blind comparative trial. *J Palliat Med.* 2007;10: 56–60.
51. Grond S, Sablotzki A. Clinical pharmacology of tramadol. *Clin Pharmacokinet.* 2004;43:879–923.
52. Mercadante SL, Berchovich M, Casuccio A, et al. A prospective randomized study of corticosteroids as adjuvant drugs to opioids in advanced cancer patients. *Am J Hosp Palliat Care.* 2007;24:13–19.
53. Saad F, et al. Long-term efficacy of zoledronic acid for the prevention of skeletal complications in patients with metastatic hormone-refractory prostate cancer. *J Natl Cancer Inst.* 2004;96:879–882.
54. O'Carrigan B, Wong MH, Willson ML. Bisphosphonates and other bone agents for breast cancer. *Cochrane Database Syst Rev.* 2017;30:10.
55. Chow E, Harris K, Fan G, et al. Palliative radiotherapy trials for bone metastases: a systematic review. *J Clin Oncol.* 2007;25:1423–1436.
56. Huo M, Sahgal A, Pryor D, et al. Stereotactic spine radiosurgery: review of safety and efficacy with respect to dose and fractionation. *Surg Neurol Int.* 2017;8:30.
57. Finnigan R, Burmeister B, Barry T, et al. Technique and early clinical outcomes for spinal and paraspinal tumours treated with stereotactic body radiotherapy. *J Clin Neurosci.* 2015;22:1258–1263.
58. Rose PS, Laufer I, Boland PJ, et al. Risk of fracture after single fraction image-guided intensity-modulated radiation therapy to spinal metastases. *J Clin Oncol.* 2009;27(30): 5075–5079.
59. Virk MS, Han JE, Reiner AS, et al. Frequency of symptomatic vertebral body compression fractures requiring intervention following single-fraction stereotactic radiosurgery for spinal metastases. *Neurosurg Focus.* 2017; 42(1):E8.
60. Vance CG, Dailey DL, Rakel BA, et al. Using TENS for pain control: the state of the evidence. *Pain Manag.* 2014;4(3): 197–209.
61. Stephenson MB, Glaenzer B, Malamis A. Percutaneous minimally invasive techniques in the treatment of spinal metastases. *Curr Treat Opt Oncol.* 2016;17:56.
62. Fourney DR, Schomer DF, Nader R, et al. Percutaneous vertebroplasty and kyphoplasty for painful vertebral body fractures in cancer patients. *J Neurosurg.* 2003;98: 21–30.
63. Dohm M, Black CM, Dacre A, et al. A randomized trial comparing balloon kyphoplasty and vertebroplasty for vertebral compression fractures due to osteoporosis. *AJNR Am J Neuroradiol.* 2014;35:2227–2236.
64. Mannion RJ, Woolf CJ. Pain mechanisms and management: a central perspective. *Clin J Pain.* 2000;16: S144–S156.

CHAPTER 14

Pain in Cancer of the Central Nervous System

ASHISH KHANNA, MD • MOHAMMAD AALAI, MD

INTRODUCTION/EPIDEMIOLOGY

Pain is one of the most common symptoms related to cancer and overall cancer treatment, and cancers of the brain and spinal cord are no exception. In fact, pain is frequently the initial presenting symptom for these types of cancers. Pain prevalence rates are about 39% after curative treatment and up to 66%–80% in advanced, metastatic, or terminal cancers. Moderate to severe pain (numerical rating scale score ≥ 5) was reported by 38.0% of all patients.[1,2] Cancer-related pain, in general, is caused by either direct tumor involvement, diagnostic or therapeutic procedures, and the side effects or toxicities of treatment. Of course, individual patients may have more than one type of cancer-related pain at the same time.[3] Painful procedures include surgery, radiation, chemotherapy, and supportive or diagnostic procedures. The different types of pain, the approach to the assessment of pain in brain and spinal cord malignancies, and the various available treatments will be discussed in this chapter.

ETIOLOGY

Types of Pain

Nociceptive

Nociceptive pain is typically what people think of when they think of pain. This is the type of pain everyone is familiar with. It is defined as pain that is triggered by the activation of the peripheral receptive terminals of the primary afferent neurons. These nociceptors fire in response to noxious irritants such as chemical, mechanical, or thermal stimuli. Unlike the other types of pain discussed in the following sections, nociceptive pain is unique in that the pain is proportional to the nociceptive input.[4]

Neuropathic

Neuropathic pain in cancer is very common, occurring in between 19% and 21% of all cancer patients who report having pain and in up to 90% of patients receiving neurotoxic chemotherapies. Neuropathic pain can have a substantial impact on quality of life of a cancer patient as it can impact activities of daily living (ADLs), ambulation, fine motor tasks, mood, and sleep. It can be challenging to manage as it is commonly just one layer in the complex pain syndromes of patients. However, neuropathic pain is a distinct entity unto its own and must be addressed as such.[5,6]

Clinical characteristics unique to neuropathic pain include sensory abnormalities such as thermal and cold allodynia, paresthesias, mechanical hyperalgesia, and dysesthesias. Pain is described as "burning", "stabbing", "numb", or "pins and needles." Severe cases can affect the motor nerves as well, resulting in weakness.[6,7] In the setting of cancer, the most common type is a painful peripheral neuropathy resulting from specific types of chemotherapies. Referred to as chemotherapy-induced peripheral neuropathy (CIPN), it is most often a dose-dependent, cumulative adverse effect of treatment with certain drugs. It usually is also length-dependent, resulting in a stocking-and-glove distribution of pain and impairment.[6]

For example, one of the most commonly used combination chemotherapy regimens in neuro-oncology is procarbazine, lomustine, and vincristine (PCV).[8] Of these, vincristine is known to result in a polyneuropathy characterized by numbness and tingling and/or burning of the hands and feet. The drug exerts its antitumor effects by disrupting microtubule structures required for mitosis and cell division. Unfortunately, these same structures are also implicated in axonal transport of nutrients, and thus we see a "dying back" effect in the damaged nerves. Vincristine can affect any nerve and so results in a mixed sensorimotor neuropathy with possible autonomic involvement.[9,10]

In another example, spinal cord gliomas are commonly treated with cisplatin and carboplatin, both members of the group of platinum chemotherapies.[11] These compounds exert their damaging effects in the dorsal root ganglia, resulting in a pure sensory neuropathy. Patients receiving this chemotherapy, unlike PCV, would not have any muscle weakness—an important clinical distinction. They can, however, have paresthesias of the hands and feet, loss of deep tendon reflexes, and impaired vibration and proprioception.[9] A unique feature of the platinum compounds is that the symptoms can continue to worsen, and even peak, weeks or months after the last dose has been administered. This phenomenon is known as "coasting." As you might imagine, this can result in undue anxiety on the part of the patient and the uninformed clinician.[12]

Myofascial

Myofascial pain is pain that arises from myofascial trigger points, which are small localized areas of taut muscle bands that are sometimes palpable. They are hypersensitive and tender to palpation, frequently reproducing a patient's pain, including any referral patterns. They frequently occur after a discrete trauma or injury but can be insidious in onset as well. In CNS cancer patients who have developed new patterns of movement, a high clinical suspicion for this type of pain should be maintained as it frequently follows postural abnormalities. The pain is regional in nature and described as a deep ache. There are many treatment options, the mainstays of which are exercise, stretching, postural/ergonomic considerations, and trigger point injections.[13]

Thalamic

Thalamic pain is a type of central pain syndrome that can be severe and difficult to treat. It typically occurs in those who sustain damage to the ventrocaudal regions of the thalamus, although it occurs from other damaged thalamic nuclei and it is difficult to predict which patients will develop it and which will not. It is generally seen in patients who have suffered a thalamic stroke and considered a type of central poststroke pain.[14] However, cancerous lesions and subsequent cancer treatments affecting the thalamus may also result in this pain syndrome. It is characterized by severe and paroxysmal pain producing a sensation described as burning. It is activated by cutaneous stimulation and changes in temperature and can be accompanied by hyperalgesia and allodynia.[15]

Funicular

Funicular pain is another type of central pain disorder that is the consequence of a lesion or disease of the ascending spinothalamic tracts. This can occur secondary to radiation to spinal lesions, for example, or secondary to mass effect resulting in compression of the tract.[16] The result of this ectopic activity in this tract is a nebulous type of excruciating pain that can be difficult to diagnose. It does not follow in any fixed dermatomal pattern and pain can be experienced anywhere in the body caudal to the lesion.[17]

SPECIFIC SYNDROMES

Malignant Spinal Cord Compression

Spinal cord or cauda equina compression as a result of mass effect is present in approximately 3%–14% of all cancer patients and is referred to as malignant spinal cord compression. After brain metastasis it is the second most common neurologic complication of cancer. It can have a major impact on a patient's quality of life—frequently resulting in not only pain but also paralysis and incontinence. Most patients who are affected by it are those with advanced cancers with limited survival. It is often considered a medical and surgical emergency.[18,19]

The spine itself is the most frequent site of osseous metastases, occurring in about 40% of patients.[20] Over half of the cases result from cancers of the breast, prostate, and lung. Other common associated cancers are lymphoma, renal cell carcinoma, multiple myeloma, melanoma, and head and neck cancers, including thyroid cancer.[21,22]

Pain is usually secondary to mass effect of a metastasis distorting the anatomy of the pedicle or vertebral body itself. This can occur independent of vertebral body collapse, which, of course, may further distort the anatomy and have its own impact on surrounding structures. Epidural compression is by far the most common cause. Either the mass grows into the epidural space and compresses the spinal cord, into the neuroforaminal space, or the metastasis results in vertebral body collapse displacing bone fragments into the epidural space.[23] Most malignant spinal cord compression occurs in the thoracic vertebra (70%), followed by the lumbar spine (20%), and then the cervical spine (10%). About one-fifth of cases will have multiple instances of compression.[24]

The vast majority of cases of malignant spinal cord compression initially present with pain (>90%). But motor weakness (76%–78%), autonomic dysfunction (40%–64%), and sensory loss (51%–80%) are also common.[23] Pain may be acute or long-standing at the time of diagnosis. The nature of this pain is variable, largely dependent on the site of compression. Pain localized to just one area is not always the case, although local tenderness is common. Spinal percussion may reproduce this local pain. Compression of the exiting nerve roots generally results in a unilateral radicular pain in the cervical and lumbar spine but is more frequently bilateral in thoracic compression. This is because the spaces available are narrower in the thoracic spine.[25] In general, there are some associated pain syndromes caused by vertebral metastases. These are outlined in the table below[26]:

Location	Bone Pain	Radicular Pain	Other Findings
Cervical spine	"Constant, aching" pain in the paraspinal area radiating to both shoulders	Unilateral radiating to the shoulder and medial aspect of the arm	Tenderness on percussion of spinous process; parestheisas and numbness in digits 4 and 5; progressive weakness of triceps and hand
Lumbar spine	"Aching" pain in the midback with referred pain to unilateral or bilateral sacroiliac joints	Pain in groin/thighs	Exacerbated by sitting or lying down, relieved by standing or vice versa
Sacral spine	"Aching" pain in sacral and/or coccygeal region	n/a	Perianal sensory loss; bowel and bladder dysfunction/ incontinence; impotence; exacerbated by sitting and relieved with ambulation
Epidural spinal cord compression	"Aching" pain and tenderness in the affected vertebrae; stocking distribution of leg pain	May or may not be present	Upper motor neuron signs; motor weakness progressing to paraplegia; sensory loss; bowel and bladder dysfunction

Meningeal Carcinomatosis

Meningeal Carcinomatosis (MC), also called leptomeningeal carcinomatosis or neoplastic meningitis, is a disease wherein intracranial primary tumors or extracranial malignant cells disseminate or focally invade into the meninges and spinal subarachnoid. It usually results from metastatic spread into the cerebrospinal fluid. Once there, the cancerous seedlings develop on the meninges of the brain and spinal cord and may invade the nearby CNS tissue as well.

Most patients with MC first present with headache, which may be severe, and associated symptoms and signs of meningeal irritation. These include nausea, vomiting, photophobia, and nuchal rigidity. Other presentations may include epilepsy, cervical radicular pain, hemiplegia, and unconsciousness. In a cohort of 60 patients with breast cancer leptomeningeal metastases, headache was the most common presenting symptom (55%), followed by various cranial neuropathies and epilepsy (50% and 12%, respectively). Vertigo presented in 12 patients (20%).[27]

Complex Regional Pain Syndrome

Complex regional pain syndrome (CRPS) is more likely a result of surgical or nonsurgical trauma as well as cervical spine or spinal cord disorders. Malignancy in general is an infrequent cause. The mechanism of the syndrome is unclear, but it is theorized to result from sympathetic nervous system hyperactivity and some degree of inflammatory response. CRPS is likely both a peripheral and central pain syndrome. The major pathologic change is thought to be the development of sensitivity of peripheral nociceptors to sympathetic stimulation. Patients frequently have spontaneous pain or allodynia/hyperalgesia not limited to the territory of one peripheral nerve. Skin changes, hair loss, sudomotor alterations, or edema are also a necessary part of making this diagnosis.[28]

Radiation Therapy Pain

Radiation-induced pain

Radiation is associated with several different types of pain syndromes. Patients may experience pain from brachytherapy, wherein radioactive seeds are placed inside the body. Positioning the body during radiation treatment and even getting onto the table for treatment may be uncomfortable. Delayed tissue damage from radiation including mucositis, mucosal inflammation in areas receiving radiation, may occur. Radiodermatitis is the skin's reaction and is frequently painful. Finally, a temporary worsening of pain in the treated area, knows as a pain flare, is a potential side effect of radiation treatment for bone metastases. Steroids, including dexamethasone, are frequently prescribed to reduce the incidence of these pain flares.[29]

Patient Assessment: The Pain History

The proper assessment of pain in the setting of cancer is frequently underperformed, which results in a high level of unnecessary distress in patients and their families. Barriers to proper assessment include patient's reluctance to discuss their pain, lack of time for the clinical encounter, low priority placed on pain, hesitancy on the part of clinician in prescribing opioids and other pain medications, and the infrequent use of standardized pain assessment tools, among others.[30]

The pain experience is the end result of a very complex, multifaceted process. The traditional biomedical model assumes a solid relationship between nociceptive pain and an underlying, organic process. Sometimes this is the case, but very frequently this view is an incomplete one. A better approach to integrating all the aspects of pain in an assessment is to address some central questions to cancer patients who report pain. The first is to assess the extent of the patient's disease or injury. This would include questions regarding nociceptive pain and the physical impairments that have resulted from their cancer or cancer treatments. The second aspect is to assess the magnitude of the illness. This would include questions regarding the extent to which the patient is suffering, disabled, and unable to enjoy their favorite activities. The third aspect is the assessment of the psychologic contribution to their pain. This is elucidated by asking about any concomitant depression or anxiety and the presence of stressful events. Studies show that at least half of all chronic pain patients suffer from depression. The last aspect of the assessment is the awareness of any pain behaviors. Pain behaviors are the way that a patient responds to pain. This can be moaning, facial grimacing, guarded movements, altered gait, etc. They also include habitual patterns such as coping behaviors and incorporate maladaptive pain behaviors, such as catastrophizing, as well.[31]

DIAGNOSTIC TESTING OF PAIN

Diagnostic testing in brain and spinal cord cancers can include electrodiagnostic testing with nerve conduction and electromyography. Aside from this, radiologic studies are a mainstay of treatment. For example, in this special cancer population, degenerative disk disease and osteoporosis are common differential diagnoses when assessing patients for possible vertebral metastasis. Radiologic differentiation is made even more difficult when the patient has vertebral body collapse. Computed tomography scans help discern among osteoporotic vertebral body collapse. In the osteoporotic collapse, vertebral end plates are intact and the collapse is likely to be more symmetric. This is in contrast to a metastatic cause of collapse wherein the vertebral endplates may be eroded, the pedicles destroyed, and the collapse asymmetric. If the clinician suspects metastasis not resulting in a structural deformity, then magnetic resonance imaging is ideal as it reflects tissue chemistry.[26,32–34]

TREATMENT

Pain in cancer patients has a reported prevalence of 39% post treatment and up to 80% in advanced cases.[1] Inadequate control of pain has been reported in up to 31% of patients.[35] Certain patients with primary bone cancers, pancreatic, lung, head, and neck are associated with increased neuropathic pain complaints; however, overall bone metastasis is the most common cause for cancer-related pain.[36]

The generally accepted guidelines for pain treatment are based on the World Health Organization treatment algorithm which separates symptoms using the 10-point visual analogue scale (VAS). These divisions are mild (VAS < 3), moderate (VAS 3–6), and severe (VAS > 6). Treatment for mild pain involves nonopioids including paracetamol and NSAIDs. The available evidence does not support the safety or superiority of any particular NSAID. Treatment for moderate pain includes mild opioids such as codeine, dihydrocodeine, and tramadol. Transdermal fentanyl and buprenorphine can also be considered. Owing to studies showing short duration of analgesia (as little as 4 weeks) with weak opioids, some authors have recommended progression to low-dose strong opioids earlier in the algorithm.[37,38]

Treatment of severe pain is much more complex and includes the use of a variety of medications. Strong opioids used in this setting include morphine, methadone, oxycodone, fentanyl, and buprenorphine. Selection of the appropriate agent should take into account the patient's age, comorbid conditions, kidney and liver function, and include a review of current medications.

Evidence shows oral morphine, hydromorphone, oxycodone, and methadone provide similar efficacy.[39] Transdermal medications may be used when opioids cannot be tolerated orally. Transdermal buprenorphine is particularly useful in patients with renal impairment, requiring no dose adjustment regardless of disease severity.[40]

Neuropathic pain, as described earlier, is a result of damage stemming from direct tumor effects or as a result of toxic sequelae due to treatments. Treatment is complicated and can involve trials of many medications, one at a time, utilizing slow titration.[41] Opioids remain as the first-line treatment for moderate to severe neuropathic pain; however, a variety of medications are generally utilized. This includes anticonvulsants such as gabapentin and pregabalin, including SSRIs, SNRIs (especially duloxetine), venlafaxine, and tricyclic antidepressants. Finally, NMDA antagonists including ketamine, corticosteroids, and local anesthetics/topical agents may be used.[42]

One of the most common treatments for neuropathic pain is gabapentin. According to the available evidence, this has a mild to moderate benefit; however, more rigorous controlled studies are required. Clinical trials have also shown some pain reduction with venlafaxine and especially duloxetine for CIPN.[43–45]

Interventional Therapies

Even with the utilization of pharmacologic therapies, up to 20% of patients have uncontrolled pain.[46] Therefore, interventional procedures remain as a major source for pain control. This includes blocking of nerve signal transmission either temporarily or permanently by destructive means. Although patient selection is critical, for those failing medical management as well as those experiencing adverse effects of medication, procedural alternatives should be offered.

Interventional therapies include peripheral nerve blocks using a combination of anesthetics and corticosteroids for temporary blockade and neurolytics for permanent blockade. These involve targeting various ganglion and peripheral nerves throughout the body including, but not limited to, Gasserian and Stellate ganglion of the head and neck, the Celiac ganglion for abdominal pain, lumbar sympathetic, superior hypogastric, and ganglion impar blocks for pain involving the lower extremities and pelvis. Celiac plexus neurolysis specifically has shown evidence for pain control.[47] It should be noted that in addition to chemical interventional treatments, radio-frequency ablation of associated peripheral nerves and ganglion can be performed for more prolonged pain control. This involves the placement of a needle near the target nerve and inducing a thermal lesion for sensory nerves and pulsed radiofrequency ablation for ganglion and motor nerves.

Other procedures include neuroaxial pumps designed to infuse medication into the epidural or intrathecal space. The goal of this is to reduce the dosage required for adequate analgesia as well as reduce associated side effects from systemic medication. This can be effective for patients with pain not responding to standard treatment as well as those intolerant of typical opioid side effects. Typical medications infused through these devices include opioids, anesthetic agents, clonidine, and ziconotide.

Vertebral augmentation, including vertebroplasty and balloon kyphoplasty, is also used to manage pain due to pathologic fracture. This procedure entails the formation of a cavity within the vertebral body and subsequent introduction of bone cement. This has the dual benefit of pain relief and increased stability. Careful patient selection is critical due to associated risks of cement leakage and subsequent sequelae.

Radiation therapy (RT) for bone pain from metastases is a commonly accepted treatment method. This involves a variety of treatment regimens varying in frequency and intensity; however, a single 8 Gy fraction is widely considered best practice.[48] Radio-frequency ablation, as described previously, is also an option for bony lesions when pain fails to respond to RT. This involves the use of heat, but cryoablation techniques are also available which utilize cooling to block painful nerve transmissions.

Management of Side Effects

Opioid treatment is associated with a number of potential side effects including gastrointestinal (constipation, nausea, vomiting), CNS (cognitive impairment, hyperalgesia, allodynia, and myoclonia), respiratory depression, and others including pruritus, dry mouth, urinary retention, hypogonadism, and immune depression. Management includes counseling and patient education, dose modification, and adjuvant therapy addition. Also considered is treatment of side effects, including management of nausea, constipation, and drowsiness.[49]

Rehabilitation therapies

The rehabilitation of the cancer patient begins with identification of impairments. In a neuro-oncology patient, this may include deficits in cognition, speech or swallow, bowel or bladder, and hemiparesis. Neuropsychologists and speech pathologists are frequently an integral part of the rehabilitation team for this reason. Patients should also be assessed for physical therapy needs such as balance and gait abnormalities and occupational therapy needs including evaluation for adaptive equipment and other strategies to improve ADLs.[50]

Appropriate goal setting is key, as the medical status of a cancer patient can deteriorate quickly. In some cases, the goal is to rehabilitate a patient to the full extent possible, whereas in other cases the goal is more palliative for those closer to the end of life. For example, rehabilitation can be used to reduce caregiver burden or for patient safety teaching. In this case, a short course of rehabilitation is more appropriate.

Psychologic approaches to cancer pain

Pain is a multifactorial problem, which includes emotional aspects that influence its character and intensity. The stress of physical illness including resultant depression can significantly alter pain perception.[51] Pain also can contribute to worsening of preexisting psychologic issues which are exacerbated by things such as stress and sleep disorders and therefore treatment should consider these factors. Treatments include cognitive-behavioral therapy, music, and exercise—all of which have shown evidence of pain mitigation.[52]

Acupuncture

Acupuncture is a form of traditional Chinese medicine that involves the placement of sterile needles into specific points on the body that are believed to have reduced bioelectrical resistance. When done correctly, it has been shown to be safe, minimally invasive, and have few adverse effects. Although the scientific evidence for acupuncture always comes with a high risk of bias, there is good evidence for its use in cancer-related nausea and vomiting. Beyond this, though, systematic reviews and meta-analyses have shown that acupuncture is also effective in relieving cancer-related pain, particularly malignancy-related and surgery-induced pain. Overall, studies suggest that acupuncture can be adopted as an appropriate adjunctive therapy for reducing cancer-related pain.[53,54]

PATIENT SAFETY CONSIDERATIONS

One of the most important jobs of any clinician in the care of patients with any type of cancer is to minimize risk by maximizing patient safety. This kind of care is done in a proactive manner. Ensuring good coordination of care among the oncology team is fundamental as these patients likely have numerous physicians, each of whom is just managing one or two specific aspects of the patient's care. Miscommunication due to physicians operating in silos can have disastrous effects.

In the CNS cancer population specifically, some common safety concerns would include appropriate prophylaxis for venothromboembolism, bowel and bladder precautions, risk of dysphagia assessment, range of motion clarification, and weight-bearing restrictions of the limbs and spine in patients with bone metastasis, to name a few. Additionally, the clinician should be cognizant regarding the side effects of the cancer treatments administered. The side effects of many medications can have serious consequences as well. For example, opioids for pain have numerous dangerous complications, as discussed earlier, including respiratory depression, which can be fatal.[50]

CONCLUSION

Adequate management of pain as a result of cancer or cancer treatments is paramount. It has numerous devastating effects on a patient's function and quality of life. Uncontrolled pain unsurprisingly is associated with an increase in emotional distress. The duration of pain and its severity have been implicated in the risk of developing a mood disorder, such as depression. The impact on quality of life is significant as well. Cancer patients are disabled an average of 12–20 days a month, with 28%–55% unable to work at all.[55] Increased distress is noted when pain becomes more permanent, unexpectedly continuing to persist long past the conclusion of their cancer treatments.[56] Between 20% and 50% of survivors experience this type of persistent pain and its associated functional impairments.[57] Beyond the patient, there are societal costs as well, including increased numbers of unnecessary hospital admissions and emergency room visits.[58]

As oncology treatments improve, the population of cancer survivors or those living with cancer will only continue to rise. These patients have numerous concerns and medical needs. One of the greatest among these is management of pain. Although pain is most certainly complex, multifaceted, and frequently difficult to treat, it is an increasingly common and very real concern for those with CNS cancers. As such, it is imperative that the clinician serving these patients is well educated on how best to do so. Only then can one say they have achieved their goal as a medical practitioner in easing the suffering of their patients.

REFERENCES

1. van den Beuken-van MHJ, Hochstenbach LMJ, Joosten EAJ, Tjan-Heijnen VCG, Janssen DJA. Update on prevalence of pain in patients with cancer: systematic review and meta-analysis. *J Pain Symptom Manage.* 2016; 51(6):1070–1090.
2. Jara C, Del Barco S, Grávalos C, et al. SEOM clinical guideline for treatment of cancer pain (2017). *Clin Transl Oncol.* 2018;20(1):97–107.
3. McGuire DB. Occurrence of cancer pain. *JNCI Monogr.* 2004;2004(32):51–56.
4. Nijs J, Leysen L, Adriaenssens N, et al. Pain following cancer treatment: guidelines for the clinical classification of predominant neuropathic, nociceptive and central sensitization pain. *Acta Oncol.* 2016;55(6):659–663.
5. Bennett MI, Rayment C, Hjermstad M, Aass N, Caraceni A, Kaasa S. Prevalence and aetiology of neuropathic pain in cancer patients: a systematic review. *Pain.* 2012;153(2): 359–365.
6. Fallon MT. Neuropathic pain in cancer. *Br J Anaesth.* 2013; 111(1):105–111.
7. Ahlawat A. Comprehensive review on molecular mechanisms of neuropathic pain. *J Innovations Pharm Biol Sci.* 2017;4.
8. Jutras G, Bélanger K, Letarte N, et al. Procarbazine, lomustine and vincristine toxicity in low-grade gliomas. *Curr Oncol.* 2018;25(1):e33.
9. Quasthoff S, Hartung HP. Chemotherapy-induced peripheral neuropathy. *J Neurol.* 2002;249(1):9–17.
10. Jaggi AS, Singh N. Mechanisms in cancer-chemotherapeutic drugs-induced peripheral neuropathy. *Toxicology.* 2012;291(1–3):1–9.
11. Vaillant B, Loghin M. Treatment of spinal cord tumors. *Curr Treatment Options Neurol.* 2009;11(4):315–324.
12. Staff NP, Grisold A, Grisold W, Windebank AJ. Chemotherapy-induced peripheral neuropathy: a current review. *Ann Neurol.* 2017;81.
13. Borg-Stein J, Simons DG. Myofascial pain. *Arch Phys Med Rehabil.* 2002;83:S40–S47.
14. Vartiainen N, Perchet C, Magnin M, et al. Thalamic pain: anatomical and physiological indices of prediction. *Brain.* 2016;139(3):708–722.
15. Wilton LM. Thalamic pain syndrome. *J Neurosci Nurs.* 1989;21(6):362–365.
16. Shoval HA, Stubblefield MD. Poster 312 radiation-induced funicular pain from treatment of a spinal metastases. *PM&R.* 2014;6(9):S292–S293.
17. Stubblefield MD. Radiation fibrosis syndrome: neuromuscular and musculoskeletal complications in cancer survivors. *PM&R.* 2011;3(11):1041–1054.
18. Kramer JA. Spinal cord compression in malignancy. *Palliat Med.* 1992;6(3):202–211.
19. Spinazze S, Caraceni A, Schrijvers D. Epidural spinal cord compression. *Crit Rev Oncol Hematol.* 2005;56(3):397–406.
20. Klimo Jr P, Thompson CJ, Kestle JRW, Schmidt MH. A meta-analysis of surgery versus conventional radiotherapy for the treatment of metastatic spinal epidural disease. *Neuro-Oncology.* 2005;7(1):64–76.
21. Gilbert RW, Kim JH, Posner JB. Epidural spinal cord compression from metastatic tumor: diagnosis and treatment. *Ann Neurol.* 1978;3(1):40–51.
22. Rajer M, Kovač V. Malignant spinal cord compression. *Radiol Oncol.* 2008;42(1):23–31.
23. Kwok Y, DeYoung C, Garofalo M, Dhople A, Regine W. Radiation oncology emergencies. *Hematol Oncol Clin.* 2006;20(2):505–522.
24. Gunderson L. *Clinical Radiation Oncology.* Philadelphia, PA: Elsevier; 2016.
25. Dunning EC, Butler JS, Morris S. Complications in the management of metastatic spinal disease. *World J Orthoped.* 2012;3(8):114–121.
26. Sykes N, Bennet M, Yuan C-S. *Clinical Pain Management Second Edition: Cancer Pain.* CRC Press; 2008.
27. de Azevedo CRAS, Cruz MRS, Chinen LTD, et al. Meningeal carcinomatosis in breast cancer: prognostic factors and outcome. *J Neurooncol.* 2011;104(2):565–572.
28. Mekhail N, Kapural L. Complex regional pain syndrome type I in cancer patients. *Curr Rev Pain.* 2000;4(3): 227–233.
29. Supportive PDQ, Board PCE. *Cancer Pain (PDQ®).* 2017.
30. Cleeland CS. Assessment of pain in cancer. *Adv Pain Res Ther.* 1990;16:47–55.
31. Turk DC, Okifuji A. Assessment of patients' reporting of pain: an integrated perspective. *Lancet.* 1999;353(9166): 1784–1788.
32. Jung H-S, Jee W-H, McCauley TR, Ha K-Y, Choi K-H. Discrimination of metastatic from acute osteoporotic compression spinal fractures with MR Imaging1. *Radiographics.* 2003;23(1):179–187.
33. Rao RD, Singrakhia MD. Painful osteoporotic vertebral fracture: pathogenesis, evaluation, and roles of vertebroplasty and kyphoplasty in its management. *JBJS.* 2003; 85(10):2010–2022.
34. Yuh WT, Zachar CK, Barloon TJ, Sato Y, Sickels WJ, Hawes DR. Vertebral compression fractures: distinction between benign and malignant causes with MR imaging. *Radiology.* 1989;172(1):215–218.
35. Rodríguez MJ, de la Torre R, Ortega JL, et al. Evaluation of the quality of care of elderly patients with chronic and breakthrough pain treated with opioids: SAND study. *Curr Med Res Opin.* 2017;34:1–9.
36. Gómez MD, Fernández ND, de Ibargüen BCS, et al. Association of performance status and pain in metastatic bone pain management in the Spanish clinical setting. *Adv Ther.* 2017;34(1):136–147.
37. Derry S, Wiffen PJ, Moore RA, et al. Oral nonsteroidal anti-inflammatory drugs (NSAIDs) for cancer pain in adults. *Cochrane Database Syst Rev.* 2017;7.

38. Ripamonti CI, Bandieri E, Roila F. Management of cancer pain: ESMO clinical practice guidelines. *Ann Oncol.* 2011; 22(suppl 6):vi69–vi77.
39. National Comprehensive Cancer N. *NCCN Clinical Practice Guidelines in Oncology: Adult Cancer Pain.* Version 2.2017. 2017.
40. Ahn JS, Lin J, Ogawa S, et al. Transdermal buprenorphine and fentanyl patches in cancer pain: a network systematic review. *J Pain Res.* 2017;10:1963–1972.
41. Vadalouca A, Raptis E, Moka E, Zis P, Sykioti P, Siafaka I. Pharmacological treatment of neuropathic cancer pain: a comprehensive review of the current literature. *Pain Pract.* 2012;12(3):219–251.
42. Beuken-van Everdingen MHJ, Graeff A, Jongen JLM, Dijkstra D, Mostovaya I, Vissers KC. Pharmacological treatment of pain in cancer patients: the role of adjuvant analgesics, a systematic review. *Pain Pract.* 2017;17(3): 409–419.
43. Bennett MI, Laird B, van Litsenburg C, Nimour M. Pregabalin for the management of neuropathic pain in adults with cancer: a systematic review of the literature. *Pain Med.* 2013;14(11):1681–1688.
44. Durand JP, Deplanque G, Montheil V, et al. Efficacy of venlafaxine for the prevention and relief of oxaliplatin-induced acute neurotoxicity: results of EFFOX, a randomized, double-blind, placebo-controlled phase III trial. *Ann Oncol.* 2012;23(1):200–205.
45. Smith EM, Pang H, Cirrincione C, et al. Effect of duloxetine on pain, function, and quality of life among patients with chemotherapy-induced painful peripheral neuropathy: a randomized clinical trial. *JAMA.* 2013;309(13): 1359–1367.
46. Ventafridda V, Tamburini M, Caraceni A, De Conno F, Naldi F. A validation study of the WHO method for cancer pain relief. *Cancer.* 1987;59(4):850–856.
47. Wyse JM, Chen YI, Sahai AV. Celiac plexus neurolysis in the management of unresectable pancreatic cancer: when and how? *World J Gastroenterol.* 2014;20(9):2186–2192.
48. Lutz S, Balboni T, Jones J, et al. Palliative radiation therapy for bone metastases: update of an ASTRO evidence-based guideline. *Pract Radiat Oncol.* 2017;7(1):4–12.
49. Paice JA, Portenoy R, Lacchetti C, et al. Management of chronic pain in survivors of adult cancers: American society of clinical oncology clinical practice guideline. *J Clin Oncol.* 2016;34(27):3325–3345.
50. Cristian A, Batmangelich S. *Physical Medicine and Rehabilitation Patient-Centered Care: Mastering the Competencies.* New York, NY: Demos Medical; 2015.
51. Syrjala KL, Jensen MP, Mendoza ME, Yi JC, Fisher HM, Keefe FJ. Psychological and behavioral approaches to cancer pain management. *J Clin Oncol.* 2014;32(16):1703–1711.
52. Sheinfeld Gorin S, Krebs P, Badr H, et al. Meta-analysis of psychosocial interventions to reduce pain in patients with cancer. *J Clin Oncol.* 2012;30(5):539–547.
53. Chiu H-Y, Hsieh YJ, Tsai P-S. Systematic review and meta-analysis of acupuncture to reduce cancer-related pain. *Eur J Cancer Care.* 2017;26(2).
54. Garcia MK, McQuade J, Haddad R, et al. Systematic review of acupuncture in cancer care: a synthesis of the evidence. *J Clin Oncol.* 2013;31(7):952.
55. Brown LF, Kroenke K, Theobald DE, Wu J, Tu W. The association of depression and anxiety with health-related quality of life in cancer patients with depression and/or pain. *Psycho-Oncology.* 2010;19(7):734–741.
56. Jim HS, Andersen BL. Meaning in life mediates the relationship between social and physical functioning and distress in cancer survivors. *Br J Health Psychol.* 2007; 12(Pt 3):363–381.
57. Harrington CB, Hansen JA, Moskowitz M, Todd BL, Feuerstein M. It's not over when it's over: long-term symptoms in cancer survivors—a systematic review. *Int J Psychiatry Med.* 2010;40(2):163–181.
58. Mayer DK, Travers D, Wyss A, Leak A, Waller A. Why do patients with cancer visit emergency departments? Results of a 2008 population study in North Carolina. *J Clin Oncol.* 2011;29(19):2683–2688.

CHAPTER 15

Attending to the Quality of Life at the End of Life. Palliative Rehabilitation Is Person-Centered Care for Patients With Advanced Cancer

MARTIN R. CHASEN, MBCHB, FCP(SA), MPHIL(PALL MED) • RAVI BHARGAVA, MD • GARY GOLDBERG, BASC, MD, FABPMR (BIM)

INTRODUCTION

The point at which active standard oncologic treatment is determined to be more likely to cause greater symptom burden than benefit for patients with advanced cancer is a critical transition which had been generally interpreted in the past within an obsolete conceptual understanding as implying the complete withdrawal of active medical care—at a particular time when, from the perspective of the patient and family, care—including rehabilitation services—may actually be most needed. This may explain the tendency toward an underutilization of cancer rehabilitation services integrated within a palliative care program.[1] However, this situation is changing rapidly as the significant benefit of interdisciplinary palliative care with embedded function-oriented rehabilitation treatment is recognized as a means of optimizing patient autonomy, self-esteem, and quality of life (QoL), as well as a measure for reducing avoidable suffering and healthcare costs, during a time when both patient and their caregiving partners have significant care needs.[2] The point at which a move toward palliation occurs is thus better viewed as a carefully guided shift in emphasis of treatment and focus of care for individuals with advanced cancer rather than as a "withdrawal" of treatment.

Palliative care[3] is defined by the World Health Organization as:

> *An approach that improves the QoL of patients (adults and children) and their families who are facing problems associated with life-threatening illness. It prevents and relieves suffering through the early identification, correct assessment and treatment of pain and other problems, whether physical, psychosocial or spiritual.*
>
> *Addressing suffering involves taking care of issues beyond physical symptoms. Palliative care uses a team approach to support patients and their caregivers. This includes addressing practical needs and providing bereavement counselling. It offers a support system to help patients live as actively as possible until death.*
>
> *Palliative care is explicitly recognised under the human right to health. It should be provided through person-centred and integrated health services that pay special attention to the specific needs and preferences of individuals.*

The American Society for Clinical Oncology (ASCO) recommends that palliative care should be combined with standard oncologic care early in the course of treatment for all patients whose cancer is considered "advanced"—typically those with identified metastatic disease and/or a high symptom burden.[4] Essential components of a palliative care program are listed in Table 15.1.

The National Comprehensive Cancer Network (NCCN) recommends that all cancer patients be repeatedly screened for palliative care needs, beginning with their initial diagnosis and thereafter intermittently as indicated.[5] Patients who screen positive for inadequately controlled symptoms, moderate to severe distress and anxiety, or otherwise serious physical, psychiatric, and/or psychosocial comorbidity, metastatic solid tumors, life expectancy of less than 6 months based on recognized indicators, patient or family concerns about the course of the disease and the associated decision-making process, or specific patient and/or

TABLE 15.1
Essential Components of a Palliative Care Program

- Building rapport, communication, and supportive relationships with patient and family caregivers
- Managing symptoms and existential distress, including but not limited to
  - Pain
  - Dyspnea
  - Fatigue
  - Sleep impairment
  - Mood and distress
  - Anxiety
  - Depression
  - Nausea
  - Constipation
- Exploration of understanding and education about illness and prognosis
- Clarification of treatment goals through ongoing communication
- Assessment and support of coping and adjustment needs for patient and caregivers
  - Complementary and integrative health interventions
  - Dignity therapy
  - Supportive counseling
  - Spirituality needs
- Assistance with medical decision-making
- Rehabilitation directed toward optimizing functionality, self-efficacy, self-esteem, and independent capability including but not limited to
  - Functional mobility and endurance
  - Physical exercise participation
  - Energy conservation and ergonomic training
  - Basic self-care training and assessment for activities of daily living equipment needs
  - Nutritional care
- Coordination of care with other healthcare providers

family requests for palliative care should receive a palliative care referral.[5]

There is mounting evidence demonstrating that participation in an integrated and appropriately timed palliative care treatment program helps to both enhance the QoL near the end of life for patients as well as their caregivers and reduce associated healthcare costs.[6–11] Cancer rehabilitation and palliative care are subspecialties that share a common holistic, person-centered philosophy of care,[12] implement comprehensive services through interdisciplinary teams, and are focused on improvement of health-related QoL, symptom-oriented management, and the lessening of caregiver burden.[1]

Cheville et al.[2] define "palliative rehabilitation" as follows:

> *Palliative rehabilitation is function-directed care delivered in partnership with other disciplines and aligned with the values of patients who have serious and often incurable illnesses in contexts marked by intense and dynamic symptoms, psychologic stress, and medical morbidity, to realize potentially time-limited goals. [p. S337]*

In some centers, palliative care and rehabilitation are each classified as components of a "supportive oncology" program where supportive oncology is identified as "the provision of the necessary services for those living with or affected by cancer to meet their informational, emotional, spiritual, social, or physical needs during their diagnostic, treatment, or follow-up phases encompassing issues of health promotion and prevention, survivorship, palliation, and bereavement." (13, p. 372).

In this chapter, we will examine the role of function-oriented, comprehensive rehabilitation treatment in the context of the palliative care of individuals with advanced cancer with special consideration to neoplasms involving the central nervous system.

THE GENERAL ROLE OF REHABILITATION IN ADVANCED CANCER

Rehabilitation derives from the Latin "rehabilitare" meaning to make fit again. Cancer rehabilitation is a process that assists the individual's physical, social, psychologic, and vocational functioning within limits imposed by the acquired pathology. The functional autonomy of patients with cancer is compromised throughout the trajectory of illness in different ways and influenced by different factors. The severity of this compromise can range from negligible to profound.

Patients with advanced cancer and their families highly value control of symptoms, maintenance of function and nutrition, and improvement in quality of life, as do their physicians.[14–16] Yet, although drug protocols for cancer are clearly outlined, formal programs addressing symptoms and the functioning of the person are not common. To achieve these goals, a multimodal approach that includes the full spectrum of rehabilitation and the involvement of a coordinated interdisciplinary rehabilitation team of professionals from the onset of advanced cancer is essential.[15,16] There is emerging clear evidence that certain dietary patterns, exercise, and a healthy psychosocial status and attitude influence cancer incidence and early progression.[17–24] "Survivorship" programs that embrace these entities are now well accepted.[25] However, few centers provide comprehensive care models that adequately address the complex needs of patients with advanced cancer, together with the needs of their caregivers.

While some patients may experience symptoms during the initial phases of diagnosis and treatment, others experience treatment-related, long-term, debilitating side effects. Following initial cancer diagnosis, patients react differently, progressing at different rates through different phases, characterized by symptoms which affect specific functional domains, requiring specific rehabilitation interventions. Post-treatment rehabilitation directed toward time-limited functional treatment goals has been shown to improve physical symptoms (such as fatigue and physical endurance), nutritional symptoms (such as poor appetite, unintentional weight loss, and nutritional deterioration), psychologic symptoms (such as anxiety, depression, and immobilizing apprehension), and overall quality of life.[26–30]

Epidemiologic Considerations

There were an estimated 14.1 million new cancer cases, 8.2 million cancer deaths, and 32.6 million people living with cancer (within 5 years of diagnosis) in 2012 worldwide. The overall age-standardized cancer incidence rate is almost 25% higher in men than in women, with rates of 205 and 165 per 100,000. It is estimated that 70% of all the patients with cancer survive for more than 5 years after the date of diagnosis and the majority of the cancer survivors are of working age (<55 years).[31] Improved outcomes with extended survival times have, therefore, created a constantly growing population of patients living with a cancer diagnosis. In 2016, there were an estimated 14.5 million cancer survivors in the United States.[32] Breast cancer survivors continue to represent the largest segment of the survivor population (23%), followed by prostate cancer survivors (21%) and colorectal cancer survivors (9%).[33] By January 1, 2026, it is estimated that the population of cancer survivors will increase to 20.3 million: almost 10 million males and 10.3 million females.[34]

Classification of Rehabilitation Needs

In 1969, Dietz introduced the first conceptual framework for designing a successful rehabilitation program triaging patients based on their rehabilitation goals and needs.[18] Owing to the nature of the cancer trajectory, rehabilitative goals have been divided into preventive, restorative, supportive, and palliative.[18]

Preventive rehabilitation aims at reducing the burden of morbidity/mortality of the disease and/or treatment. Rehabilitation interventions include education concerning the functional impact of the treatment, specifically preserving social function and activities of daily living (ADLs).

Restorative care aims to return the individual with minimum functional impairments to their premorbid state. Postoperative range-of-motion (ROM) exercises for patients undergoing reconstructive surgery for head and neck cancer represent this category of care.

Supportive efforts seek to reduce functional difficulties and compensate for permanent deficits. An example of this approach would include the multimodal techniques used to rehabilitate patients after amputation. Rehabilitation intervention aims at developing a program to restore mobility and management of symptoms that can occur as a result of the primary disease as well as treatment effects.

Palliative treatment aims to eliminate or reduce complications, especially pain and any other symptoms associated with impaired functioning. Emotional support at this stage is also clearly important. Prevention of bedsores can be achieved by education of caregivers. Existential issues can also be addressed sensitively by clergy and other palliative care team members. Rehabilitation intervention for this phase focuses on educating the patient and their caregivers on how to conserve energy and optimize physical capability in the face of the pathophysiologic effects of advanced cancer.

PSYCHOSOCIAL INTERVENTIONS IN PATIENTS WITH ADVANCED CANCER

Psychosocial problems and psychologic distress are common consequences of cancer and its treatment and can often become a major issue in palliative care as existential concerns emerge. The term "distress" refers to emotionally difficult experiences that may be in response to psychologic, social, spiritual, or other sources of suffering linked to existential uncertainty. Distress becomes a significant clinical concern when it precipitates significant disturbance and disorder interfering with one's ability to engage socially or function in daily life.

In cancer care, this may manifest as difficulties engaging constructively with clinicians, seeking appropriate medical or supportive care, adhering to treatments, coping with losses, or adjusting to the existential uncertainty that accompanies advanced cancer. Interventions can help patients attend to factors of distress that interfere with their functioning or QoL. In addition to helping patients address distress, psychosocial clinicians embedded in the rehabilitation team can also help patients improve other physical difficulties, such as pain,[35] sleep,[36] fatigue,[37] or other debilitating physical concerns. Canadian psychosocial scientist-practitioners spearheaded efforts to successfully have distress recognized as the sixth vital sign in cancer care.[38,39] In 2008, screening for distress became an accreditation standard for all Canadian cancer programs under Accreditation Canada.[40] In the United States, the American College of Surgeons' Commission on Cancer (CoC) adopted a similar screening policy in 2016 for all CoC-accredited cancer programs.[41] The consensus report issued by the US Institute of Medicine (IOM) specified processes that need to be in place to (1) identify distressed patients; (2) link patients and families to needed psychosocial services; (3) support patients and families in managing the illness; (4) coordinate psychosocial and biomedical care; and (5) follow up on care delivery to monitor the effectiveness of services provided and make modifications if needed. These recommendations are similar to those contained in the Clinical Practice Guidelines for Management of Distress developed by the US NCCN.[42] Similar to the IOM report, the NCCN guidelines recommend that all patients be routinely screened with validated measures to identify the level and sources of their distress. This could be accomplished using the single-item "Distress Thermometer"[43] and the accompanying problem checklist described in the guidelines. Canadian guidelines recommend the Edmonton Symptom Assessment System (ESAS) and the problem checklist as the minimal toolkit. The ESAS provides nine single-item scales that screen for the severity of nine common symptoms, including depression and anxiety.[44] A published randomized trial has demonstrated the benefits of an approach to psychosocial care similar to that described in the NCCN guidelines.[45] In this study, cancer patients found to have major depressive disorder through a screening process were randomly assigned to usual care or usual care plus a collaborative care intervention, termed "Depression Care for People with Cancer," delivered by a specially trained oncology nurse. Findings showed significantly lower scores on a measure of depression 3 months post randomization for patients who received the collaborative care intervention. The beneficial effects of the collaborative care intervention observed at 3 months were still evident at 6-month and 12-month follow-up assessments.[45] Emotional distress manifests at different points of the cancer clinical trajectory in different forms. Anxiety is frequently observed in association with the diagnostic phase, whereas depressive symptoms are more insidious and are seen in higher incidence later in the clinical course of the disease.[46]

Another more recent study investigated the factors associated with psychologic distress in advanced cancer patients under palliative treatment.[47] Patients with high and low distress were compared according to the Hospital Anxiety and Depression Scale. Based on the development of a multivariate prediction model, the authors concluded that "high levels of hopelessness, impaired emotional functioning and body image distortions are the main factors associated with psychologic distress in patients with advanced cancer." [47, p. 608] Potential interventions to modify these specific factors in palliative care units are then presented by the authors.

A recent randomized clinical trial with results presented at the ASCO conference in 2017 suggests that a brief structured psychologic intervention, called "Managing Cancer and Living Meaningfully" (with the assigned acronym CALM), could help significantly relieve distress in patients with advanced cancer.[48,49] CALM is a psychologic intervention that consists of three to six 45- to 60-min sessions delivered over three to 6 months by trained healthcare professionals, such as social workers, psychiatrists, psychologists, palliative care doctors and nurses, and oncologists. The sessions focus on four broad domains: (1) symptom control, medical decision-making, and relationships with healthcare providers; (2) changes in self-concept and personal relationships; (3) spiritual well-being and the sense of meaning and purpose in life, and (4) future-oriented concerns, hope, and questions about mortality. In this study, at both 3 and 6 months, the CALM treatment group was better prepared for the end of life and they had greater ability to express and manage their feelings about it. At 6 months these effects were strengthened, and the CALM group was more prepared to deal with changes in relationships due to the cancer, and they were also able to better clarify and articulate their values and beliefs.[49]

Important work has also been done on developing a systematic brief psychotherapeutic intervention designed to address the challenge of helping persons with advanced cancer who are nearing the end of life maintain a sense of dignity in the face of significant uncertainty about their future and to attempt to mitigate the distress precipitated by such uncertainty.[50,51] Chochinov et al. have developed a dignity model of palliative care directed toward decreasing suffering, enhancing QoL, and augmenting a sense of meaning, purpose, and dignity through the offering of opportunities to address concerns that are of greatest meaning and significance to the patient as well as the chance to speak about how they would most want to be remembered by those who survive them. Dignity Therapy also provides for encouragement to recognize and take pride in various accomplishments and to cherish their legacy. The patient is provided with an edited transcript of these guided discussions with the therapist that they are then encouraged to share with friends and family as a precious bequest. Themes that guide these sessions include generativity, continuity of self, role preservation, maintenance of pride, hopefulness, aftermath concerns, and care tenor.[51] While a controlled trial of the described dignity-focused therapy did not demonstrate a significant reduction per se in patient distress, those provided with this form of psychotherapeutic intervention reported an improved QoL and sense of dignity as well as improvement in family relationships.[52]

Another approach to the treatment of intractable depression and existential psychospiritual distress or "spiritual pain"[53]—defined as "pain caused by extinction of the being and the meaning of the self" [53, p. 15] evaluated according to the three dimensions of temporality, relationship, and autonomy—has been the application of hallucinogenics in combination with an intensive single session of supportive psychotherapy while the patient is experiencing the hallucinogenic effects of the drug.[54,55] A randomized double-blind controlled trial in 51 advanced cancer patients using high- versus low-dose psilocybin, a serotoninergic classic hallucinogen derived from mushrooms, demonstrated large and sustained decreases in clinician- and self-rated reports of depressed mood and anxiety together with improved quality of life, life meaning, and sense of optimism in the high-dose group.[54] The authors postulated that the beneficial effect of high-dose psilocybin was mediated by "mystical-type psilocybin experience" occurring during the closely monitored single-treatment session on the day of drug administration. In reviewing their experience with this form of treatment, Grob and Griffiths[55] made the following statement:

> *A unique aspect of utilizing a classic hallucinogen (e.g. psilocybin) to treat the severe psychologic demoralization and existential anxiety seen in life-threatening medical illness is its seeming capacity to facilitate powerful states of spiritual transcendence that exert in the patient a profound therapeutic impact with often dramatic improvements in psychologic well-being. For a patient population struggling with often overwhelming levels of existential anxiety and demoralization, such a therapeutic intervention may have the capacity to re-infuse a sense of meaning and purpose into their lives. [p. 305]*

Future research into this potentially powerful and promising approach to the management of existential anxiety and demoralization, as well as intractable depression in patients with advanced cancer is clearly warranted.

Another emerging approach to management of anxiety and mood disorders in patients with advanced cancer are mindfulness-based interventions (MBIs). A recently published literature review examining the value of MBIs in the treatment of psychologic concerns in both patients and caregivers in the scenario of advanced cancer suggests that MBIs can be beneficial to the advanced cancer population with an associated improvement in quality of life, together with acceptance of their cancer situation and associated reduction in depression and anxiety.[56] In their extensive review of the research literature, Rouleau et al. note that, although accumulating evidence suggests that participation in an MBI may contribute to reductions in psychologic distress, sleep disturbance, and fatigue, while promoting personal growth in areas such as QoL and spirituality, care must be taken to balance these potential benefits against the limited scientific evidence supporting their measurable impact on specific clinical outcomes.[57]

SURVIVORSHIP AND REHABILITATION

A new model to describe palliative care was recently introduced; one that prepares the patients for the worst (death), but still allows hope for the best (cure). It helps illustrate the possibility of dying at a time when patients'/families' thoughts may be occupied by hope of cure. The model consists of two overlapping triangles resembling a bow tie (Fig. 15.1). The first triangle represents disease management and the second triangle is palliative care. The base of the palliative care triangle (end of the model) includes both death and survival as possible outcomes. The arrow, pointing from left to right, signifies this dynamic process with a gradual switch in focus. Survivorship, a unique aspect of this model, is included as a possible outcome. It may be used to illustrate where the various components of modern supportive and palliative care might fit into the patient's journey along with anticancer treatments.[58]

COMMUNICATION AND CLARIFICATION REGARDING END-OF-LIFE PREFERENCES

One of the most challenging areas in which clinicians are involved when treating individuals with advanced cancer is ensuring that communication about

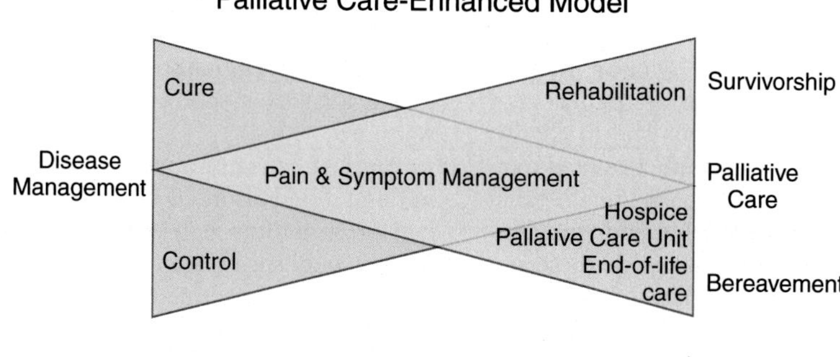

FIG. 15.1 Bow-tie palliative care—enhanced model. (Courtesy Dr. Philippa Hawley.)

end-of-life preferences is clear and established relatively early in the process. This is of particular concern when cancers involve the brain and thus may significantly impact the cognitive capacity and judgment of the person and affect their ability to communicate lucidly and make clear and definitive judgments about decisions and directions that are emotionally charged and of existential consequence. This issue becomes an increasingly significant issue as the cancer progresses. It is also important that a clear consensus about personal preferences is established among the communication partners of the person and that the wishes of the person be respected and supported by all concerned. Communication with patients and families presents a number of difficult challenges including the need for a clear and direct discussion of prognosis and about what can be expected as the cancer advances; the challenges encountered in managing emotionally charged situations, questions, and concerns related to the nurturing of hope; and the recognition of the central importance of culturally dependent factors such as religious belief and spirituality. This can thus frequently be a complex and exacting task, and it will not be dealt with in detail here. The reader is referred to a monograph on the topic produced by an expert panel convened by the Institute on Medicine and published by the National Academies Press.[59]

This summary of this influential report[59] concludes as follows:

> *In sum, the committee believes that a patient-centered, family-oriented approach to care near the end of life should be a high national priority and that compassionate, affordable, and effective care for these patients is an achievable goal. [p. 20]*

PALLIATIVE REHABILITATION AS IMPLEMENTED AT THE ÉLISABETH BRUYÈRE HOSPITAL—AN INNOVATIVE TEAM APPROACH

One of Dietz' cancer rehabilitation categories listed above, palliative rehabilitation, was largely neglected until approximately the past decade.[18] Palliation and rehabilitation both focus on QoL and daily functionality as opposed to cure or survival. As noted earlier, they are both person-centered, involving the patient, the family, and other relevant aspects of the environment.[12] They incorporate the expertise of multiple specialized professionals and accordingly both have biopsychosocial traditions.[60,61] Together, palliation and rehabilitation stand to improve function and QoL for patients with complex or advanced cancer. The Élisabeth Bruyère Palliative Rehabilitation Program (PRP) in Ottawa, Canada, was modeled after the McGill Cancer Nutrition and Rehabilitation program with some notable differences. The PRP specifically took a palliative rehabilitation approach, targeting patients with complex cancer. Patients of the PRP were adults with diagnosed incurable advanced heterogeneous cancers, typically classified as stage 3 or 4. Patients had completed their cancer treatments, were medically stable, were motivated to participate in the program, and were experiencing symptomatology and limitations that impaired their ability to engage in a productive daily life (e.g., physical dysfunction, malnutrition, mental health concerns). They needed to have a Palliative Performance status of 50% or greater.[62] By the time that the program discontinued, 366 patients had successfully completed the 8-week program. Pilot data[63] acquired and compiled in 2013 revealed that with interdisciplinary palliative rehabilitation, patients reported improvements in physical function (increased endurance, mobility, balance, and decreased fatigue), nutrition, severity of burden of multiple symptoms, and reduced symptom interference in several domains of daily life (mood, enjoyment, general activity, and work). Patients did not report improvements in pain, shortness of breath, or mental fatigue. Longitudinal follow-up revealed that, despite indications of progressing neoplastic disease, many of the gains reported earlier were maintained. These included reduced symptom interference with walking, enjoyment in life, as well as improvements in nutrition, and reported "anxiety." The approach of the PRP team is one of empowerment and emphasis on personal capability, bolstering the patients' perception of their ability to deal with the multiple stressors faced (i.e., general self-efficacy),[64] which are inherent in the challenging experience of living with advanced cancer.

Palliative care programs should be expanded to include formal exercise and nutrition components. From the point of diagnosis, patients with advanced cancer should have access to palliative care. Further research is needed to determine whether rehabilitation will improve survival in patients with advanced cancer although the primary focus of concern is substantial and meaningful improvement of QoL.

ELEMENTS OF A MEANINGFUL AND EFFECTIVE PALLIATIVE REHABILITATION PROGRAM

Physical Exercise

Physiologic changes associated with exercise provide a rationale for its use throughout the progression of cancer, both to alleviate symptoms and possibly to prolong life.[65–67] These include a reduction in the chronic inflammatory state associated with a poor prognosis, a reduction in muscle proteolysis, and an improvement in muscle synthesis, thus reducing cancer cachexia. Improvement of the patient's physical condition, functional capacity, and ability to carry out daily activities are the main goals. Through exercise programs and other physical goal-directed functional activities, the building of strength, improvement of endurance, and reduction of fatigue results in improved mobility for the patient.

The physical therapists on the team provide assistance with ADLs that may be difficult to continue because of the effects of the advanced disease or the chemotherapy.[68,69] In doing so, the patient gains greater patient autonomy and self-efficacy and reduces dependency on the caregiver. The physical therapist initially evaluates the patient's muscle strength, mobility, and joint ROM. The treatment interventions that the physical therapist provides include therapeutic exercises to maintain or increase ROM, endurance, and mobility training (for example, transfers, gait, stair climbing).[69] A systematic review[19] of exercise in a palliative care population found six clearly interpretable studies, one a randomized controlled trial (RCT).[20] Only 84 patients were enrolled in the six trials. The authors concluded that there was evidence that patients in palliative care are willing and able to tolerate physical activity interventions, and that the modest but promising reported outcomes should encourage more feasibility studies. In an RCT on exercise in a mixed population of 231 patients with an estimated survival of 2 years or less, the authors concluded that exercise may sustain function in patients with advanced cancer.[20]

Early-phase rehabilitation therapy aims to preserve muscle function, prevent disuse atrophy, preserve joint ROM, and prevent contractures with passive stretching exercises. Severity of the clinical problems in the acute stage is related to the severity and distribution of muscle weakness. If weakness is confined to the shoulder and hip girdle muscles and if 50% of normal strength is preserved, patients require minimal assistance with ambulation and ADLs. Rehabilitation therapy should focus on work amplification, pacing physical activities, gait training, use of assistive devices to reduce fall risk, and instruction for an active and passive daily stretching exercise routine to preserve ROM and prevent contractures. With more widespread involvement of functional muscle groups and with the development of profound weakness, patients lose functional independence and require substantial assistance with eating, grooming, transfers, dressing, and bathing, and they become nonambulatory.

Support of Mobility and Self-Care

An occupational therapist's goal is to maximize a person's independence in all aspects of daily functioning. The occupational therapist evaluates a patient's ability to carry out ADLs such as washing, dressing, preparing meals, working, driving, or performing leisure activities.[68] A Simmonds Functional Scale Assessment, which allows for a better understanding of the day-to-day functional ability of the patient, is performed.[70] On the basis of the assessment, occupational therapists decide on an intervention plan that has demonstrated effectiveness (which may include either preparatory skills or engagement in various purposeful activities).

Education regarding energy conservation strategies, including the use of compensatory techniques, how to plan and set priorities, and the use of adaptive equipment are part of the therapeutic armamentarium. Patients are also supported and assisted, when feasible and appropriate, in developing new vocations or returning to previous employment, albeit with assistance that may be temporary or permanent.

Occupational therapists help patients to overcome deficits in distal upper-extremity sensation, allowing them to execute the many fine motor tasks required for basic self-care. Reliance on visual rather than tactile feedback is stressed for hand positioning and task sequencing. Patients are taught compensatory strategies to monitor the amount of pressure exerted during activities requiring pinch and grasp. Many modified utensils for performing ADLs are available with ergonomic alterations that neutralize sensory deficits. Providing patients with such adaptive equipment and assistive technology is perhaps the most beneficial intervention in restoring autonomy with home activities and self-care.

Nutrition

Appropriate diet and adequate nutrition are important factors in a patient's rehabilitation. Weight loss in a patient with cancer carries with it the consequences of poorer prognosis, increased toxicity from chemotherapy, increased fatigue, and breakdown in social communication, especially at mealtimes. These effects can substantially influence the patient's overall quality of life. The dietitian's role is to evaluate the patient's current nutrition status and to provide recommendations regarding specific dietary needs. Many patients need to identify the foods and smells that cause adverse symptoms such as nausea. Adequate education regarding the prevention and treatment of constipation is also a vital function, as is appropriate mouth care. Dietary supplements and alternative foods are discussed and prescribed. Dietitians also teach family members about the importance of appropriate diet in successful rehabilitation.[71,72]

Critical interpretation of nutrition studies can be challenging. A plethora of nutritional guidelines exist, with conflicting recommendations, and the degree of dietitian input and compliance of patients and families are not usually quantified. However, nutrition has long been acknowledged as an important issue in the recovery of people with head and neck cancer. In cancers of the central nervous system as well, dysphagia due to impairment of the swallowing process can also become a major nutritional challenge. It is increasingly recognized as an important concern following treatment for other cancers as substantial weight loss occurs in approximately 1/3 of survivors.[73,74,75] With regard to issues related to eating following head and neck cancer, in one recent RCT,[76] patients who received 12 sessions of structured swallowing training following tongue resection had higher scores on the M.D. Anderson Dysphagia Inventory immediately following the completion of this intervention than patients who did not receive this training. With regard to more general nutrition needs, two systematic reviews[77,78] were located. Both dealt with dietary intervention to decrease cancer recurrence. One recommended a low-fat diet for breast cancer survivors with estrogen-receptor-positive disease. The other reported three studies which found no benefit of low fat or flaxseed diets after prostate cancer. Two RCTs were located. Bourke et al.[79] found an increase in fiber and vitamin C intake following a 12-week home-based supervised exercise program that included dietary advice for colon cancer survivors. However, other nutritional outcomes did not change. Von Gruenigen et al.[80] demonstrated a 4.5 kg average weight loss among overweight and obese endometrial cancer survivors following 6 months of education and counseling compared with usual care. One review of guidelines was identified.[81] These researchers based their recommendations on the American Cancer Society and World Cancer Research Fund/American Institute for Cancer Research guidelines for dietary strategies for the prevention of cancer,[82] which are also recommended for cancer survivors. The resulting recommendations included achieving and maintaining a healthy weight, engaging in regular physical activity, ensuring adequate consumption of vegetables, fruit, and whole grains, and limiting intake of meat and alcohol.

DOES REHABILITATION MAKE A DIFFERENCE IN PALLIATIVE CARE?

A randomized trial evaluated the clinical and cost effectiveness of a mixed rehabilitation intervention for patients with advanced cancer.[83] Forty-one participants were enrolled; 36 completed the trial. The primary outcome was the psychologic subscale of the Supportive Care Needs Survey (SCNS). The intervention arm showed significant improvement in the SCNS psychologic, physical, and patient care subscales and self-reported health state.[83] In an Australian nonrandomized study, 25 of 41 enrolled patients with advanced cancer who remained in the combined program for 2 months showed improved nutritional and functional status, endurance and strength, with a decrease in reported symptoms.[84] The limited rehabilitation team in this study included a palliative care physician, dietitian, and physical therapist. After baseline assessment, patients received individualized nutritional interventions, exercise programs, and symptom management and were followed prospectively for up to 6 months. The exercise program was undertaken either in the physical therapy gym at the hospital or at home with monthly reviews. Patients performed a combination of endurance and strengthening exercises. Measures were determined at baseline and on reviews at 1, 2, 3, and 6 months. The 2-month follow-up visit was the principal end-point of the study.[84] Researchers at the MD Anderson Cancer Center reported on 151 participants assessed at a cachexia clinic.[85] Fifty-nine patients did not return for follow-up. All patients with cancer received dietary counseling by a dietician and standard exercise recommendations. A combination of simple pharmacologic and nonpharmacologic interventions significantly improved appetite and increased weight in one-third of patients who were able to return for follow-up. No functional outcomes were reported. In 2003, a multidisciplinary program was launched at McGill University and the Jewish General Hospital in Montréal based on the premise that nutritional counseling together with an exercise program and detailed symptom control could improve QoL for patients and families and slow loss of function.[86–91] The program was conceived as a model for the application of palliative care early in the course of a predictably fatal cancer. Core team members include the patient and family, a nurse specialist, a dietitian, an allied health professional, palliative care physicians, a social worker and a clinic coordinator. Patients manage their own nutritional, exercise, and symptom therapies with guidance from team members. Later, similar programs were launched at the Royal Victoria Hospital in Montréal and the Élisabeth Bruyère Hospital in Ottawa. Reviews of results achieved at the Royal Victoria Hospital have been published in a number of reports. Recently, outcome data from programs at the Royal Victoria Hospital and the Élisabeth Bruyère Hospital have been published.[87–91]

Among 67 patients who completed the 2-month program at the Élisabeth Bruyère Hospital, significant improvements with moderate effect sizes, shown in parentheses, were seen in physiologic performance, nutrition (0.46), symptom severity (0.39–0.46), symptom interference in functioning (0.38–0.48), fatigue and physical endurance, mobility, and balance/function (0.45–0.61). Patients who completed the program at the Royal Victoria Hospital experienced strong improvements in the physical and activity dimensions of fatigue (effect size 0.8–1.1).[91] They also had moderate reductions in the severity of weakness, depression, nervousness, shortness of breath and distress (effect size 0.5–0.7), and moderate improvements in 6-min walk distance, maximal gait speed, coping ability, and QoL (effect size 0.5–0.7). Furthermore, 77% of patients either maintained or increased their body weight.[91] In a recent report on the program at the Jewish General Hospital, Parmar et al. concluded that weight gains are associated with subjective improvements in physical functioning and that changes in perceived physical strength are consistently correlated with quality of life.[92] A recently published result of a retrospective analysis of QoL in patients with advanced cancer, referred for the management of cachexia by a specialized multidisciplinary clinic, suggests that those patients who gained weight and increased their 6 min walk test (6 MWT) had the greatest improvements in QoL.[92,93]

Challenges to Implementing Palliative Rehabilitation

Early evidence suggests that a comprehensive cancer care program should incorporate rehabilitation services with drug and radiotherapy treatment throughout the span of care. Numerous pronouncements and consensus statements call on physicians to treat the "whole person" in a person-centered care approach[12] and to introduce palliative care principles early on in the treatment process following diagnosis rather than transitioning from active to palliative treatment at the point at which active medical treatment of the cancer is no longer considered justifiable.[4,5,14–16] A new ASCO clinical practice guideline summarizes the medical literature documenting the significant benefits of concurrent palliative and standard oncology care over usual oncology care alone.[94] Some of these benefits include a better QoL, improved symptom management, reduced anxiety and depression, reduced caregiver distress, more alignment of care with patient wishes, and less unwanted aggressive end-of-life care. The guideline also provides direction regarding how to implement concurrent palliative care and standard oncology care using the TEAM approach as follows:

1. Time set aside and dedicated to structured palliative team care;
2. Education about prognosis, symptom management, and facilitated communication with the palliative care team regarding realistic options, formal goal-setting, and discussion of advanced directives;
3. Assessment of patient-reported symptoms, spiritual health, and psychosocial status; and

4. Management using set protocols and an experienced interdisciplinary team to give people knowledge of their realistic options and an agreed-upon plan of action developed through shared decision-making.

One of the most challenging areas of palliative care is finding ways to maintain effective, open, and direct communication between clinicians and patients and their caregivers regarding goals of treatment, incorporating a model of shared decision-making such that patients, surrogates, and healthcare team members all remain aligned regarding agreed-upon medical goals in conjunction with a shared understanding of the patient's hopes, values, and preferences—ensuring that the "goals of medicine" are consistent with the patient's "goals of care," taking into account what is most important to the patient.[95] An ASCO consensus guideline providing guidance for "effective communication to optimize the patient-clinician relationship, patient and clinician well-being, and family well-being" has recently been published.[96] The guideline includes recommendations that address specific topics such as discussion of goals of care and prognosis, review of treatment options and available clinical trials, discussing end-of-life care, facilitation of family participation in care, effective communication in the face of barriers to communication, meeting the needs of underserved populations, and clinician training in communication skills. Strategies for implementation of the provided recommendations are also suggested.

Furthermore, accessing and responding to patient-reported concerns in real time can serve as an important operational link between the patient and palliative care providers. A recently reported RCT involving 766 patients demonstrated that a simple web-based tool enabling patients to report occurrence of significant symptoms in real time, triggering alerts to clinicians, can result in major benefits.[97,98] Patients with advanced cancer who used the tool to regularly report their symptoms while engaged in active treatment lived a median of 5 months longer than those who did not use this tool.

We can learn from geriatricians, cardiologists, and pulmonologists, who have incorporated successful rehabilitation programs to add function-oriented treatment into their care programs, ideally working in tandem with physiatrists and coordinated interdisciplinary rehabilitation teams. The pathophysiology of existential distress in patients with advanced cancer and the various functional challenges faced by this population is not dissimilar from those affecting frail elderly patients with end-stage chronic medical conditions, patients with advanced coronary artery disease, and those with chronic obstructive pulmonary disease. There may be a common neurobiologic pathway through which the existential uncertainty that undermines QoL under such circumstances precipitates distress and associated pathophysiologic disturbances that lead to a disordering of life, social withdrawal, and suffering.[99] This suggests the possibility that some common principles of effective, pragmatic treatment including function-oriented rehabilitation may well apply under such difficult clinical circumstances. However, given the central role the brain plays in coordinating the response to stress,[100] cancers that affect the brain directly and precipitate cognitive and communication impairment may present additional complications and challenges over and above those issues that arise in conjunction with advanced cancers that primarily involve other organ systems.

PALLIATIVE REHABILITATION SPECIFIC TO NEOPLASMS OF THE CENTRAL NERVOUS SYSTEM

The need for rehabilitation to address functional concerns in patients with neoplasms involving the central nervous system reflect those encountered in other pathologies impacting the function of the brain and spinal cord. These include problems involving both physical mobility and basic self-care, as well as general cognition, information processing, judgment, emotional regulation, insight, and problem-solving, among other potential functional concerns. Dysphagia can also develop and interfere with adequate nutritional maintenance, precipitating clinical decision-making around the need to move to enteral hydration and nutrition. Impaired cognition may be secondary to treatment-related effects on brain function, paraneoplastic consequences, as well as direct effects of the cancer. Patients with advanced forms of brain cancer may also experience changes in sensorium and level of consciousness, increased risk of intractable seizures, delirium, agitation, and episodic confusion, and emotional lability, which may become more frequent and increasingly problematic and disruptive as the cancer advances. The major difference between most other acquired pathologies and neoplastic disease relates to prognosis and expected clinical course. Patients with advanced cancer may also have a lower tolerance for physical activity due to generalized fatigue and deconditioning as well as limitation due to pain. Care must be taken to structure treatment around patient's desires and preferences in terms of choosing activities that they determine to be of value and meaningful in order to encourage participation and maximize benefit. Goals should be constructed to be achievable and realistic and approached in a stepwise fashion. Care must be taken not to overchallenge the patient's current capabilities. Teaching energy conservation as well as methods and means for accomplishing goals that minimize the required effort and physical energy expenditure should receive high priority. Empathic communication and the provision of sincerely communicated positive feedback for effortful participation in therapy are important interactional imperatives. Whenever possible, instruction for caregivers in how best to assist the patient while minimizing risk of injury or exhaustion should be a key component of rehabilitation treatment. A holistic systemic approach to treatment should recognize and address the overall functionality of the patient-caregiver system in context, as a whole. Physical function and autonomy should be maintained as long as reasonably possible to improve patients' QoL and to reduce the burden of care for caregivers.

Relatively little research is currently available on the palliative rehabilitation benefits and care requirements of patients with primary central nervous system cancers such as high-grade glioblastoma in spite of the fact that such patients and their caregivers clearly have significant supportive and palliative care needs. One exception is a recently published study from a neuro-oncology research team in VIC, Australia, that proposes a systematic, evidence-based, collaborative framework for such care that is "responsive, relevant, and sustainable."[101] Another study of home-based palliative care for glioblastoma multiforme in a sample of 122 patients documented the positive impact of home-based rehabilitation care in 92% of cases with 72% demonstrating a significant improvement in patient and caregiver reported QoL scores secondary to rehabilitation treatment. End-of-life palliative sedation with midazolam was required in 11% of cases to obtain adequate control of florid delirium, agitation, death rattle, or refractory seizures. The authors noted that, with a well-trained, dedicated, interdisciplinary neuro-oncology team involved in the management of neurologic deterioration, addressing clinical complications, rehabilitation needs, and psychosocial issues, improper and expensive hospitalizations can be avoided and families, patients, and caregivers can be assisted in navigating through a difficult and trying situation.[102]

CONCLUSION

Advances in screening as well as better healthcare and cancer treatments have led to significantly improved survival rates in patients with cancer. Consequently, patients are expected to live longer with the physical, psychosocial, and other impairments that result from their disease and/or its treatment. Cancer rehabilitation empowers individuals to regain strength, preserve function, and improve QoL. In fact, people can benefit from rehabilitation treatment throughout their illness as a component of "integrative oncology."[103–105] Rehabilitation improves self-esteem, self-efficacy, and patient's perceptions of themselves and equips them with the tools necessary for successful social reintegration and community participation. To effectively improve the care and management of the patients, it is crucial to educate and create greater awareness among healthcare professionals and rehabilitation specialists themselves regarding the significant benefits that can be attained through judicious deployment of rehabilitation services for patients with advanced cancer. The importance of developing and implementing recommendations and guidelines, incorporating psychosocial rehabilitation, and a comprehensive, "whole-person" plan carried out by an interdisciplinary team must be emphasized and put into effect early in the course of the disease process. Best practice involves a palliative care approach operating concurrently with standard oncology care so that patients and caregivers can be prepared well in advance for eventual contingencies. A well-functioning interdisciplinary team operating in the context of a transdisciplinary model of person-centered healthcare is vital to achieving these objectives.[12,106–109]

REFERENCES

1. Silver JK, Raj VS, Fu JB, et al. Cancer rehabilitation and palliative care: critical components in the delivery of high-quality oncology services. *Support Care Cancer.* 2015:3633–3643.
2. Cheville AL, Morrow M, Smith SR, Basford JR. Integrating function-directed treatments into palliative care. *PM&R.* 2017;9:S335–S346.
3. Palliative Care Fact Sheet No. 402. World Health Organization. Available at: http://www.who.int/mediacentre/factsheets/fs402/en/.
4. Ferrell BR, Temel JS, Temin S, et al. Integration of palliative care into standard oncology care: American Society of Clinical Oncology Clinical practice guideline update. *J Clin Oncol.* 2017;35:96–112.
5. NCCN Clinical Practice Guidelines in Oncology. Palliative Care. Version 1. Available at: http://www.nccn.org/professionals/physician_gls/pdf/palliative.pdf.
6. Grudzen CR, Richardson LD, Johnson PN, et al. Emergency department-initiated palliative care in advanced cancer: a randomized clinical trial. *JAMA Oncol.* 2016;2:591–598. https://doi.org/10.1001/jamaoncol.2015.5252.

7. Greer JA, Tramontano AC, McMahon PM, et al. Cost analysis of a randomized trial of early palliative care in patients with metastatic nonsmall-cell lung cancer. *J Palliat Med*. 2016;19:842–848.
8. Kavalieratos D, Corbelli J, Zhang D. Association between palliative care and patient and caregiver outcomes: a systematic review and meta-analysis. *JAMA*. 2016;316: 2104–2114.
9. Bakitas MA, TOsteson TD, Li Z, et al. Early versus delayed initiation of concurrent palliative oncology care: patient outcomes in the ENABLE III randomized controlled clinical trial. *J Clin Oncol*. 2015;33:1438–1445.
10. Temel JS, Greer JA, Muzikansky A, et al. Early palliative care for patients with metastatic non-small cell lung cancer. *N Engl J Med*. 2010;363:733–742.
11. Dalal S, Bruera E. End-of-life care matters: palliative cancer care results in better care and lower costs. *Oncologist*. 2017;22:361–368.
12. Entwistle VA, Watt IS. Treating patients as persons: a capabilities approach to support delivery of person-centered care. *Am J Bioeth*. 2013;13:29–39. https://doi.org/10.1080/15265161.2013.802060.
13. Hui D. Definition of supportive care: does the semantic matter? *Curr Opin Oncol*. 2014;26:372–379.
14. Smith T, Temin S, Alesi E, et al. American Society of Clinical Oncology provisional clinical opinion: the integration of palliative care into standard oncology care. *J Clin Oncol*. 2012;30:880–887.
15. Peppercorn JM, Smith TJ, Helft PR, et al. American Society of Clinical Oncology statement: toward individualized care for patients with advanced cancer. *J Clin Oncol*. 2011;29:755–760. https://doi.org/10.1200/JCO.2010.33.1744.
16. ASCO-ESMO consensus statement on quality cancer care. *Ann Oncol*. 2006;17:1063–1064. https://doi.org/10.org/10.1093/annonc/mdl152.
17. Fearon KC. Cancer cachexia: developing multimodal therapy for a multidimensional problem. *Eur J Cancer*. 2008;44:1124–1132. https://doi.org/10.1016/j.ejca.2008.02.033.
18. Dietz JH. Rehabilitation of the cancer patient. *Med Clin North Am*. 1969;53:607–624.
19. Lowe SS, Watanabe SM, Coumeya KS. Physical activity as a supportive care intervention in palliative cancer patients: a systematic review. *J Support Oncol*. 2009;7: 27–34.
20. Oldervoll LM, Loge JH, Lydersen S, et al. Physical exercise for cancer patients with advanced disease: a randomized controlled trial. *Oncologist*. 2011;16:1649–1657. https://doi.org/10.1634/theoncologist.2011-0133.
21. Baldwin C, Spiro A, Ahern R, et al. Oral nutritional interventions in malnourished patients with cancer: a systematic review and meta-analysis. *J Natl Cancer Inst*. 2012; 104:371–385. https://doi.org/10.1093/jnci/djr556.
22. Champ CE, Mishra MV, Showalter TN, et al. Dietary recommendations during and after cancer treatment: consistently inconsistent? *Nutr Cancer*. 2013;65:430–439. https://doi.org/10.1080/01635581.2013.757629.
23. Payne C, Larkin P, McIlfatrick S, et al. Exercise and nutrition interventions in advanced lung cancer: a systematic review. *Curr Oncol*. 2013;20:e321–337. https://doi.org/10.3747/co.20.1431.
24. Artherholt SB, Fann JR. Psychosocial care in cancer. *Curr Psychiatry Rep*. 2012;14:23–29.
25. Howell D, Hack TF, Oliver TK, et al. Survivorship services for adult cancer populations: a pan-Canadian guideline. *Curr Oncol*. 2011;18:e265–e281.
26. Chasen M, Bhargava R. Gastrointestinal symptoms, electrogastrography, inflammatory markers, and pg-sga in patients with advanced cancer. *Support Care Cancer*. 2011;20:1283–1290. https://doi.org/10.1007/s00520011-1215-8.
27. Spence RR, Heesch KC, Brown WJ. Exercise and cancer rehabilitation: a systematic review. *Cancer Treat Rev*. 2010;36:185–194. https://doi.org/10.1016/j.ctrv.2009.11.003.
28. Isenring EA, Capra S, Bauer JD. Nutrition intervention is beneficial in oncology outpatients receiving radiotherapy to the gastrointestinal or head and neck area. *Br J Cancer*. 2004;91:447–452. https://doi.org/10.1038/sj.bjc.6601962.
29. Isenring EA, Bauer JD, Capra S. Nutrition support using the American Dietetic Association Medical Nutrition Therapy Protocol for radiation oncology patients improves dietary intake compared with standard practice. *J Am Diet Assoc*. 2007;107:404–412.
30. León-Pizarro C, Gich I, Barthe E, et al. A randomized trial of the effect of training in relaxation and guided imagery techniques in improving psychological and quality-of-life indices for gynecologic and breast brachytherapy patients. *Psychooncology*. 2007;16:971–979.
31. Wolff SN. The Burden of Cancer Survivorship: a pandemic of treatment success. In: Feuerstein M, ed. *Handbook of Cancer Survivorship*. New York: Springer; 2007:P7–P18.
32. Miller KD, Siegel RL, Lin CC, et al. Cancer treatment and survivorship statistics 2016. *CA Cancer J Clin*. 2016;66: 271–289. https://doi.org/10.3322/caac.21349.
33. Ries LAG, Melbert D, Krapcho M, et al. *SEER cancer statistics review, 1975–2005*. Bethesda, MD: National Cancer Institute; 2008. http://seer.cancer.gov/csr/1975_2005/. Based on November 2007 SEER data submission, posted to the SEER web site.
34. American Cancer Society. *Cancer Treatment & Survivorship Facts & Figures 2016-2017*. Atlanta: American Cancer Society; 2016.
35. Darnall BD, Scheman J, Davin S, et al. Pain psychology: a global needs assessment and national call to action. *Pain Med*. 2016;17:250–263. https://doi.org/10.1093/pm/pnv095.
36. Howell D, Oliver TK, Keller-Olaman S, et al. A Pan-Canadian practice guideline: prevention, screening, assessment, and treatment of sleep disturbances in adults with cancer. *Support Care Cancer*. 2013;21:2695–2706. https://doi.org/10.1007/s00520-013-1823-6.
37. Kangas M, Bovbjerg DH, Montgomery GH. Cancer-related fatigue: a systematic and meta-analytic review of

non-pharmacological therapies for cancer patients. *Psychol Bull.* 2008;134:700−741. https://doi.org/10.1037/a0012825.

38. Bultz BD, Groff SL, Fitch M, et al. Implementing screening for distress, the 6th vital sign: a Canadian strategy for changing practice. *Psychooncology.* 2011;20: 463−469. https://doi.org/10.1002/pon.1932.
39. Howell D, Keshavarz H, Esplen MJ, et al. *On Behalf of the Cancer Journey Advisory Group of the Canadian Partnership against Cancer. A Pan Canadian Practice Guideline: Screening, Assessment and Care of Psychosocial Distress, Depression, and Anxiety in Adults with Cancer.* Toronto: Canadian Partnership Against Cancer and the Canadian Association of Psychosocial Oncology; July 2015.
40. Accreditation Canada. *Qmentum Program 2009 Standards: Cancer Care and Oncology Services.* Ottawa, ON: Accreditation Canada; 2008. Ver. 2.
41. Commission on Cancer. *Cancer Programs Standards: Ensuring Patient-centered Care.* Chicago, IL: American College of Surgeons; 2016.
42. NCCN practice guidelines for the management of psychosocial distress. *Oncology (Willist Park).* 1999;13: 113−147.
43. National Comprehensive Cancer Network. Distress management clinical practice guidelines. *J Natl Compr Cancer Netw.* 2003;1:344−374.
44. Bruera E, Kuehn N, Miller MJ, Selmser P, Macmillan K. The Edmonton Symptom Assessment System (ESAS): a simple method for the assessment of palliative care patients. *J Palliat Care.* 1991;7:6−9.
45. Strong V, Waters R, Hibberd C, et al. Management of depression for people with cancer (SMaRT oncology 1): a randomised trial. *Lancet.* 2008;372(9032):40−48. https://doi.org/10.1016/S0140-6736(08)60991-5.
46. Li M, Boquiren V, Lo C, Rodin G. Depression and Anxiety in Supportive Oncology. In: Davis M, Feyer P, Ortner P, Zimmerman C, eds. *Supportive Oncology.* Philadelphia: Elsevier; 2011:528−540.
47. Diaz-Frutos D, Baca-Garcia E, García-Foncillas J, Lopez-Castroman J. Predictors of psychological distress in advanced cancer patients under palliative treatments. *Eur J Cancer Care.* 2016;25:608−615. https://doi.org/10.1111/ecc.12521.
48. OncLive. *CALM Psychotherapy Eases Depression and Distress in Patients with Advanced Cancer. [online]*; 2018. Available at: http://www.onclive.com/conference-coverage/asco-2017/calm-psychotherapy-eases-depression-and-distress-in-patients-with-advanced-cancer.
49. Rodin G, Lo C, Rydall A, et al. Managing cancer and living meaningfully (CALM): a randomized controlled trial of a psychological intervention for patients with advanced cancer. *J Clin Oncol.* 2017;35(suppl_18). https://doi.org/10.1200/JCO.2017.35.18_suppl.LBA10001.
50. Chochinov HM. Dignity-conserving care: a new model for palliative care. *JAMA.* 2002;287:2253−2260.
51. Chochinov HM, Hack T, Hassard T, et al. Dignity Therapy: a novel psychotherapeutic intervention for patients near the end of life. *J Clin Oncol.* 2005:5520−5525.
52. Chochinov HM, Kristjanson LJ, Breitbart W, et al. The effect of dignity therapy on distress and end-of-life experience in terminally ill patients: a randomised controlled trial. *Lancet Oncol.* 2011;12:753−762.
53. Murata H. Spiritual pain and its care in patients with terminal cancer. Construction of a conceptual framework by philosophical approach. *Palliat Support Care.* 2003;1: 15−21.
54. Griffiths RR, Johnson MW, Carducci MA, et al. Psilocybin produces substantial and sustained decreases in depression and anxiety in patients with life-threatening cancer: a randomized double-blind trial. *J Psychopharmacol.* 2016; 30:1181−1197.
55. Grob C, Griffiths RR. Uses of the classic hallucinogen psilocybin for treatment of existential distress associated with cancer. In: Carr BI, Steel J, eds. *Psychological Aspects of Cancer.* Springer Science+Business Media; 2013: 291−308.
56. Zimmermann FF, Burrell B, Jordan J. The acceptability and potential benefits of mindfulness-based interventions in improving psychological well-being for adults with advanced cancer: a systematic review. *Complement Ther Clin Pract.* 2018;30:68−78. https://doi.org/10.1016/j.ctcp.2017.12.014.
57. Rouleau CR, Garland SN, Carlson LE. The impact of mindfulness-based interventions on symptom burden, positive psychological outcomes, and biomarkers in cancer patients. *Cancer Manag Res.* 2015;7:121−131.
58. Hawley P. The bow tie model of 21st century palliative care. *J Pain Symptom Manage.* 2014;47(1):e2−5. https://doi.org/10.1016/j.painsymman.2013.10.009. Epub 2013 Dec 8.
59. Committee on Approaching Death: Addressing Key End-of-Life Issues. *Dying in America. Improving Quality and Honoring Individual Preferences Near the End of Life.* Washington DC: National Academies Press; 2015.
60. Delbruck H. Structural characteristics and interventions in the implementation of rehabilitation and palliation. In: Delbruck H, ed. *Rehabilitation and Palliation of Cancer Patients.* Paris, France: Springer; 2007:3−26.
61. Kim A, Fall P, Wang D. Palliative care: optimizing quality of life. *J Am Osteopath Assoc.* 2005;105:S9−S14. Retrieved from: http://www.jaoa.org.
62. Victoria Hospice Society. *Palliative Performance Scale (PPSv2): Version 2: Victoria Hospice Society*; 2001. Retrieved from: http://www.npcrc.org/files/news/palliative_performance_scale_PPSv2.pdf.
63. Chasen MR, Feldstain A, Gravelle D, MacDonald N, Pereira J. Results of an interprofessional palliative care oncology rehabilitation program. *Curr Oncol.* 2013;20: 301−309. https://doi.org/10.3747/co.20.1607.
64. Feldstain A, Lebel S, Chasen MR. An interdisciplinary palliative rehabilitation intervention bolstering general self-efficacy to attenuate symptoms of depression in patients living with advanced cancer. *J Support Care Cancer.* 2016;24:109−117.
65. Lenk K, Schuler G, Adams V. Skeletal muscle wasting in cachexia and sarcopenia: molecular pathophysiology

and impact of exercise training. *J Cachexia Sarcopenia Muscle*. 2010;1:9–21.
66. Fanzani A, Conraads VM, Penna F, et al. Molecular and cellular mechanisms of skeletal muscle atrophy: an update. *J Cachexia Sarcopenia Muscle*. 2012;3:163–179.
67. Handschin C, Spiegelman BM. The role of exercise and PGC1alpha in inflammation and chronic disease. *Nature*. 2008;454:463–469.
68. van Weert E, Hoekstra–Weebers JE, Grol BM, et al. Physical functioning and quality of life after cancer rehabilitation. *Int J Rehabil Res*. 2004;27:27–35.
69. Schneider CM, Hsieh CC, Sprod LK, Carter SD, Hayward R. Exercise training manages cardiopulmonary function and fatigue during and following cancer treatment in male cancer survivors. *Integr Cancer Ther*. 2007; 6:235–241.
70. Simmonds MJ. Physical function in patients with cancer: psychometric characteristics and clinical usefulness of a physical performance test battery. *J Pain Symptom Manage*. 2002;24:404–414.
71. American Dietetic Association (ADA) Home page [Web resource]. Chicago: ADA; n.d. Available at: www.eatright.org.
72. National Cancer Institute. *Eating Hints: Before, During, and After Cancer Treatment* [online]. 2018.
73. Bozzetti F, Mariani L, Lo Vullo S, et al. The nutritional risk in oncology: a study of 1,453 cancer outpatients. *Support Care Cancer*. 2012;20:1919–1928.
74. Chasen MR, Dippenaar AP. Cancer nutrition and rehabilitation – its time has come! *Curr Oncol*. 2008;15:2–7.
75. Mariani L, Lo Vullo S, Bozzetti F. Weight loss in cancer patients: a plea for a better awareness of the issue. *Support Care Cancer*. 2012;20:301–309.
76. Zhen Y, Wang JG, Tao D, et al. Efficacy survey of swallowing function and quality of life in response to therapeutic intervention following rehabilitation treatment in dysphagic tongue cancer patients. *Eur J Oncol Nurs*. 2012; 16:54–58.
77. Demark-Wahnefried W, Jones LW. Promoting a healthy lifestyle among cancer survivors. *Hematol Oncol Clin North Am*. 2008;22:319–342.
78. Pekmezi DW, Demark-Wahnefried W. Updated evidence in support of diet and exercise interventions in cancer survivors. *Acta Oncol*. 2011;50:167–178.
79. Bourke L, Thompson G, Gibson DJ, et al. Pragmatic lifestyle intervention in patients recovering from colon cancer: a randomized controlled pilot study. *Arch Phys Med Rehabil*. 2011;92:749–755.
80. von Gruenigen V, Frasure H, Kavanagh MB, et al. Survivors of uterine cancer empowered by exercise and healthy diet (SUCCEED): a randomized controlled trial. *Gynecol Oncol*. 2012;125:699–704.
81. Robien K, Demark-Wahnefried W, Rock CL. Evidence-based nutrition guidelines for cancer survivors: current guidelines, knowledge gaps, and future research directions. *J Am Diet Assoc*. 2011;111:368–375.
82. Kushi L, Doyle C, McCullough M, et al. American cancer society guidelines on nutrition and physical activity for cancer prevention [Internet] *CA Cancer J Clin*. 2012;62:30–67. https://doi.org/10.3322/caac.20140/full.
83. Jones L, Fitzgerald G, Leurent B, et al. Rehabilitation in advanced, progressive, recurrent cancer: a randomized controlled trial. *J Pain Symptom Manage*. 2013;46: 315–325.
84. Glare P, Jongs W, Zafiropoulos B. Establishing a cancer nutrition rehabilitation program (CNRP) for ambulatory patients attending an Australian cancer center. *Support Care Cancer*. 2011;19:445–454.
85. Del Fabbro E, Hui D, Dalal S, et al. Clinical outcomes and contributors to weight loss in a cancer cachexia clinic. *J Palliat Med*. 2011;14:1004–1008.
86. Eades M, Murphy J, Carney S, et al. Effect of an interdisciplinary rehabilitation program on quality of life in patients with head and neck cancer: review of clinical experience. *Head Neck*. 2013;35:343–349.
87. Eades M, Chasen MR, Bhargava R. Long-term physical and functional changes following treatment. *Semin Oncol Nurs*. 2009;25:222–230.
88. Townsend D, Accurso-Massana C, Lechman C, et al. Cancer nutrition rehabilitation program: the role of social work. *Curr Oncol*. 2010;17:12–17.
89. Lemoignan J, Chasen MR, Bhargav R. A retrospective study of the role of an occupational therapist in the cancer nutrition rehabilitation program. *Support Care Cancer*. 2010;18:1589–1596.
90. Chasen MR, Bhargava R. A rehabilitation program for patients with gastro-esophogeal cancer — a pilot study. *Support Care Cancer*. 2010;18(suppl 2):S35–S40.
91. Gagnon B, Murphy J, Eades M, et al. A prospective evaluation of an interdisciplinary nutrition-rehabilitation program for patients with advanced cancer. *Curr Oncol*. 2013; 20:310–318.
92. Parmar MP, Swanson T, Jagoe TR. Weight changes correlate with alterations in subjective physical function in advanced cancer patients referred to a specialized nutrition and rehabilitation team. *Support Care Cancer*. 2013; 21:2049–2057.
93. Parmar MP, Vanderbyl BL, Kanbalian M, et al. A multidisciplinary rehabilitation programme for cancer cachexia improves quality of life. *BMJ Support Palliat Care*. 2017;7:441–449. https://doi.org/10.1136/bmjspcare-2017-001382.
94. Smith CB, Phillips T, Smith TJ. Using the new ASCO clinical practice guideline for palliative care concurrent with oncology care using the TEAM approach. *Am Soc Clin Oncol Educ Book*. 2017;37. Accessed at: https://meetinglibrary.asco.org/record/137931/edbook/.
95. Moses BD. Incorporating the 'goals of medicine' with the 'goals of care'. *ASCO Post*; June 25, 2017. Accessed at: http://www.ascopost.com/issues/june-25-2017/incorporating-the-goals-of-medicine-with-the-goals-of-care/.
96. Gilligan T, Coyle N, Frankel RM, et al. Patient-clinician communication: American Society of Clinical Oncology Consensus guideline. *J Clin Oncol*. 2017;35: 3618–3632.

97. Basch E, Deal AM, Kris MG, et al. Symptom monitoring with patient-reported outcomes during routine cancer treatment: a randomized controlled trial. *J Clin Oncol.* 2016;34:557–565.
98. *Web-Based System for Self-reporting Symptoms Helps Patients Live Longer; Study Supports Increased Use of Patient-reported Outcomes in Oncology*; June 4, 2017. https://www.asco.org/about-asco/press-center/news-releases/web-based-system-self-reporting-symptoms-helps-patients-live/.
99. Peters A, McEwen BS, Friston K. Uncertainty and stress. Why it causes diseases and how it is mastered by the brain. *Prog Neurobiol.* 2017;156:164–188.
100. McEwen BS. Physiology and neurobiology of stress and adaptation: central role of the brain. *Physiol Rev.* 2007; 87:873–904.
101. Philip J, Collins A, Brand C, et al. A proposed framework of supportive and palliative care for people with high-grade glioma. *Neuro Oncol.* 2018;20: 391–399.
102. Pompili A, Telera S, Villani V, Pace A. Home palliative care and end of life issues in glioblastoma multiforme: results and comments from a homogeneous cohort of patients. *Neursurg Focus.* 2014;37:E5. https://doi.org/10.3171/2014.9.FOCUS14493.
103. Loughran K, Rice S, Robinson L. Living with incurable cancer: what are the rehabilitation needs in a palliative setting? *Disabil Rehabil.* 2017;29:1–9.
104. Wittry SA, Lam NY, McNalley T. The value of rehabilitation medicine for patients receiving palliative care. *Am J Hosp Palliat Care*; 2017:1049909117742896. https://doi.org/10.1177/1049909117742896.
105. Lopez G, Mao JJ, Cohen L. Integrative oncology. *Med Clin North Am.* 2017;101:977–985.
106. Van Bewer V. Transdisciplinarity in health care. A concept analysis. *Nurs Forum.* 2017;52:339–347. https://doi.org/10.1111/nuf.12200.
107. Mueller SK. Transdisciplinary coordination and delivery of care. *Semin Oncol Nurs.* 2016;32:154–163. https://doi.org/10.1016/j.soncn.2016.02.009.
108. Polley MJ, Jolliffe R, Boxell E, Zollman C, Jackson S, Seers H. Using a whole person approach to support people with cancer: a longitudinal, mixed-methods service evaluation. *Integr Cancer Ther.* 2016;15:435–445.
109. Grassi L, Mezzich JE, Nanni MG, Riba MB, Sabato S, Caruso R. A person-centred approach in medicine to reduce the psychosocial and existential burden of chronic and life-threatening medical illness. *Int Rev Psychiatry.* 2017;29:377–388. https://doi.org/10.1080/09540261.2017.1294558.

Index

Note: Page numbers followed by "f" indicate figures and "t" indicate tables.

Printed in the United States
By Bookmasters